The Embodied Brain and Sandtray Therapy

The Embodied Brain and Sandtray Therapy invites readers to absorb the magic and mystery of sandtray therapy through a collection of stories.

Woven throughout these pages is the neurobiological foundation for the healing and transformation that takes place during deep encounters with sand, water, and symbolic images. Such scientific grounding provides the basis for clinicians to understand how sandtray therapy supports their healing work. In addition to client stories, the authors have also bravely shared their personal experiences, both challenging and rewarding, of being sandtray therapists.

Clinicians who are considering becoming sandtray therapists are given an inside peek into the learning journey and its many benefits. Those who are already practicing sandtray therapy will find this book both supportive and affirming.

Rita Grayson created the body–brain approach to sandtray therapy by combining her deep understanding and experience of sandtray with emerging knowledge in the field of relational neuroscience.

Theresa Fraser is the owner/director of the Maritime Play Therapy Centre in Nova Scotia, Canada. She provides neurobiologically informed play therapy training internationally.

The Embodied Brain and Sandtray Therapy

Stories of Healing and Transformation

**Edited by
Rita Grayson and Theresa Fraser**

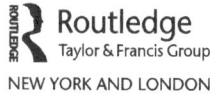

Routledge
Taylor & Francis Group

NEW YORK AND LONDON

First published 2022
by Routledge
605 Third Avenue, New York, NY 10158

and by Routledge
2 Park Square, Milton Park, Abingdon, Oxon, OX14 4RN

Routledge is an imprint of the Taylor & Francis Group, an informa business

Library of Congress Cataloging-in-Publication Data
A catalog record for this book has been requested

ISBN: 978-0-367-50780-0 (hbk)
ISBN: 978-0-367-50779-4 (pbk)
ISBN: 978-1-003-05580-8 (ebk)

DOI: 10.4324/9781003055808

Typeset in Bembo
by Apex CoVantage, LLC

To the courageous souls who bring hands and heart to the sand in the hope of rediscovering what may have been lost or forgotten.

Contents

Acknowledgments

We would like to acknowledge the work of our chapter contributors. Without them, this book would not exist. Their love and respect for working in the sandtray kept them going in the midst of a worldwide pandemic. They faced many challenges, including locked-down offices and lack of access to sandtray materials and client files. We are endlessly grateful for their persistence fueled by a deep passion to bring their experiences of the sacred nature and healing power of sandtray therapy to others.

The cover photo is used with permission of the Lowenfeld Trust and the family of Dr. Margaret Lowenfeld. A child built this world in Lowenfeld's clinic. At the time, hand drawings were used to document sandtray creations.

The picture of Dr. Margaret Lowenfeld in Figure 1.2 is used with permission of the Lowenfeld Trust and the family of Dr. Margaret Lowenfeld.

Figures 3.1 and 3.2 are from THE HEART OF TRAUMA: HEALING THE EMBODIED BRAIN IN THE CONTEXT OF RELATIONSHIPS by Bonnie Badenoch. Copyright © 2018 by Bonnie Badenoch. Used by permission of W. W. Norton & Company, Inc.

Foreword

In all the versions of Children's Secret Garden stories, one must find a key to a secret door that leads to a magical world that lies within a beautiful garden. The key is invisible to many, especially adults, but if you want to gain entrance, you must be courageous and find the key that will unlock the hidden door. Once inside the secret kingdom, however, you will find special freedom for magic with fairies, wise gnomes, gold, jewels, and many other wondrous treasures. There also are dangers, ogres, and wicked spells in this world, but if you are virtuous and you know the rules of this magic kingdom, you will not get hurt. You will be able to do whatever you wish – find new friends, play to your heart's content, create fantasies, make wishes come true. Best of all, you will be able to return to your ordinary world with these gifts, new discoveries, and special energies in hand.

Grown-ups usually do not know about the garden or that there is a secret door. Nor do they even imagine what would be inside. The door can only be opened at midnight, and unbeknownst to their parents, children can leave their ordinary homes for a little while to inhabit this magical kingdom.

Margaret Lowenfeld, originator of sand therapy in the late 1920s, turned to the Secret Garden stories in an attempt to describe her ideas about a region in the brain that was distinct from ordinary cognitive and rational processes. She struggled to articulate what she was observing in the treatment process of the children in her clinic who were using small trays of sand, water, and miniature figurines to reveal their inner worlds. Although she was trained as a pediatrician in the rigors of the physical and biological sciences, there was no language or knowledge in Lowenfeld's time to help her explain what she was observing, so she turned to the secret garden metaphor to describe the difference between the magical realm and the ordinary garden that the children also inhabited. These two spaces sound remarkably close to how Iain McGilchrist's work (2009) has helped us picture the two hemispheres of the brain. They each perceive the world differently yet are essential and complementary to one another. Lowenfeld (1979/1993) imagined the Secret Garden as "a well-defined region" with a "wall" separating it from the home garden. She said,

> The rules of conduct and the type of event that occurs on one side of the wall are different from those on the other side. What is expected

in one garden does not happen in the other, and in the magic garden almost anything can come about. (p. 17)

Lowenfeld went on to explain that time and space were different, essentially limitless, in the Secret Garden. She said that those who ventured inside were changed and brought the treasures they discovered into the home garden to transform daily life.

Without the benefit of our current neuroscience, Lowenfeld understood intuitively that this area of the brain, if accessed, could be instrumental in healing children's trauma. What we know now is that Lowenfeld was pointing to the richly symbolic right-mode processes of the divided brain. This is the home of embodied implicit memory, the storehouse of the felt sense of traumas. The timelessness she pointed to is because implicit memories carry no sense that they happened in the past. When they wake up, they fill our bodies with the sensations and perceptions from the original experience as though it is happening now. Sand and miniatures can open this realm so that it can be embraced in the healing energies of the therapeutic relationship. Once the memories are held in this way, the sandtray maker can begin to develop a coherent story, fostering further integration of this trauma.

Lowenfeld's felt sense about sand therapy has stood the test of time in terms of its effectiveness as a treatment modality. However, because there was no way for her and those who followed to explain the process in scientific terms, the legitimacy of using this modality has been called into question until very recently. Beautifully articulated, this book that you are holding in your hands comes to us as a bridge between the magical experiences of playing in the sand and the solid research and scientific knowledge now available to help us understand, to a great extent, how sandtray therapy can access this mysterious part of the brain for healing purposes. Remarkably, this group of authors has managed this task without losing the power of the mystery and the inexplicable aspect of what it means to immerse ourselves in the integrating experience of sand, play, miniatures, and personal storytelling. They offer the KEY to invite left mode and right mode processes to be equally honored.

It is often so tempting to take an easy path that leads either left *or* right. Without realizing it, we can mistake leaning one way or the other as the truth because it simplifies the task of welcoming what seems to be contradictory. The left hemisphere may encourage us to simply create a manual defining the symbolic figures, writing a script, and organizing a set of rules for therapists to use in order to direct the process. With manualized treatment, we can measure, and science is certainly mandated to measure. Unfortunately, our comfort with being able to predict and measure outcomes omits the ingenuity, mystery, depth, and inner knowing of the human beings who put their hands in the sand to experience their own unique ways of healing. On the other hand, we can lean the opposite way toward only the magic of healing, reciting the well-worn phrases that we just need to trust and to follow our guts. That path, unfortunately, also falls short of what sandtray therapy really is. Worse, this path has sometimes led to disastrous clinical harm to patients who trusted and were then betrayed by a therapist who relied solely on magical thinking without the science or proper training. Instead, we want to hold the complementarity of right *and* left, mystery *and* science, parts *and* wholeness.

Dora Kalff, revered teacher of the Jungian-based sandplay modality, understood its healing power, and equally important, she knew the potential for harm that could be done with the sandtray modality. She addressed these issues in her book, *Sandplay: A Psychotherapeutic Approach to the Psyche*. On the first page, she wrote a short paragraph entitled "Caution," expressing her concerns.

Caution

In the hands of a properly prepared therapist, sandplay is a powerful, invaluable modality. The operative word is "powerful." To the extent that any method can heal, so can it do harm. Therefore, I urgently advise that even a psychotherapist highly experienced in other methodologies, who contemplates practicing sandplay, should have had a deep personal experience doing a sandplay process as a patient with a qualified sandplay therapist and an extended period of careful supervision – anything less would be irresponsible. (Kal, 1980, 1st English translation published by Sigo Press)

These words, standing alone on a single page, at the beginning of her book, right before the prologue, underscore Kalff's high regard for the healing power of this modality. Having studied intensively with Margaret Lowenfeld, she understood ethically and intuitively the very tender territory that sandtray therapy can open and therefore the need to respect its power by carefully preparing our own inner world before inviting others to enter theirs in our care.

The authors of this current book have given us an essential guide pointing the way to ethical practice through deepening our understanding of the process and by offering us a KEY for bridging and integrating mystery and science. With intention, they have presented in this book their personal clinical experiences alongside leading-edge neuroscience concepts and research. They are showing us an integrated path that will enhance our capacity to see how, even when we invite and allow our right-mode processes to lead "as if" we were fully inside a wondrous magical kingdom, the left mode is constantly stabilizing us with solid scientific information. It may feel "as if" we have left behind the tedious and challenging ways the left often uses because the right mode has the capacity to integrate what the left brings simultaneously and seamlessly and with such speed that it feels like magic instead of science.

A foundation for this extraordinary integration of left and right modes was developed by McGilchrist (2009), who combined science and metaphor to describe the complex relationship of our two hemispheres. He drew from a large body of experimental research and philosophical traditions to explain how, through human understanding, human values, and intention, we can nurture and welcome both modes. *The Embodied Brain and Sandtray Therapy* includes this kind of current neuroscience to demonstrate the potential that lies in sand therapies when used consciously and intentionally to promote healing through integration of the opposing yet complementary forms. This book will help us continue to develop the supporting left-based knowledge while inspiring us to cherish and welcome the mystery of the Secret Garden's healing realm in the sandtray images arising in the right. This book is inviting us to find and use the invisible KEY.

Theresa A. Kestly

References

Kalff, D. (1980). *Sandplay: A psychotherapeutic approach to the psyche.* Sigo Press. (Original English version, no longer in print).

Lowenfeld, M. (1993). *Understanding children's sandplay: The world technique.* Margaret Lowenfeld Trust. (Original work published in 1979).

McGilchrist, I. (2009). *The master and his emissary: The divided brain and the making of the Western world.* Yale University Press.

Preface

The seed for this book was planted back in 2006 when Rita and Theresa met for the first time at a Level 2 sandtray-worldplay training. It was the beginning of a relationship that would strengthen as we studied and practiced the art of sandtray therapy under the tutelage of Dr. Gisela Schubach De Domenico. Each year, we met for another level of training, and our friendship deepened, as did our passion for sandtray therapy. In 2010, we completed Gisela's six-level training program and went our separate ways for a while: Theresa returned to Ontario, Canada, to help build a trauma-focused Play Therapy Center and Rita continued to hone her sandtray skills in her clinical practice in Georgia, USA. The years that followed found our paths crossing here and there, mostly on social media. It was always good to connect and catch up.

In 2018, the conversation began to change. By that time, both Rita and Theresa were offering training in sandtray therapy, and we found ourselves wishing there was a book that captured the sacred nature of the process. The awareness of sandtray therapy and the builder–witness relationship as sacred was always central in our experiences with Gisela. Our training began with a head-first dive into the numinous, followed by learning how to invite and hold healing space for another, which was a wise and wonderful departure from traditional training methods. It is also an approach that cannot be adequately captured in words. This book is our attempt to do just that, and we offer it with all humility, knowing it will fall short. To truly understand the power of sandtray therapy, you must dig in and give it a chance to work its magic on you. In recent years, we have also become increasingly concerned about the growing popularity of sandtray as a treatment modality in play therapy. You may be wondering why this would be of concern, but for us, it seemed to bring with it a proliferation of one- or two-day trainings that profess to equip therapists to use this process that, we believe, requires years of study, practice, and personal experiences of healing in the sand.

Wishing for a different kind of book on sandtray therapy did not cause one to appear out of the ether, so it was time to roll up our sleeves and get to work. As we envisioned this book, we searched out sand therapists who share our passion and understanding of the depth offered by sand, water, and symbolic figures within the container of a reverent relationship. Because we believe sandtray is best learned "from the inside out," we wanted to convey the essence of sandtray's power via stories that could be taken in rather than studied. We are endlessly grateful to our chapter authors who share their experiences of magic, mystery, and healing.

The contract for this book was signed in February of 2020. Little did we know that a few weeks later, the World Health Organization would declare a global pandemic caused by the novel coronavirus SARS-CoV-2. In spite of the upheaval in our personal and professional lives, this book continued to call our fingers to our keyboards, demanding its story be told. What is that story? We invite you to share in the experiences recounted on these pages and allow sandtray therapy to reveal itself to you.

About the Editors and Contributors

Jacqueline Aldridge, MA, LCMHCS, NCC, RPT-S, PSC, has more than 15 years of experience working with children, adolescents, adults, and families. Holding a Master of Arts degree in counseling from Appalachian State University, Jacqueline is a North Carolina Licensed Clinical Mental Health Counselor Supervisor, a National Certified Counselor, a Registered Play Therapist Supervisor, and a Professional School Counselor. Jacqueline has trained extensively and is certified in play therapy, sandtray-worldplay, and EMDR. In addition, she has presented on play therapy and supervision at the North Carolina Play Therapy Conference, on EMDR at the North Carolina Counseling Association Conference, and on sandtray therapy at the Licensed Professional Counselor Association of North Carolina Clinical Supervision Workshop. She also facilitated a discussion of mental health issues pertaining to student athletes at the Southern Conference Student Athlete Leadership Conference.

Bonnie Badenoch, LMFT, therapist, mentor, teacher, and author, has spent the last 17 years integrating the discoveries of relational neuroscience into the art of therapy. In 2008, she co-founded the nonprofit agency Nurturing the Heart with the Brain in Mind to offer this work to the community of therapists, healthcare providers, and others interested in becoming therapeutic presences in the world. For 25 years, she has supported trauma survivors and those with significant attachment wounds to reshape their neural landscapes for a life of meaning, resilience, and warm relationships. These days, Bonnie takes joy in offering immersion trainings for therapists and others. These year-long groups cultivate the capacity for presence through the development of deep listening and the embodiment of the principles of interpersonal neurobiology. Her conviction that wisdom about the relational brain can support healing experiences for people at every age led to the publication of *Being a Brain-Wise Therapist: A Practical Guide to Interpersonal Neurobiology* in 2008 and *The Brain-Savvy Therapist's Workbook* in 2011. Bonnie's latest writing is *The Heart of Trauma: Healing the Embodied Brain in the Context of*

Relationships (2018). These books seek to build a bridge between science and practice with clarity, compassion, and heart.

Theresa Fraser CYC-P, CPT-S, RP, MA, RCT, works as a clinician in Nova Scotia, Canada. She is the owner/director of the Maritime Play Therapy Centre and teaches play therapy workshops around the world. She has published books, book chapters, peer-reviewed journal articles, magazine and newspaper articles on play therapy, adoption/foster care, trauma, and child and youth work. Sandtray has enhanced her personal and professional experiences for almost twenty years. She is the current president of the Canadian Association for Play Therapy and the vice president of the World Association of Sand Therapy professionals Theresa is currently completing her Ph. D. in sandtray with the University of South Wales.

Rita Grayson, LCSW, RPT-S, is the founder of SageSource Learning Center, a training facility for sandtray therapy. Combining her deep knowledge and experience of sandtray therapy with emerging knowledge in the field of relational neuroscience, she created the body–brain approach to sandtray therapy. She is also the owner of Johns Creek Counseling, LLC where she has offered to join with children, adolescents and adults on their healing journeys for over 20 years. She is a Registered Play Therapist Supervisor with the Association for Play Therapy and serves on the advisory board of the World Association of Sand Therapy Professionals.

Rosalind Heiko, PHD, RPT-S, ISST, NCSP, is a psychologist, a Registered Play Therapist-Supervisor (RPT-S) with the Association for Play Therapy in the U.S. and a Sandplay Teacher with the International Society of Sandplay Therapists (ISST) and the Sandplay Therapists of America (STA), and holds national certification in school psychology. She trains therapists nationally and internationally. Dr. Roz is an executive board member of the World Association of Sand Therapy Professionals (WASTP.org) and has been an executive board member of STA. She has worked clinically with children and families for almost 40 years. She has published chapters in books edited by Eliana Gil and Eric Green, as well as being an author of several articles in the *Journal of Sandplay Therapy®*. Her most recent book is *A Therapist's Guide to Mapping the Girl Heroine's Journey in Sandplay* (2018), published by Rowman & Littlefield. She was published most recently in an article on Jungian play therapy for the *APT Play Therapy Magazine*.

Aimee L. Jennings, LMHC, RPT-S, is a licensed mental health counselor, RPT-S, and certified sandtray therapist and has been in the field 30 years. She is the program coordinator of a private grant funded school-based counseling program and operates a full-time private practice.

Aimee utilizes expressive arts within counseling. Though she works with a variety of clients, she has a deep interest in working with highly sensitive individuals.

Sean P. Jennings, Psy. D., RPT-S, is a licensed psychologist and certified sandtray therapist and has been in the field for 33 years. He is a tenured professor of psychological science at Valencia College and operates a full-time private practice. Sean utilizes expressive arts within therapy and is currently pursuing his credentials in psychodrama.

The Jenningses have been practicing nondirective/noninterpretative sandtray for more than 20 years and teaching sandtray for over ten years. They consider themselves fortunate to be co-therapists with couples, co-facilitate sandtray workshops, and co-teach a graduate class in expressive arts therapies at Stetson University.

Caron J. Leader, LCSW, ACSW, is a licensed clinical social worker who has been practicing for 25 years. She has been a private practice owner for 17 years and currently co-owns a practice in Evansville, Indiana called Within Sight. Caron treats all ages but especially loves working with children. She has done extensive training focused on children's needs including sandtray-worldplay, EMDR, and somatic experiencing, with special emphasis on trauma and attachment issues. Caron's experience extends to public speaking and writing. She has spoken at many conferences on various mental health subjects. Caron also has written several articles for publications and books on sandtray, EMDR, and mental health issues.

MereAnn Reid, LPC, RPT, is a child and family therapist specializing in adoption and parenting support. Her path as a play therapist was shaped early by somatic approaches and relational neuroscience, explored through studying complex trauma and child development, yoga and mindfulness practices, attachment-focused parenting, and extensive training at the Sandtray Training Institute of New Mexico. MereAnn leads experiential workshops for therapists, parents, educators, and adoption professionals on topics of attachment, regulation, social-emotional skills, grief, and trauma. She runs a private counseling practice in Portland, Oregon, working with young children and adults.

Barbara Jones Warrick, RP, CPT-S, is a play therapist and supervisor for the Canadian Association of Play Therapy (CAPT) with a longtime interest in sandtray therapy. She has completed the sandtray-worldplay training (with creator Dr. Gisela De Domenico) and uses this extensively in her practice with children and families as well as her work in adult mental health with survivors of sexual violence. Barbara has also completed training in the Erica method (with Margareta Sjolund) and the EMDR sandtray protocol (with creator Ana Gomez). Barbara developed a group sandtray approach as part of her work with bereaved families, where she has offered children's grief groups and professional consultation. She has written about and adapted this approach for use in schools and workplaces and for community building. Barbara teaches the two-day Introduction to Sandtray as part of the CAPT Foundations program. When she isn't working as a psychotherapist, Barbara enjoys playing in her garden, creating in her kitchen, reading, cycling, and birding. Barbara is the 2019 award winner of the Monica Herbert Award for her work in Child and Family Mental Health in Canada.

Joanne Marie Wicks, PhD, RPT-S, MACA, is an Australian Registered Play Therapist Supervisor and Registered Counsellor Supervisor. For more than a decade, Joanne has worked with children and families in a variety of settings including Aboriginal communities, private practice, government agencies, not-for-profit organizations, and immigration detention centres in Darwin and on Christmas Island. Her areas of expertise include child-centered play therapy (CCPT), developmental trauma, therapeutic parenting, multicultural counselling, and counselling through interpreters. Dr. Wicks's PhD project focused on an intensive variant of CCPT for children who have experienced significant adversity in Aboriginal and non-Aboriginal communities. Joanne is a recipient of the United States Association for Play Therapy 2019 Student Research Award of Excellence, awarded in Dallas, Texas.

Elaine Wittmann, MAEd, NCLCMHCS, NCC, RPT-S, ACS, holds a master's degree in clinical counseling from Wake Forest University and has been practicing for more than 35 years. Her private practice, Pathways Counseling and Wellness, is located in Banner Elk, North Carolina, where she provides psychotherapy for children, adults, and families. Elaine also hosts retreats and provides supervision and training for professionals at Rainbows End in Beech Mountain. As a North Carolina Licensed Clinical Mental Health Counselor Supervisor, Registered Play Therapist Supervisor, and Approved Provider for play therapy training, Elaine has presented at national and state conferences on a variety of subjects associated with sandtray therapy. Elaine found the power of sand and figures in the sacred space of the tray and incorporated other mediums – art, dreamwork, and EMDR (eye movement desensitization and reprocessing) – to increase the potential for insight and movement. Elaine continued to learn, experience, and appreciate the depths and heights of these powerful interventions for herself and with clients, students, and those she supervises.

Part 1

Introduction

1 Playing in the Sandbox

The Birth of a Healing Tool

Theresa Fraser and Caron J. Leader

In the Beginning With the Wells Family

Looking at the picture, you can't actually see my shiny body, but I am right behind a building made of blocks. I have no soldier friends beside me. The boys put me here and move me from time to time. I stand in silence, watching how buildings are created. The dad gets on the floor too and curiously looks around to view what has changed day to day. The mother human looks my way at times as well but often spends time in a room down the hall. I have lots of other toy friends here. Many look different than I. The boys use the train sometimes to move toy friends from one end of the room to the other. I stand in anticipation, ready to serve. I don't have an earnest need to join a war, but if the boys need me to, I am ready. I overheard the dad tell a friend that.

> upon such a floor may be made infinite of imaginative games, not only keeping boys and girls happy for days together but building up a framework of spacious and inspiring ideas in them for life. The men of tomorrow will gain new strength from nursery floors. (Wells, 1911, p. 49)

I have watched these boys grow. When they were younger, they spent much time on the floor, but as they have gotten older, they leave the toys on the floor and run outside whenever they have a chance. It was no surprise that one day the mom human packed me up in a box and took me to a store.

Margaret Lowenfeld: Off to London to Help Children

I love this photograph of Dr. Lowenfeld. She saw the photos of me and my friends in the book written by the father. She found me at a charity shop[1] and took me to her office with loads of other toys including soldiers like me. I overheard her tell a woman in a green smock that toys reflect the thoughts and feelings of children. I felt very important and wondered when I would

DOI: 10.4324/9781003055808-2

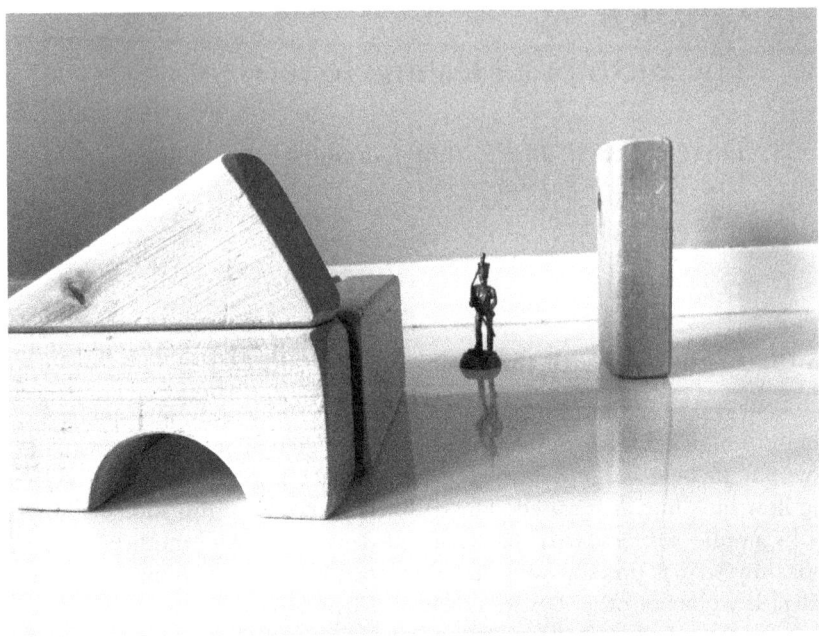

Figure 1.1 Toy soldier as might be used in floor games described by H.G. Wells.

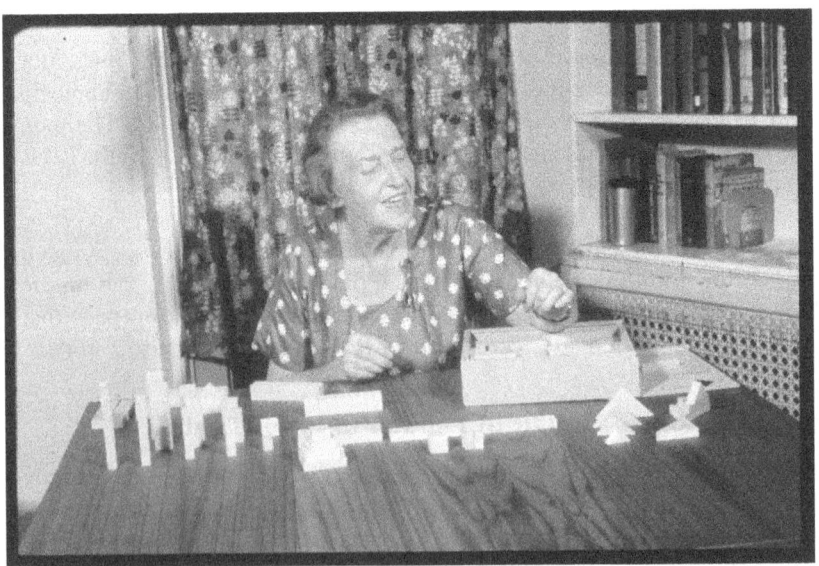

Figure 1.2 Margaret Lowenfeld.

Source: Photo courtesy of Dr. Margaret Lowenfeld Trust

be lifted out of my drawer to be used by a child. Would it be a young child or an older child? What feeling would I express for them?

One day, I did get lifted out. The young girl picked me up and eyed me from side to side and top to bottom. She then smooshed me into soft sand. I couldn't see those behind me, as I was almost in the middle of this wooden tray box, but I could see what lay in front of me. There was a tree and a cow underneath the tree. The sand had been moved away to uncover a blue bottom. A boat sat on this bottom that looked like water. This was a different view than I am accustomed to. I am not on the floor. In fact, when I look around, there are walls keeping the sand in one place. I see the body of a female human sitting beside the child. She isn't looking at the child or even talking. She is looking straight at me!

The little girl is humming now and adding more toy friends to this world. When she is finished moving her hands, she sits down beside the adult and talks about me and what I am protecting. I feel very, very important. After a while, she leaves the room, and two ladies with green smocks come in and move me and the other toys back to drawers. I heard them talking about how many of us lived in the wonder box. One of the green-smock ladies was called Dora. When she left the clinic, Dr. Lowenfeld gave me to her as a goodbye gift. Now I am on another adventure, and I end up going all the way to Switzerland.

Dora Kalff: Standing at Attention on a Shelf

Dora took me to her home office. Her office had white shelves, and I found my place on a shelf and could see the whole space. When others visited this space, she would ask them if they would like to make a sand picture. I once heard her tell another big person that "what we want to mediate for others should emerge from our own experience. This means that the therapist/counselor should possess an openness that is the fruit of an open encounter with one's own dark and unknown sides" (Sandtray Therapists of America, 1991).

The Beginning of Sandtray Therapy

Margaret Lowenfeld discovered combining sand and play was much more natural to children than talk therapy (Homeyer, 2019). Lowenfeld is generally accepted as the first clinician to use a tray, sand, water, other toys, and art materials as she treated children in the late 1920s. Lowenfeld initially used these items in sessions with children who were displaced in the First World War. She recalled a book she had read written by H.G. Wells entitled *Floor Games* (1911). This book described using small toys and objects with children as they created scenes on the floor (De Domenico, 1995).

Dr. Lowenfeld recognized that a child does not think the same way as an adult and that their emotional expressions seem complete to them. Children can react impulsively without thinking of consequences; therefore, Lowenfeld elected to work with an apparatus to better give children a means to express their feelings and ideas. This apparatus was a tray with sand, and as she described,

> My own endeavor in my work with children is to devise an instrument with which a child can demonstrate his own emotional and mental state without the necessary interventions of an adult either by transference or interpretation, and which will allow of a record being made of such a demonstration. (Lowenfeld, 2007, p. 3)

Lowenfeld believed a sandtray would provide a method of accessible expression for children, and it did not require learning any special skills before use. She further described that the apparatus "must allow for representation of movement and yet be sufficiently circumscribed to make a complete whole, must combine elements of touch and sensation, as well as of sight, and be entirely free from a necessary relation to reality" (Lowenfeld, 2007, p. 4).

Lowenfeld decided to call this therapeutic method "The World." The nickname formally evolved to be known as The World Technique (Lowenfeld, 2007). She refined her method when she provided specific criteria for the tray size, discussed how much sand to use in the trays, suggested tables of varying heights, and detailed the types of materials to use with the sand. Lowenfeld fostered the richness of creative expression this method invites as she described obtaining a variety of sand toys, tools, natural items, and miniature objects that included:

> *Living creatures:* ordinary men, women and children; soldiers; entertainers; people of other races; wild and domestic animals.
> *Phantasy and folk-lore:* figures; animals, including prehistoric and space specimens.
> *Scenery:* buildings of any kind, trees, bushes, flowers, fences, gates and bridges.
> *Transport:* for road, rail, sea and air.
> *Equipment:* for road, town, farms and gardens, playground and fairs, hospital, school, etc.
> *Miscellaneous objects:* which may be anything at any time obtainable in shops. (Lowenfeld, 2007, p. 5)

As sandtray therapists, we know the seemingly endless array of objects that can be collected for use in sandtray and can get quite excited when we add something new to our collections, ensuring that we "select not collect" (Landreth, 2002, p. 133).

Not only did Lowenfeld provide the specifics for the tray, sand, and what objects to use in it, but she also provided a protocol for how to introduce the method to children, how to allow for other types of creative expression to accompany sandtray, how to record sandtray sessions, and how to discover what each object placed in the tray means to the child. Her focus was not to interpret but rather to assist the child in exploring their experiences that manifested in the tray. At the time of her work and research, the sandtrays were recorded as a drawing, which allowed for continuation of the work from session to session (Lowenfeld, 2007). She later added therapists dressed in green smocks who may not even work with the same child upon their return to the playroom. The play was considered the most important part of the process versus the relationship with the therapist.

The miniatures and objects used in the sand became an accepted way for children to express themselves non-verbally. They would choose these objects and begin playing in the sand, using their innate senses to guide them as they assembled their world. The play unfolded visually and in real time, allowing the child's inner experiences to manifest and be explored with the help of the therapist's observation and inquiry about the play. Through this process, the therapist could gain further understanding of the emerging world, which reflected the inner and outer experiences of the child (Lowenfeld, 2007).

Lowenfeld's development of The World Technique sparked many other clinicians' interest in using the sandtray, leading to more research and models, each adding their unique spin to her original method. One of these was a student of Lowenfeld's named Dora Kalff (1904–1990), a Swiss child psychoanalyst (Homeyer, 2019). Kalff merged her influences of C.G. Jung, Margaret Lowenfeld, and Eastern contemplative traditions into her method of sandtray psychotherapy, which she called sandplay (Kalff, 2020). Kalff emphasized the importance of the therapist to "create a free and, at the same time, protected space for the child within our relationship," which served as the foundation for building a trusting relationship in which the child could feel a safe connection with the therapist, allowing them to express "whatever is moving within" (Kalff, 2020, p. 5).

The main difference between Kalff's method of sandplay and Lowenfeld's World Technique was the emphasis on Kalff's view of how to help children obtain a developed self through the archetypal understanding and use of symbols. Her understanding of children's play, art, and language was through the use of symbols as ancient and universal images of wholeness. Taking Lowenfeld's work as the foundation for her sandplay model, Kalff felt the symbol played a major role in the building process of sandtray work and informed her analysis. She described her work as the "innate healing forces within the unconscious, the transference connection between the client and therapist, delayed interpretations, and the evolution of trays over time" (De Domenico, 1995).

If someone visited the play space of Dora Kalff, they would find sandtrays that could hold both sand and water. The individual therapist decided the best categories of figures or symbols, which were typically displayed on open shelves and represented archetypal and universal symbols in miniature form. While she also used sandplay with adults, her focus was on using this method specifically with children. She stated, "the child plays out an unconscious problem like a drama in the sand. He or she transposes the conflict from the inner world into the outer world and makes it visible" (Kalff, 2020, p. 7). Dora Kalff's value was to hold a "free and protected space" (Kalff, 2020, p. 16) for the child. She also viewed the analyst's space as a part of the treatment. This meant that the child was welcomed into her home and invited to explore and make decisions about how the therapy time would unfold (Kalff, 2020).

This very brief overview of Margaret Lowenfeld's World Technique and Dora Kalff's sandplay is just a cursory background for understanding the beginnings of sandtray as a psychodynamic process for children. In the opinions of Lowenfeld, Kalff, and the authors and editors of this book, each sandtray session centers around the building of a sacred world, one with (or without) images that depict the child's psyche as they are allowed to freely create and integrate their being in the here and now.

Others came after Lowenfeld and Kalff. Homeyer (2019) shares that some therapists/researchers used miniatures and the sandtray to assess what the builder was thinking. The sandtray equipment became a diagnostic tool for Bühler, Bolgar, Fischer and others where the child would be asked to create a picture about a specific topic (Homeyer, 2019). These clinicians/researchers clearly used the sandtray process for the purpose of assessment, which the editors of this book distinguish as using the sandtray equipment versus engaging in sandtray therapy. In fact, according to Friedman and Mitchell (1994), Lowenfeld was concerned "that my whole research and therapeutic method should not be misunderstood or distorted when part of the equipment is borrowed and adapted to a different purpose" (p. 12). This purpose being to give the builder a sacred space to manifest inner and outer thoughts, feelings, and ideas. Since the days of Lowenfeld and Kalff, there have been numerous influential trainers in sandtray therapy who seek to preserve the nondirective essence of the original method.

For all of our differences, we share commonalities. Respect for the contribution of our elders in our learning is cited in our writing about sandtray, and we need to continue to be generous with each other as we continue to learn and practice.

Thank you to all of the clients that bravely use these healing tools.

Thank you to the teachers who inspire therapists to learn.

Thank you to our colleagues who are as passionate about this work as we are. It is a privilege to stand alongside you in the sand.

Note

1. This is a fictitious reflection imagining the transition of toys from Margaret Lowenfeld's play therapy space to Dora Kalff's.

References

De Domenico, G. (1995). *Sand tray world play: A comprehensive guide to the use of the sandtray in psychotherapeutic and transformational settings.* Vision Quest Images.

Friedman, H. S., & Mitchell, R. R. (1994). *Sandplay: Past, present and future* (1st ed.). Routledge.

Homeyer, L. (2019). *History of sand therapy.* World Association of Sand Therapy Professionals. https://worldsandtherapy.org/history-of-sand-therapy

Kalff, D. (2020). *Sandplay: A psychotherapeutic approach to the psyche.* Analytical Psychology Press. (Original work published in 1966).

Landreth, G. (2002). *The art of relationship.* Brunner-Routledge.

Lowenfeld, M. (2007). *Understanding children's sandplay: Lowenfeld's world technique.* Sussex Academic Press. (Original work published in 1997).

Sandtray Therapists of America. (1991). *Introduction to sandplay therapy.* Sandplay Therapists of America. https://static1.squarespace.com/static/55c0d233e4b0ae953a80a086/t/5ce6b9adf9619a605a61e28f/1558624687801/Sandplay+Therapy.pdf

Wells, H. G. (1911). *Floor games.* Frank Palmer.

2 Drawn to the Sand

Becoming a Sandtray Therapist

Rita Grayson and Theresa Fraser

Drawn to the Sand: Becoming a Sandtray Therapist

Sandtray is a compelling medium. The very presence of sand, water, and symbolic figures whispers an invitation that can be felt in our bodies. A simple blue, rectangular tray filled with sand offers a safe, contained space to play. An attuned companion witnessing the playful creation adds to the alchemy, opening the door to transformative experiences. You may be reading this chapter because you want in on the magic. We welcome you with open arms! In this chapter, we share our stories of becoming sandtray therapists. While our stories are different, there are a surprising number of themes in common. We both felt drawn to the sandtray in a way that was difficult to deny. The drive to learn about sandtray therapy did not come from an analytical, left hemisphere–driven place. It came from the inherent drive toward healing that keeps implicitly held experiences of pain and fear available for modification (Badenoch, 2018). We were both drawn to a therapy that could bring experiences to life without relying on words. We recognized the power inherent in sandtray therapy and wanted to bring this to our work as therapists. It quickly became clear to us that sandtray therapy is more an art and less a technique. This meant seeking a teacher and mentor who could guide us in our craft, much like an apprentice learns from a skilled craftsman. As luck would have it, we both landed in the same cohort of students learning the sandtray-worldplay method under its creator, Gisela Schubach De Domenico. We settled in for 6 years of learning, practicing, engaging in our personal sandtray processes, and transforming, both personally and professionally. Here are our stories.

Rita's Story

The Motivation to Study Sandtray

Do any of us fully understand why we make the choices we make and do the things we do? We may think we know at the time, but for me, it is only after time has passed that the less obvious influences can be seen. This

DOI: 10.4324/9781003055808-3

seems particularly true as I reflect on my motivation to become a sandtray therapist. My stated motivation at the time was to learn a new therapeutic modality that would be accessible to both children and adults and would not rely on words or cognitive gymnastics. The deeper, truer yearning was an implicitly held drive toward my own personal healing. I believe a wall of sandtray images beckoned my implicit world the very first time I encountered them. It is less accurate to say I was motivated to learn sandtray therapy than to say sand, water, and symbolic images drew me to them. The parts of me that longed for healing responded, even though my conscious mind remained unaware.

I vividly recall the moment I fell in love with sandtray therapy. It was 1995, and I was a middle-aged woman pursuing a graduate degree in social work after leaving the corporate world. I was working in my first internship when a local sand therapist invited us to a lunch-and-learn about sandplay therapy. I had no clue what sand therapy was about, but I was being invited to learn of a therapeutic technique, and I was all in.

The meeting took place in the sandplay therapist's office and, as I entered, I was thunderstruck by a wall of bookshelves containing thousands of figures, small and large. I wanted to explore them all! Instead, as a dutiful student, I took my place on the couch and settled in to listen and learn. He showed slide after slide of sandtray creations and told stories of discovery and healing. I was mesmerized! I left the office with a vision that someday I, too, would have a wall of bookshelves holding figures large and small and would have slides of sandtray creations and stories of healing. At the time, I believed those stories would belong to the clients I would one day serve. I had no idea that the healing stories would also be deeply personal.

Ten years passed before I found my teacher. During that time, the notion of doing sandtray therapy slowly simmered on the back burner of my professional aspirations. My second internship brought me under the tutelage of a seasoned cognitive behavioral therapist in a busy mental health clinic. Being someone with a robust left hemisphere, I took to CBT like a duck to water! I was good at detecting dysfunctional thought patterns and offering possible reframes. I honed my skills and ultimately carried CBT, and a few other therapeutic interventions I picked up along the way, with me into private practice. In those early years, I noticed that many of my clients found our work together helpful, but a deeper resolution of the challenges that brought them to therapy seemed elusive. I began to sense a distinction between helping and healing. I knew I was helping, but I longed to be a healing presence for those who sought my assistance. It became apparent that to make the leap from helper to healer, I needed to broaden my skills. What I didn't understand at the time was that I needed to broaden myself. Sandtray therapy was calling me louder than ever!

It was 2005 when I learned that Dr. Gisela Schubach De Domenico, creator of the sandtray-worldplay method, was presenting at our local play therapy conference. I had researched other trainers and training programs, but none were within driving distance of my home. As a self-employed businesswoman, I had rules about managing my continuing education expenses. In the world of health insurance reimbursement for psychotherapy, it was clear to me that a well-trained therapist was reimbursed at the same rate as a poorly trained one. While I wanted to be well trained, my left-hemisphere narrative was that the financial return on my training investment was lacking. Add travel expenses and lost private practice income to the equation and it became financially foolhardy. Ultimately, I settled on the strategy of investing in high-quality training as long as it was local. Finally, a master of sandtray therapy was coming to town!

Walking into the hotel ballroom on the first day of the two-day conference was like walking into sandtray heaven! Tables lined the room, and therapists were busy setting out sandtray images they had brought with them from their collections. We all brought our own sandtrays and placed them on the tables in front of us. I was a bit apprehensive about what these two days would bring, but I was mostly excited and eager to learn. We dove in, creating our own worlds and sharing them with whoever was seated nearby. I was fortunate to be seated next to an experienced sandtray therapist, and with her gentle witnessing, I had my first taste of the power of sandtray.

When I arrived at my seat on the second day, I found a flyer sitting on top of my sandtray. Gisela was offering the first level of her six-level training program in Lansing, Michigan, that September. It was a five-day immersive experience, which would necessitate a plane flight, hotel reservations, and a week away from my practice. I recall reading the details and saying to myself, "Well, it looks like I'm going to Michigan!" This would not be the last time the call from my implicit world would blow right through the well-thought-out rules created by my left hemisphere. It was the beginning of a journey that took me to Michigan every year for the next five and a half years, where I met my co-editor, Theresa, along with a loving group of people I came to call my "Michigan family." It was also the beginning of an immensely healing personal journey that would alter the course of my life.

Personal Transformation in the Sand

I have spent a fair amount of my life with my left hemisphere leading the way. I grew up in a family in which intelligence and intellect were highly valued, while displays of so-called "negative" emotions were generally discouraged. Over time, I adapted by placing more trust in the workings of my left hemisphere and less in the wisdom of my body-brain.

One challenge to left-hemisphere dominance is that it seeks a settling explanation for life experiences. In my case, for as long as I could remember, I carried within me a pervasive sense of inadequacy. Experiences of social acceptance had to be earned and felt tenuous at best. Given what I knew about my childhood, there was no reasonable explanation for feeling this way. I was raised by two loving parents and was well aware of my favored status as the baby of the family. Where could these feelings of never-good-enough possibly come from? In the absence of a true explanation, my left hemisphere sought a settling strategy. For me, the solution was to minimize or deny the uncomfortable feelings. If there was no explanation for them, they must not exist, right?

Fortunately, through my study of neurobiology, I have come to understand the power of implicit memories created in our earliest days. Although I will never know the actual circumstances, I trust there must have been conditions in my family when I was born that temporarily impeded secure attachment and embedded an anticipation that unconditional acceptance was not my birthright. The single greatest toehold into the world of being "good enough" centered around my intelligence. In a bid for acceptance, I put my intelligence forward for all the world to see while keeping other parts of me safely tucked away most of the time. A good bit of energy went into keeping my less-desirable traits under wraps, creating a space between my inner self and the outward persona I presented. Needless to say, my know-it-all behaviors were often off-putting and only served to reinforce the inner sense of inadequacy. Because my wounding happened when I had no ability to form explicit memories, my healing process would have to invite what was alive implicitly in my body. It is no wonder I was so drawn to sandtray therapy.

Gisela offered to facilitate private sandtray sessions for her students. While this may seem like a boundary issue to some, blurring the line between teacher and personal therapist, for me, it was the perfect opportunity to learn sandtray from the inside out with a master practitioner. Each year, when I traveled to Michigan, I scheduled a private session. The sandtrays I created during the course of the training deepened self-awareness and offered healing experiences. The relational bonds with my Michigan family that continued to strengthen over the years offered an atmosphere of safety and trust. The individual sessions I had with Gisela during these times often went deep, and some were profoundly transformative. What follows is the story of one such session that literally changed my life.

By the time I arrived at the session I'm about to describe, I was several years into my training and personal sandtray journey. My body-brain was well connected with my skull-brain, and I had developed a deep trust in its wisdom. Some years, when I arrived for the training, a particular life challenge was alive in my body and brain; other times, the personal growth would be sparked by something I experienced during the training itself. This was one of those times. That year, on the first day, we worked with a partner and witnessed each other's sandtray creations. As I listened to the story of my partner's world, I can only imagine that a part of her story must have touched some bit of unhealed implicit pain I was holding. As a protection against feeling that pain, my know-it-all persona arrived on the scene, and I offered an I-understand-this-better-than-you-do statement. My partner called me out on my arrogance, and I descended into an all-too-familiar shame spiral. I recall heading to the restroom on the next break and, after safely locking myself in a stall, I burst into tears. I cried because I had hurt my partner, and I cried because I knew better. I had made a mistake, and the self-loathing was palpable. My inadequacy was on display for all to see. Behind the initial wave of distress came the exhaustion. I was so tired of feeling this way about myself. (As an aside, my partner's act of claiming her truth about the tray instead of deferring to my interpretation turned out to be a healing experience for her, so we both ultimately, albeit painfully, benefited from my misstep.)

That night, I had a private session scheduled with Gisela. I was uncharacteristically nervous about what might transpire. As we began, I told Gisela I was sick of my self-loathing. I wanted to fall in love with myself, and I wanted it to happen that night. No pressure! I chose my sandtray and started to select images from the shelves. My eyes landed on a figure I had brought with me to my first training in Michigan. It was a woman with a sassy look who was wearing hiking clothes and boots. Her arms and legs were made of wire, with the rest of her made of resin. I love to hike and had added her to my collection some years before. One of the sponsors of the training had frequently used her, and I felt prompted to gift her as a token of my appreciation for the hard work hosting the training. It was this colleague's collection Gisela used for her private sessions. What a pleasant surprise to see Hiker Woman beaming at me from the shelves! After selecting her, I went on to collect the rest of the images I needed and got to work creating my sandtray world. I arranged all the figures except Hiker Woman, who didn't seem to have a place in the tray but who couldn't be left out either, so I put her in an upper corner.

My work in the sandtray that night focused on two beings in the center. One I referred to as Butterfly Woman was lying down and couldn't get up. The other was standing nearby, looking both beautiful and frozen with her arms glued to her sides. The one on the ground felt like my authentic self that wanted to stand on its own. The other one felt like the persona I showed to the world. As I sat with the tray, I was acutely aware of a sensation of space within my own body separating my inner self and my outer façade. Butterfly Woman needed assistance to get up, and yet the frozen one was unable to help. My entire awareness of the world was reduced to these two beings. The situation felt dire and a bit hopeless. I voiced the dilemma, "She can't help her up. She is frozen in place. Her arms can't move. Butterfly Woman can't get up without help. They are both stuck." As I heard myself speak the words, I could hear desperation creep into my voice. This was not lost on Gisela, and in her quiet, wise way, she softly asked, "Who in this world has arms that can bend to help Butterfly Woman stand up?" Hiker Woman! In an instant, the frozen one moved out of the way, and Hiker Woman swept in from her corner, lifting Butterfly Woman and wrapping her bendable arms around her. Simultaneously, I felt the space inside me close. I had a visceral sensation of something shifting inside my body. I have no explanation for the physical sensation, but afterward, I felt comfortable in my own skin for the first time in my life.

Since that session, my mistakes may amuse me or they may embarrass me, but they no longer have the power to send me into a shame spiral. I am better able to offer myself authentically in both my personal and professional lives. I can take more risks and spend less energy in self-protective behaviors. Without the profound change that took place that night, I would never have been able to offer myself as a teacher of sandtray, and I would not

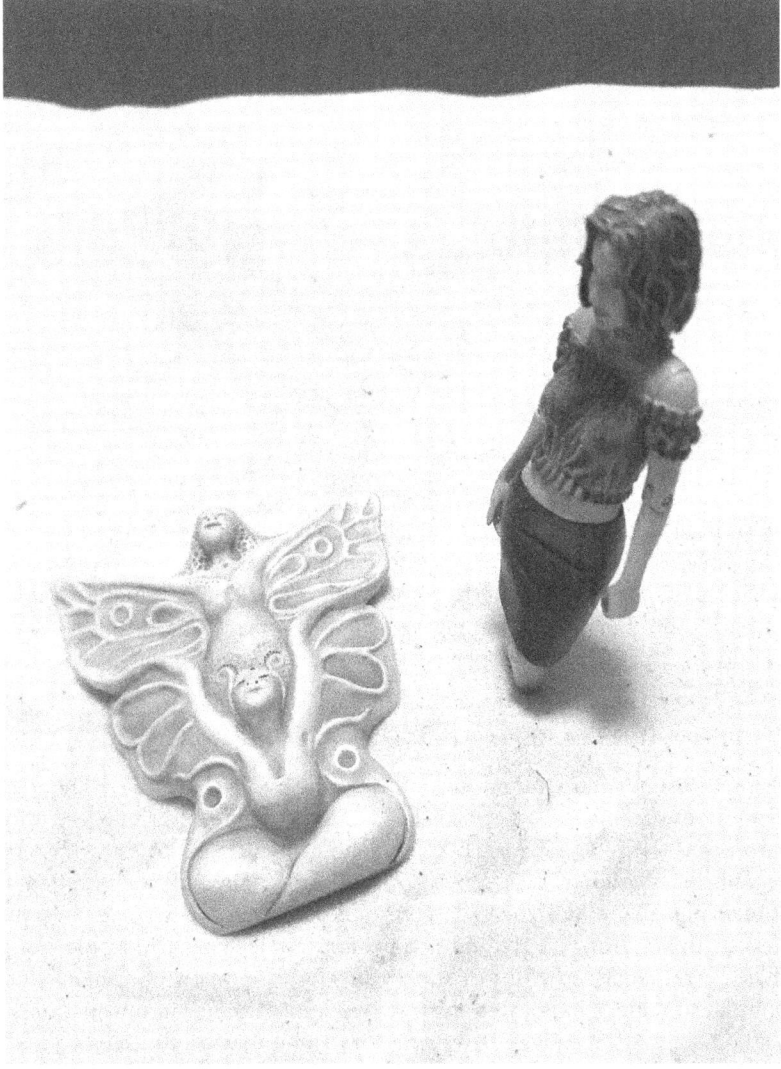

Figure 2.1 Butterfly woman needs assistance, but the frozen one is unable to help her.

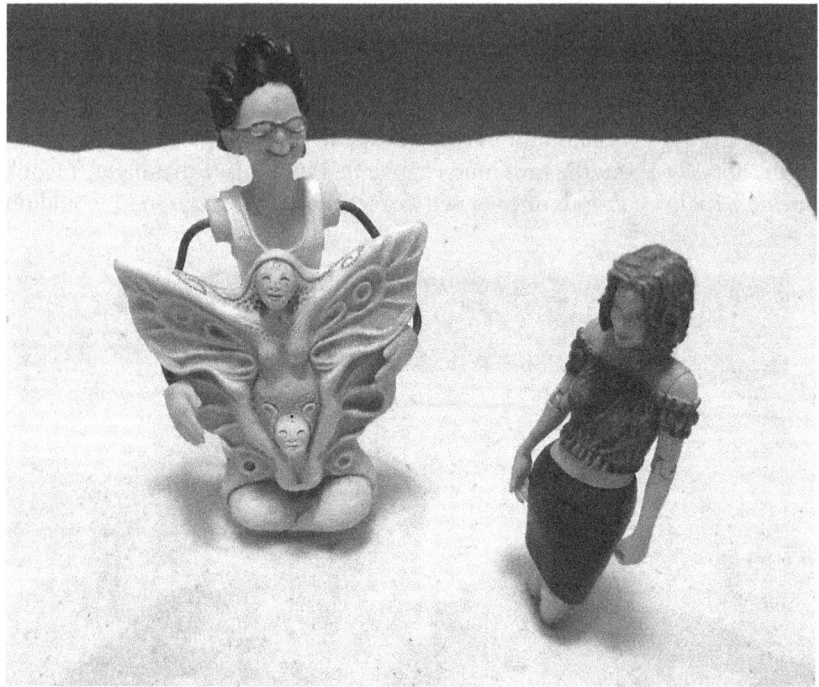

Figure 2.2 Hiker Woman to the rescue!

be writing this chapter. My personal sandtray journey is far from over, but I am able to explore parts of myself with more courage and less fear about what I will discover. And perhaps most important of all, I am better able to sit with other humans, holding their personal journeys, with the rock-solid confidence that they can experience profound healing in the sand.

On Being a Wounded Healer

Prior to the pivotal sandtray session described above, I carried my confusion about feeling "less than" in the context of a life of privilege with me into my work as a therapist. I recall feeling ill equipped to sit with people recounting stories of overt abuse or neglect, as I could not point to any similar personal experiences. I often believed I had no right to bear witness to their pain, that I could not possibly understand it. I could not see that my pervasive sense of inadequacy (in this case, that I was not wounded enough to understand others' pain) was creating distance in my relationships with clients, when in fact, it was the very thing that could have brought us together on the level playing field of human frailty. Fortunately, this paradox did not escape one of the wise women who mentored me for a time. During one of our consultation sessions, with my inadequacy on full display, she looked at me with kind eyes and said, "Welcome, wounded healer." I still recall the emotions and sensations that ran through my body. Could this be true? Could I be wounded in the absence of any explicit explanation? Could I embrace the wounded parts of myself and use them as a bridge to join with the struggles of my clients? Accepting that the pain I felt was valid, even if I couldn't explain it, paved the way for the deep healing I experienced in the sandtray session described earlier.

A personal sandtray journey is a fluid, nonlinear process. As I look back on my early years working in the sand, I can trace three phases that some-times followed one another and often overlapped, dancing back and forth between the themes. The first was exploring and accepting the validity of the pain and fear expressed in my sandtray worlds. This phase brought with it a loosening of the protective strategies of perfectionism and intel-lectual showmanship. The work of the second phase was a gradual shifting from dependence on my robust left hemisphere to getting in touch with right-hemisphere processes and the wisdom of my body. Sand and symbolic images offered a direct invitation to my body-brain that quieted my left hemisphere. Over time, the third phase settled in with a deepening trust that my right hemisphere and my body-brain could lead the way, and my left hemisphere could use its prowess in a supportive role. My healing journey will be with me until my last breath; however, it is from this more-healed place that I welcome my clients these days. Below are some of the ways learning and engaging with the sandtray have changed my clinical work.

Validating. Over the years, I have worked with many clients who feel shame around their personal suffering, as if it is silly or childish to feel the way they do. Because of my own experiences with the sandtray, I can assure clients that the pain and fear they are experiencing is valid and does not need to be justified or explained. We can simply trust it and welcome it into the healing process.

Compassion. Resting on the foundational belief that my clients' struggles are valid, we are able to join together to offer compassion to the parts that got hurt or frightened. This is especially available in sandtray therapy, as these parts are often sitting in the tray in front of us.

Empowering. When I'm engaged in sandtray therapy with a client, I step into the role of witness, empowering them to take the lead in their indi-vidual healing process. Because of my own reparative experiences with the sandtray, I have unshakable trust in the promptings of the implicit to know the path and guide the journey.

Nonpathologizing. Trusting my clients' implicit world to guide the healing frees me from the role of "expert," which implies taking charge of the treat-ment. My numerous experiences working with sand, water, and symbolic images have opened body-based and right-hemisphere channels, which allows me to experience a deep presence as I accompany my people on their unique journeys.

Empathy. Perhaps the most important contribution my personal sandtray journey has made to my work as a therapist is an increase in my capacity to empathize with my clients. This came, first, from healing my own wounds that spawned protective strategies aimed at distancing me from others' pain and fear. In their place grew the capacity for deep connection that comes when we walk familiar paths together. I know, experientially, of the courage mustered each time a client approaches the sandtray with an open mind, inviting implicitly held memories to surface.

Self-awareness. As sandtray therapists, we provide containment for our clients' work. My ongoing commitment is to be the biggest container possible; to offer an expansive space for healing. With each session, I strive to notice the places in me that want to contract or pull away from the pain and fear being expressed. If I can sense the pull and hold it with tenderness and curiosity, it may lead to a bit of healing work, which, in turn, creates more room in the container.

As therapists, our professional development rests on our own experiences of healing as much as if not more, than the education we receive. Therapy is an intensely personal experience and it calls on us to offer our full presence to our clients. The more we heal our own implicit pain, the more we can release self-protective strategies in favor of right hemisphere–to–right hemisphere connection. The need to do our own personal work never ends. As we continue to heal, we may notice the capacity for our clients' healing also expands. Through time and experience, I have come to value presence over procedure, trust over explanations, and welcoming wounded parts over fixing them.

Theresa's story

A Lifetime in the Making

The safety provided by sandtray therapy (Kalff, 1980) is palpable, even for clients who may not have experienced safety in other spaces. For me, working in the sand has also been a source of wisdom and reflection. These three qualities were foundational in my journey of self -discovery as a therapist as well as the many other roles I have experienced in life including professor, foster parent, wife, mom, daughter, friend, and wounded child.

Sandtray taps into the therapeutic powers of play (Schaefer & Drewes, 2013), and I have certainly had deeply healing experiences along the way, but I have also learned that each witnessed sandtray does not have to have an immediate cathartic outcome. Sometimes, trays appear to hold insight if not mystery. Some trays appear to be a simple story. Yet every sandtray creation is meaningful. Even trays that do not take a lot of time or energy to create can have significant therapeutic value (Garrett, 2015). Eliana Gil (Homeyer & Sweeney, 2017, p. XII) affirms that suitable preparation is required by therapists who are interested in learning this method of psychotherapy. In my case, I feel like I have been preparing to be a sandtray therapist my whole life.

Safety

Childhood experiences that included birth at 30 weeks' gestation, sexual abuse, suicide attempts before the age of 5, surviving two fires, homelessness, and foster care connected me to formal helpers throughout my childhood. None of these helpers asked the "why" question: Why does a preschool child want to die? Nor did they provide me with the tools I needed to process and understand behaviors rooted in low self-esteem and past trauma. Various therapists coached me in day-to-day coping strategies but never investigated the experiences that I can only describe as my growing-up passport. I entered into all of my relationships feeling ill equipped to engage in the life experiences that others seemed to navigate effortlessly. I felt like I was "less than" those around me, feeling deeply broken and assuming that anyone looking at me could see this. Like many trauma victims, I believed that if this brokenness was not seen immediately, it would be recognized eventually.

When I was 11, my family lived in a townhouse unit after a fire destroyed all we owned. I created my own home with an empty shoebox and wallpaper samples. I was using play to create a safe home for myself, intended to hold all the worries and stories, but mostly the hopes for my family's future.

In my late 20s, I began to collect miniatures for dollhouses. These weren't the same dollhouse toys that I made sure our two sons and our foster children had for their play. These were the intricate miniatures utilized in decorative dollhouses. I had gathered quite a collection by the time my husband and I decided to move houses. The children were older, we had suspended fostering, and I was heading back to school. A friend encouraged me to purge things we didn't need in order to make the move easier. I decided to donate all my miniatures to a charity shop, because by then, I knew the 11-year-old me, who had lived in public housing, and the adult me, who had created a home and a family of her own, didn't need them anymore.

Wisdom

A few years after this move, I sat in my first play therapy training. It was here that I came to a deeper understanding of why I had been collecting vast numbers of toys over the years. They weren't exclusively for our children. They were also for my own healing. They were toys that helped me figure out how to be a survivor instead of a victim. These were toys that helped me feel empowered about creating my own home because I knew what homelessness felt like. These were toys that helped me express feelings of loss and rejection. The more I learned about play therapy, the more deeply I understood the role toys had played in my personal healing. This understanding drove the need to learn more about the sandtray. If toys could be that meaningful on their own, offering them the containment of the sandtray was likely to be more powerful.

I began reading anything I could find about sandtray therapy, researching tray dimensions and teaching programs. While doing this research, I encountered the name Gisela De Domenico over and over again. I eventually gathered the courage to phone her at her California office so I could purchase a tray from her. To my surprise, she answered her own phone and encouraged me to attend a training in Michigan, USA, which was a 6-hour drive from my Canadian home. With the encouragement of my husband, I headed to Michigan to attend this first level of sandtray-worldplay training and purchase my own sandtray. On the first day, Gisela opened the training with a mindfulness prayer, and I experienced the feeling of finding my place. Her approach supported using the sandtray with adults as well as children. I felt like all my lived experiences up to this point had brought me to this place of learning and healing.

The sandtray therapist in me had found a home, and I continued with the 6-year sandtray-worldplay training program while also pursuing the three-year play therapy training program with my Canadian Association for Play Therapy. In all, I completed 200 hours of supervision, much of which focused on my sandtray practice, and more than 2,000 hours of clinical work, as well as hundreds of my own trays. Some of these were witnessed by others and some I simply sat with and reflected on their possible meaning. Marrying education with reinforced practice helped me to learn what having a deep experience witnessed by a sandtray therapist felt like.

I am indebted to Gisela for sharing her wisdom. I often see her words in books, even those that are recently published. She was truly ahead of her time, and I am grateful for her wise mentorship. I am in awe of the insight she possessed and shared about the healing power of the sandtray. Her training rested on the foundation of her study under John Hood Williams (a student of Margaret Lowenfeld) and her own research in sandtray with children, as well as her experience training hundreds of therapists and witnessing thousands of sandtrays.

During one of our five-day trainings in Michigan, a building near where we met caught fire. I was hijacked by emergency vehicle sirens and the smell of fire that surrounded me. Panic arose in my body. I was right back in the experience of the fire that destroyed my home and precipitated my sister and me being placed in foster care. My fight-or-flight instincts were activated, and all I wanted to do was escape. I proposed that we consider evacuating the building housing our training. Gisela reassured us that it was safe to stay put, which ran contrary to my felt sense of the moment. She must have noticed the panic in my voice and encouraged me to breathe. While I sat in silence, smelling the smoke, I became aware of sensations arising in my body. I continued breathing and listening inside, then my hands went to the sand.

The sandtray world that emerged didn't focus solely on the fire and its attendant fear but also included the hopeful aftermath. As we know, after a forest fire, there are fast-germinating leafy plants that grow and produce a new generation of seeds. Sitting with the sandtray world I created with the trauma of my childhood fire experiences awake in my body, I was able to see the bridge from the sad and scary trauma to the potential for future growth. Fences were placed to contain experiences that were truly in the past, releasing my body from having to hold the fear that came with them. I included a wire stand that stood over all of the sandtray images and held an angel positioned so she could oversee the world. I didn't label her as God or a loved one already passed over but rather as a positive spirit that was always with me, encouraging me to bravely utilize sandtray images to overcome past adversity.

To this day, I vividly remember my sandtray creation, the compassionate witnessing of my practice partner, and the healing that came with it. The nearby fire awakened implicit memories of a traumatic childhood experience. With this trauma awake in my body and brain, my sandtray world offered a bigger picture. The fire was there, but it sat alongside the resilience and recovery that followed. This bigger, more balanced picture invited my nervous system to settle rather than remain stuck in the terror.

Reflection

Sandtray, at its core, teaches both the builder (client) and the witness (sandtray therapist) that growth is continuous. When we engage the body, we actually invite implicit memories to arrive, and they bring with them the actual feelings we were experiencing when the memory was formed. Once these feelings are alive in our bodies in present time, we can "process" them, which really is the possibility of a disconfirming experience or the integration with an associated explicit memory so that we can then experience them as belonging to the past. I continue to learn, teach, share, and apply what I have learned with those I support as well as the learners who come to me. Over the years, I have witnessed the trays of builders who, like myself, found healing through accessing implicit memories and processing them with miniatures, sand, and the sandtray instead of with words.

My motivation to be a play therapist and sandtray therapist is to share these amazing healing tools with others. I am also motivated to help other therapists obtain the skills they need to support the people they serve. Each year, back when I was studying under Gisela, I knew I would experience both personal and professional change with each subsequent training, although I rarely knew what form that change would take. I trusted it was always for the better, although it often brought with it the personal challenge to confront past experiences that were negatively influencing present-day functioning in any or all of my many life roles. Healing these painful and frightening traumas, and using the sandtray to do so, was an integral part of *my becoming*.

It Starts With Me

When we engage in a sandtray process, we allow our implicit world to take the lead, which is very different from using the sandtray as a tool to meet a specific goal. We are opening ourselves to what arises and allowing ourselves to be vulnerable and truly reflect on what sits before us. How can we ask our clients to summon the courage to engage in this way if we have not prepared ourselves through extensive training and a deep personal experience of sandtray therapy? Engaging with the sandtray offers a powerful invitation to our implicit world. It is my belief that we must meet depth with depth. Once you taste the healing potential offered through this medium, it becomes impossible to offer it in a superficial manner. At this point, you will begin to sense the depth and breadth of your own journey to become a sandtray therapist.

Throughout my personal sandtray journey, created worlds have brought forth past experiences of trauma alongside experiences of resilience, allowing me to take in the whole. While I often feel the pull to focus on the brokenness, putting these experiences in the sandtray inevitably reminds me that I am neither solely broken nor am I fully healed, but in all of the mess, I am exquisitely human.

> As we experience the integrity, wholeness and wisdom that result from such play, we become more rooted in ourselves and more interested in living in a familial global community with one another and the earth. We learn how to embrace and support others on their transformational healing journey. (De Domenico, 2002, p. 0)

Beginning the Journey

Sandtray May Choose You

As Rita and Theresa's stories illustrate, sandtray may choose us rather than the other way around. As you will learn in Rita's chapter on neurobiology, our bodies and brains possess an inherent wisdom that seeks healing for past traumas. Outside of any conscious awareness, for both Theresa and Rita, this inner wisdom sensed that encounters with sand, water, and symbolic images, along with the accompaniment of a caring other, could offer a pathway to healing. Not everyone reading this book will feel drawn in such a powerful way, as if the sandtray is choosing them, but many will. It is a call worth heeding. Becoming a sandtray therapist can be transformative, both personally and professionally.

Becoming Versus Learning

Our use of the phrase "becoming a sandtray therapist" rather than "learning how to do sandtray therapy" is intentional. Becoming someone who can create and hold healing space for those you serve is vastly different from gathering the equipment and learning a set of steps, which often begin with an offer of direction from the therapist. We make a distinction between entering into a sandtray process alongside your client versus using the sandtray in a more directed therapeutic intervention. In the first, your role is to support the inherent drive toward healing, allowing your client to set the pace and direction of the journey. There is no intended intervention beyond offering the experience along with your deep, supportive presence. Not everyone uses sandtray this way, but we want you to know it is available. And we want you to understand that supporting clients in an open sandtray process necessitates getting your own hands sandy. You will read in some of the following chapters how the sandtray was used to support a particular therapeutic intervention, such as eye movement desensitization reprocessing (EMDR) or in a children's grief group. Those are examples of using the sandtray equipment as a tool in your therapy practice. However, in each of those chapters, you will also see that the therapist is extensively trained and equally capable of holding an open, nondirective sandtray therapy process. The use of the sandtray as a tool in a directed activity is best grounded in a personal experience of its power.

Training Requirements

You may be wondering what this process of becoming a sandtray therapist involves. Let's first look at sandplay, which is a defined way of using the sandtray and symbolic images and is grounded in a Jungian theoretical orientation. Because there is a cohesive theoretical framework in sandplay, it is more accessible to define a process that qualifies one to use this method. According to the Sandplay Therapists of America (STA), to become a Certified Sandplay Therapist (CST), you must engage in an intensive therapeutic process with a minimum of 40 sessions using the sandtray, attend a minimum of 120 hours of sandplay education, and complete a minimum of 80 hours of sandplay case consultation along with several other preconditions (Sandplay Editor, n.d.). It is clear from these requirements that learning to use sand, water, and symbolic images as part of a healing process involves extensive study, practice, and experience.

The picture is not as clear with sandtray therapy. As we saw in the previous chapter, different ways to use the sandtray developed from varying theoretical orientations. Margaret Lowenfeld, the originator of sandtray therapy, states her desire that creations in the sandtray speak for themselves.

> My own endeavor in my work with children is to devise an instrument with which a child can demonstrate his own emotional and mental state

without the necessary intervention of an adult either by transference or interpretation, and which will allow of a record being made of such a demonstration. My objective is to help children to produce something which will stand by itself and be independent of any theory as to its nature. (Lowenfeld, 1979, p. 3)

However, as is human nature, practitioners who introduced the sandtray in their clinical practices naturally made modifications, big and small, to fit their ways of working. As a result, there are different approaches to using the sandtray along a continuum from highly structured and directed by the therapist to the more open invitation into sacred space described in many chapters of this book.

At the time of this writing, there are no guidelines on training that unite the variety of applications and sandtray training programs in existence. A new organization, the World Association of Sand Therapy Professionals, still in its infancy as we write this, seeks to develop key competencies and recommendations for how to become qualified in the use of sandtray in clinical practice. Until such recommendations are established, all we can offer is our opinions, based on personal learning experiences, years of practice, and time spent teaching the nondirective use of sandtray.

For us, there are four essential components to becoming a sandtray therapist. They are:

- a commitment to receive adequate training.
- a commitment to doing your own sandtrays – lots and lots of them – to deeply experience the power sandtray offers.
- a commitment to supervision/consultation while you are learning.
- a commitment to mindfully build the vocabulary – a collection of sandtray images – for the clients you serve.

Commitment to Learning

How much training is adequate? Both Rita and Theresa completed Gisela De Domenico's six-level training in sandtray-worldplay. We spent 32 full days learning and practicing newly acquired skills over a period of 6 years. Pacing the learning in this way meant we learned the basics then returned home to create our own trays and begin to practice with clients. By the time the next year's training rolled around, we had a sense of what we didn't know and where we needed to practice and grow, both personally and professionally. Each year, we arrived ready and eager to deepen into the next level. For Rita, a sense of mastery began to emerge roughly two-thirds of the way through the 6 years. It took a bit longer for Theresa, who felt more confident after completing the training and spending 2 years practicing the art of witnessing. Theresa spent a lot of time using the sandtray to work out how old hurts impacted life experiences. Additionally, there wasn't a large sandtray community in Canada to consult with or play with. All told, Rita and Theresa each have more than 250 hours of training in sandtray therapy. The entire process moved us from learning it to living it.

Commitment to Doing Own Trays

Sandtray therapy is best learned from the inside out. You may have heard the saying "you can only take clients as far as you have gone yourself." This is particularly true when it comes to honing the art of creating and holding sacred space with sandtray. Over the course of their training, Rita and Theresa created more than a hundred personal sandtrays. In the beginning, they found it helpful, nearly necessary, to have a witness support the work. With time and experience, it became easier to process their own trays. To this day, every sandtray we witness is a gift to us, offering a potential avenue for self-reflection, as well as a gift to the recipient of our attuned witnessing. These days, our sandtrays and collections of images stand at the ready to help guide us through any personal and professional challenges that come our way.

Commitment to Supervision/Consultation

As with any therapeutic technique, supervision or consultation is a must. There is so much to absorb, it is unrealistic to think you can get it all the first time it is presented. Having a safe and nurturing relationship with a sandtray expert provides the opportunity to make corrections and deepen your confidence in your ability to hold this sacred space for those you serve. For Rita, more than 25 hours of individual case consultation with Gisela laid a solid foundation, and now she engages in peer consultation when cases are challenging. For Theresa, she engaged in more than 200 hours of supervison with a few different Registered (American) or Certified Play Therapy Supervisors (Canada) that used sandtray to varying degrees in their practice. She also seeks out peer consultation as needed.

Commitment to Curating a Collection

We like to refer to the process of acquiring your sandtray vocabulary as curating rather than collecting. It is a mindful exercise that takes time, and as you deepen into your own relationship with the sandtray, your collection will also deepen. You will expand and refine it until you have a vocabulary of symbolic images that honors the healing path of those you serve. At first, you will work toward covering the basics, as discussed in Linda Homeyer and Daniel Sweeney's sandtray manual (2017). You will also be drawn to images that will play a role in your own healing journey. If the life of a sandtray therapist beckons you, be prepared: you will likely always want to add to and refine your sandtray vocabulary. To underscore the importance of the collection, we turn to the words of Gisela Schubach De Dominico.

> You are creating a dormant storehouse of human experiences. If you provide a carelessly arranged, haphazard, and impoverished storeroom of pictographic vocabulary, you are expecting an impoverished language to be spoken. Such an impoverished language leads to impoverished possibilities and impoverished creations. (De Domenico, 1995, p. 44)

Conclusion

While it might calm your inner student if we offered a roadmap to becoming a sandtray therapist, we can't do that. What we can offer is our own stories of how things went for us. Each encounter with the sand is unique, and each learner has their own path. While we all appreciate having the surety of steps and timelines for reaching our personal and professional goals, learning to sit in the mystery of not knowing how things will go is an important capacity every sandtray therapist would do well to develop. The advice we offer is to follow your heart (De Domenico, 2002) and trust your gut. Listen inside. Deeply. As you evaluate available trainings, notice what you are drawn to. There is no need to know where you will end up before you begin. Take the first step. Get your hands in the sand. Allow it to work its magic on you and be open to where it takes you. Understand that you will need more than a few days of training to feel comfortable and practice ethically. However, a few days is an excellent start. And once you take that first step, the second often reveals itself. If it isn't clear, keep doing your own trays and attend another training, perhaps with a different trainer. Do your research about the people you learn from. Who trained them? What is their theoretical orientation, and does it fit with yours? How long have they been working in the sand? At some point, you will likely find your teacher – a sandtray therapist who holds the sandtray as a sacred healing tool and offers a deeper level of learning. At this point, you may want to settle in for a while and enjoy the journey. If you commit to this path, the day will come when you know you've arrived, knowing that sandtray is now in your bones. You will have become a sandtray therapist.

References

Badenoch, B. (2018). *The heart of trauma: Healing the embodied brain in the context of relationships*. W. W. Norton & Company, Inc.

De Domenico, G. S. (1995). *Sandtray-worldplay: A comprehensive guide to the use of sandtray in psychotherapeutic and transformational settings*. Vision Quest Images.

De Domenico, G. (2002). Sandtray-worldplay: A psychotherapeutic and transformational sandplay technique for individuals, couples, families and groups. *The Sandtray Network*, 6(1), 1–19. www.visionquestintosymbolicreality.com

Garrett, M. (2015). A sandtray a day keeps the doctor at play: Using sandtray for personal and professional development. *Journal of Creativity in Mental Health, 10*(4), 522–532, DOI: 10.1080/15401383.2015.1009605

Homeyer, L., & Sweeney, D. (2017). *Sandtray therapy: A practical manual*. Routledge.

Kalf, D. (1980). *Sandplay: A psychotherapeutic approach to the psyche*. Sigo Press.

Lowenfeld, M. (1979). *The world technique*. George Allen and Unwin.

Sandplay Editor. (n.d.). *STA/ISST certified member (CST)*. Sandplay Therapists of America. Retrieved October 28, 2020, from www.sandplay.org/membership/certified-member/

Schaefer, C., & Drewes, A. (2013). *The therapeutic powers of play: 20 core agents of change*. Wiley.

3 Healing the Embodied Brain

The Neurobiology of Sandtray Therapy

Rita Grayson

When Talking Isn't Enough: Why We Need Experiential Therapies

If you have ever had the experience of trying to convey the magnitude of a big life event, like the birth of a child or a spiritual awakening, you know firsthand that words can be inadequate. The greater the intensity of emotion associated with an event, the more difficult it can be to put into words. There is a reason the phrase "words don't do it justice" is in our lexicon. The heart of psychotherapy is the cultivation of a safe space for people to explore painful and frightening life experiences (Geller, 2018). What happens if these difficult experiences are outside the realm of words? As therapists, we need to offer our clients alternative ways to "speak" of what troubles them when words fall short. The offer of sand, water, and symbolic images[1] along with the containment of a tray and the accompaniment of a trusted other, can invite wordless experiences into a healing process.

Recent findings in the field of interpersonal neurobiology (IPNB) have illuminated the extent to which our lived experience is governed by the unconscious workings of our brains and our bodies. Stephen Porges (2004) suggests that behavior is biologically driven. He points to the influence of our autonomic nervous system (ANS) on our behavioral responses as well as our drive to connect with one another. In this chapter, we will look closely at what transpires in the brain and body of both client and therapist during a sandtray therapy session. Before we do, it will be helpful to have a foundational understanding of two concepts in IPNB: the workings of the ANS and the way memories are created, stored, and retrieved. As we explore these topics, we will gain an appreciation of just how deeply our sense of well-being is influenced by the workings of our brains and nervous systems. Sandtray therapy, which taps bodily held pathways, offers a way to bring these influences into awareness and into the therapeutic process.

Explicit and Implicit Memory

Our clients come to us for help when past experiences create present-day challenges. It is helpful to understand the concepts of explicit and implicit

DOI: 10.4324/9781003055808-4

memory to get a feel for the way events that happened in the past can continue to live inside us and influence our present-day experiences.

Let's begin our exploration with explicit memory, the type of memory that is most familiar to us. Explicit memory can be divided into episodic memory, which includes autobiographical events and experiences, and semantic memory, which is the recall of general facts like multiplication tables (Dahlitz, 2017). Explicit memory requires conscious awareness to encode (Squire et al., 1993). The brain structures involved in the encoding of explicit memory are not developed at birth. Generally, we begin to form bits of this type of memory when we are 12 to 18 months of age, but we are about 4 to 5 years old before we begin to remember whole stories (Badenoch, 2011). This is why we may have difficulty recalling events from our toddler or preschool years. In general, the recall of an explicit memory is what we associate with the act of remembering, "I remember writing the title of this section about two minutes ago." I am telling the story of something I know happened in the past. This is not the case with implicit memory.

When implicit memory is recalled, it feels in our bodies as though it is happening right now. I remember a playful encounter with a friend's puppy. Explicit memory knows this happened some time ago. Implicit memory brings the felt sense of joy to my chest, a smile to my face, and an overall sense of well-being that is vivid in this moment. For people who have experienced trauma, this kind of memory may trouble their lives every day.

Components of implicit memory may include our emotional reactions, behavioral urges, bodily sensations, and possibly sensory fragments or perceptions we experienced in response to what was happening at the time (Siegel, 2020). It is generally believed this is the only kind of memory encoded for the first 12 to 18 months of life. Because implicit memories do not carry a timestamp, when they are awakened, they bring with them the felt sense of the original experience. Because there is no timestamp, we are likely to attribute the emotions, behavioral urges, bodily sensations, sensory fragments, and perceptions to what is happening in the present moment.

Implicit memory differs from explicit memory in other ways too. Implicit memory does not require conscious awareness to encode, so we make many more of these than explicit memories. We are also able to create this type of memory before we are born (Siegel, 2020). Unlike explicit memory, when an implicit memory is recalled, we do not have the sense we are remembering something. As we become familiar with the workings of implicit memory, we can understand how our present-day response may be largely influenced by something we experienced in the past (Siegel, 2020).

A memory, either explicit or implicit, awakens when something happening in the present holds a familiar quality of a past experience. For example, a song that was popular when I was in high school comes on the radio. My mind quickly jumps to a picture of my friends and me dancing to that song. This is an explicit memory opening up. At the same time, I notice my body wanting to move, and I begin to sway in my seat. I feel a flutter of excitement in my belly and warmth in my heart area. A smile finds its way to my face, and I have a general notion that life is fun and exciting. My mood elevates as I ride the sensations of the implicit memory that awakens alongside the explicit memory of enjoying that song when I was younger. Because the explicit and implicit memories of this particular past event have arrived in close proximity to one another, I know what I am feeling in the present is related to how I felt in the past.

Our capacity to encode implicit memory far outstrips our ability to encode explicit memory (Riener, 2011). We have a vast sea of implicit memories that can be touched and awakened without the accompaniment of an associated explicit memory. When this happens, sensations arise in our bodies without the understanding that we are responding to something from the past. When the sensations are pleasant, we may just enjoy them. When they are unpleasant, even distressing, we may attempt to explain or even justify them based on what is happening in the present moment. Let's imagine an example of how this might work. I'm in line at the local bakery to pick up a favorite dessert for a family gathering. I notice they are running low and start to feel tension in my body along with a bit of wariness directed at the customer in front of me. "She had better not buy the last piece of my favorite dessert!" Which, of course, she does. My fists clench, my belly tightens, frustration rises, and my mind starts to formulate how I am going to complain to the man behind the counter, chastising him for not doing a better job managing the inventory. Fortunately, knowing what I know about implicit memory, rather than act on my impulses of the moment, I take a breath and wonder if my mind and body may be experiencing the arrival of an implicit memory. Almost immediately, I sense the presence of a much younger version of myself. As the youngest member of my family, I often felt circumstances unfairly favored my older siblings. They were bigger and stronger and had more privileges than I did. I can feel the younger me wanting to stomp her foot and exclaim, "That's not fair!" Understanding that the magnitude of what I am feeling in the bakery line is more a response to past experiences and less about the sold-out dessert, I am able to right the ship, order a different dessert, and get on with my day. But what if I had no idea that my clenched fists, tightened belly, rising frustration, and blaming thoughts were in response to an implicit memory awakening? In all likelihood, my left hemisphere would have come up with a narrative that justified everything I was feeling, and I may have left the bakery convinced it was the worst bakery in the world and determined to never return. Enough of these kinds of experiences, and I might even find myself looking for a therapist who could help me feel less frustrated and get more enjoyment out of life!

The Role of Implicit Memory in Attachment

When we arrive in the world, our brains are a sea of neurons that are largely unconnected (Cozolino, 2016). There is a saying in neuroscience that what fires together wires together (Hebb, 1949). Through our earliest relational experiences, neurons begin to connect, and patterns wire into our brains and bodies (Cozolino, 2016). An infant born into a family in which the caring adults are attentive, relatively unstressed, and supported by others to meet the challenges of early parenthood is likely to experience life as safe and relationships as dependable. Repeated experiences of care and connection encode implicitly and form an expectation of how life will go. Bonnie Badenoch (2018) calls these embodied anticipations. We might be tempted to think of embodied anticipations as core beliefs, but it goes deeper than that. An embodied anticipation is more of a bodily held perceptual bias that is so intricately woven into the fabric of our life that we don't even know it is there most of the time. For the little one with responsive, attuned adults, the embodied anticipation is that needs can be expressed, and caring others will respond. You may recognize this relational pattern as an element of secure attachment.

If an infant's early experiences are more along the lines of abuse or neglect, the learning will be quite different. Such an infant may come to anticipate a world in which relationships are unreliable or perhaps even frightening and may develop adaptive strategies to support survival in these circumstances. This baby may learn to suppress cries of distress because such cries have failed to reliably summon care and may have even brought harsh treatment. Our early patterns can stay with us throughout life, but they are also available for modification thanks to neuroplasticity (Doidge, 2007), a term that refers to the brain's ability to create or reorganize synaptic connections. Repeated nourishing relational experiences can modify our initial attachment experiences toward what is called earned security (Roisman et al., 2002).

Let's pause for a moment to consider the importance of inviting implicitly held pain and fear into the therapy process, along with the associated challenge that arises when the difficulties were experienced early in life, before there was any capacity to form explicit memory. Malcom's parents brought him for play therapy when he was 7 years old. He was having difficulty managing his anger when things didn't go his way. Malcom enjoyed using the sandtray, and his sandtray worlds often reflected social challenges, such as waiting for one's turn and deciding who gets to be in charge of the games being played out in the sand. In my playroom, I keep a bucket half filled with water for anyone who wants to wet the sand or incorporate water play into their sandtray process. One day, Malcom placed the bucket next to his sandtray and lined up animals in the tray, announcing that they would all have to wait their turn to go for a swim in the water bucket. As he placed the lead animal in the water, his entire body stiffened. With arms straight at his sides, fists clenched, and panic in his voice, he announced the water was too cold. I could sense that Malcom was working hard to maintain control. I calmly offered to replace the cold water with warm, and Malcom stiffly nodded. Together, we went to the sink, waited for the water to reach just the right temperature, and refilled the bucket. Malcom's body visibly relaxed, and he resumed his play.

As I thought about his session later that day, I realized Malcom's stiff body posture seemed familiar. In short order, a memory of my daughter as an infant, arms stiff at her sides, in the grip of pain from colic, came to mind. I also recalled Malcom's intake, when his parents informed me that he had suffered from severe, unresolvable belly pain for the first six months of his life. Although I will never know for sure, it makes sense to me that something about the cold water in my office woke up an implicit memory of belly pain along with the experience of caring adults nearby who could not bring relief. My ability to meet his need for warm water offered what is called a disconfirming experience (Ecker et al., 2012) that may have touched the original wound with a bit of comfort. It also provided insight into what implicitly might be going on inside Malcolm's brain and body when things didn't go his way. Armed with this possible explanation, I talked with his parents about an alternative explanation for his challenging behavior that did not define Malcom as a difficult or strong-willed child but rather as a child suffering the after effects of traumatic early life experiences. This new possibility freed Malcom's parents to respond to his anger a bit differently.

The Role of Implicit Memory in Trauma

Three conditions increase the likelihood an experience will be remembered, either explicitly or implicitly. The first two are repetition and emotional intensity. The third is the process of myelination, which we will touch on a bit later when we discuss the autonomic nervous system. As we discussed, repetitive early-life experiences can engrain implicit memories that can become embodied anticipations that color our life experiences. Repetition also comes in handy when we are learning our multiplication tables. But we don't always need repetition to create memory. The emotional intensity we experience at the time of an event can also contribute to its neural strength. A bride doesn't have to get married over and over to remember her wedding day! The influence of emotion on memory depends on the intensity. Too little emotion and the experience is less likely to be remembered. A moderate amount of emotion and the likelihood increases. But if the emotion becomes overwhelming, protective mechanisms in the brain are activated, and explicit memory may not encode, while the implicitly held part of the experience may embed as a trauma (Siegel, 2020).

Bonnie Badenoch (2018) offers a definition of trauma based on how an experience is encoded rather than on the qualities of the experience itself. Badenoch states, "Any experience of fear and/or pain that doesn't have the support it needs to be digested and integrated into the flow of our developing brains" (p. 23) can result in an embedded trauma. As we can see from this definition, trauma has less to do with the nature of the event itself and more to do with the neural encoding process. This is not to minimize the terrifying and agonizing experiences that are generally considered traumatic but rather to include experiences of pain and fear that one might dismiss as too minor to have lasting impact. For Badenoch, the pathway for an experience to embed as a trauma is often connected to our sense of being alone with the experience. Humans are exquisitely designed to seek out and maintain connection with other humans (Porges, 2015). Badenoch (2018) tells us the key to an experience encoding as trauma has more to do with our sense of who is with us before, during, and after the event than the nature of the event itself.

When trauma embeds, the implicit memory holding our bodily sensations, behavioral impulses, emotional surges, sensory fragments, and perceptions is stored in subcortical circuits in the brain and in the body. The associated explicit memory of the event, if one is formed, may not be integrated with the implicitly held part. In the same way implicitly encoded early attachment experiences that have no associated explicit memory can influence our present-day experiences, so too can embedded traumas. Even when there is an explicit memory of the traumatic event, the implicit and explicit memories may not be integrated, which allows the bodily held implicit memory to awaken without the associated explicit memory. Because implicit memories have no timestamp, we may not understand that what we are experiencing in the present is tied to a past event.

However, there is good news in all of this. When the implicit memory of pain or fear awakens in our brains and bodies, it is available for modification. If the present situation offers a disconfirming experience, the felt-sense quality of the original trauma can change. An experience can be disconfirming when it offers what was needed but not available at the time of the trauma. Badenoch (2018), drawing on the work of Bruce Ecker and his colleagues (2012), tells us the key to healing "is the arrival of two embodied experiences at the same time: the awakening of the implicit memory and the offering of what is called a mismatch or disconfirming experience" (p. 175). It is also possible for an explicit memory to arrive without the associated implicit memory. When this happens, our clients might describe a traumatic event without experiencing any emotion or bodily response, and we are likely to sense the detachment of the person from the event. In these moments, the trauma is not available for healing because it is not alive in the body. Sandtray therapy offers a safe way to invite embodied trauma, opening the possibility of disconfirmation.

Returning to the story of Malcolm, when he experienced belly pain as an infant and his cries brought his caregivers to him, but they were unable to bring any comfort, it is possible his little system became overwhelmed, and the experience embedded as a trauma in subcortical circuits and in his body. Years later, the sensation of cold water may have been familiar enough to awaken this implicitly held trauma. At that moment in my office, we can imagine he felt frightened and alone and probably had little confidence that the caring adult nearby (me) would be able to do anything to relieve his distress. I was able to respond with calm care and offer a solution that relieved his discomfort while the neural net holding the original pain and fear was open and receptive to modification. Some hours later, through the process of memory reconsolidation (Ecker et al., 2012), the now-modified neural net closed, holding the new possibility that caring others can, in fact, offer relief from distress. After I coached Malcom's parents to respond to him a bit differently when he got upset, they could continue to offer him repeated disconfirming experiences that, over time, could modify the original embodied anticipation away from a sense of being alone in his pain toward one of being cared for and helped in connection with another.

Giving Voice to the Implicit World Through Sandtray Therapy

Riener (2011) tells us we can encode 6 to 50 bits of information per second consciously, while our capacity to encode sensory information implicitly is on the order of 11 million bits per second. These numbers can give us a sense of the depth and breadth of what may be referred to as our implicit world. Louis Cozolino (2016) sums it up nicely when he says, "Explicit memory is the tip of our experiential iceberg; implicit memory is the vast infrastructure below the surface" (p. 70).

Given the vastness of our implicit world, the way it shapes our foundational expectations (particularly with regard to relationships), and the understanding that our most painful and frightening life experiences may be held implicitly, it becomes clear that we need a way to invite these memories into therapy. Because they are outside of conscious awareness, they are not easily accessed via cognitive processes. We must invite them and wait patiently for their arrival. The sense of safety, connection, and presence within the therapeutic relationship creates a welcoming environment for the arrival and healing of implicitly held pain and fear. Sandtray therapy offers a broad invitation, tapping into bodily held pathways, which we will explore in more detail later in this chapter. For now, it is enough to note that bodily sensations and behavioral impulses, two components of implicit memory, come alive in the sandtray therapy process. Transmissions from these and other body-based pathways ultimately gather in the limbic system of the right hemisphere, which is the seat of our relational world and the neural real estate where healing in therapy happens (Badenoch, 2018).

The Autonomic Nervous System

As we saw with implicit memory, much of our lived experience is influenced by forces outside our conscious awareness. This is particularly true when it comes to the workings of our autonomic nervous system (ANS).

Moment to moment, the state of our ANS influences whether we move to connect with others or to protect ourselves (Dana, 2018). Because effective therapy rests on the connection between therapist and client, it is helpful to bring an awareness of ANS states into our work. Creating safety in the environment and in the therapeutic relationship is foundational (Porges & Dana, 2018). Sandtray therapy in particular, with its powerful invitation to open and explore implicitly held experiences, requires clients to have unshakable confidence that we, as co-journeyers, can safely accompany them on their healing journey.

The Polyvagal Theory

Stephen Porges's polyvagal theory provides us with a lens through which we can view the struggles our clients bring to therapy, as well as a guide to how we might join with them to cultivate a space in which they can heal. There are three main principles of the polyvagal theory: neuroception, hierarchy, and co-regulation (Dana, 2018). We will look at each one and how they inform our work, particularly when we are using the sandtray.

Neuroception

Stephen Porges (2004) coined the term "neuroception," which is a neural process, distinct from perception, whereby neural circuits distinguish whether conditions, either environmental or visceral, are safe, dangerous, or life-threatening. Because neuroception takes place in primitive parts of the brain, it is outside conscious awareness. Long before any cognitive evaluation takes place, a neuroception of danger will have already set in motion adaptive strategies of fight, flight, or immobilization. From a survival perspective, a few seconds taken to think about whether to fight or flee could cost us our lives. Bonnie Badenoch (2018) refers to our ANS as the guardian of safety, as it is constantly scanning the environment, both external and internal, for threats to our safety. As therapists, our first order of business is to create an environment, physically and interpersonally, in which our clients' nervous systems neuroceive safety. Without that, as we will see in the following discussion, our clients will be unable to settle into relationship with us.

The Hierarchy of the Autonomic Nervous System

The ANS is made up of the sympathetic and parasympathetic nervous systems. A primary process of the sympathetic nervous system is to govern our fight-or-flight response. The parasympathetic nervous system, sometimes referred to as the rest-and-digest system, has a down regulating effect. A main component of the parasympathetic nervous system is the vagus nerve, sometimes referred to as the wandering nerve, because it "wanders" throughout the body, from our head down into our abdomen. These vagal pathways can be divided into the ventral vagal complex which innervates primarily above the diaphragm, and the dorsal vagal complex, which innervates primarily below the diaphragm. Thus, we have three distinct states of the ANS: sympathetic, ventral vagal parasympathetic (also known as our ventral state), and dorsal vagal parasympathetic (also known as our dorsal state).

An important tenet of the polyvagal theory is that the ANS is hierarchical in nature. Porges (2001) discovered that the ventral branch of the vagus nerve is myelinated, which greatly increases the speed of neuronal firing. Based on this finding, he deduced that when the ventral vagal complex is activated, we are in our preferred state of social engagement and can connect with one another. When there is the neuroception of threat, alongside a sense that we can do something about it, our ANS calls on the sympathetic nervous system, and we shift into the mobilization strategy of fight or flight. In the event the threat is experienced as overwhelming and there is a sense of helplessness, the dorsal vagal branch of the parasympathetic nervous system takes over, and we move toward immobilization. This is the "playing possum" strategy of feigning death to avoid death (Siegel, 2020). In this state, heart rate and breathing slow, and metabolic resources are conserved to be available in the event we don't die. Experiences of shame, humiliation, and dissociation are associated with the dorsal vagal collapse (Badenoch, 2018).

Let's look at what happens when we move into and out of our preferred ventral state. When my ANS has a neuroception of safety, the muscles around my eyes soften, my voice takes on a comforting tone, my ears tune to hear your voice, and my heart rate calms. In this state, my ANS sends a message to your ANS that it is safe for us to engage with one another. Your system responds by settling into a sense of safety and connection. If, on the other hand, my ANS has a neuroception of threat, coming from either the external environment or my own internal state, the softness of my eyes disappears as I focus sharply on possible sources of danger, my voice loses its pleasing tone, my heart rate increases, and my ears tune away from your voice and toward predatory sounds. Your ANS, in turn, may respond with a neuroception of threat and orient toward survival and away from connection with me. All of this happens outside our conscious awareness.

Co-regulation

Co-regulation means that we are constantly influencing the state of each other's nervous systems (Dana, 2018). When our ANS neuroceives safety, we are in our ventral state and inside our window of tolerance. Others' systems will feel the influence and move to follow us if they can. Additionally, if we are in ventral, our system can move toward sympathetic in states of play and excitement without activating our fight-or-flight response or toward dorsal for deep rest without collapsing. Let's take a minute to sit with Badenoch's (2018) diagram of the window of tolerance shown in Figure 3.1.

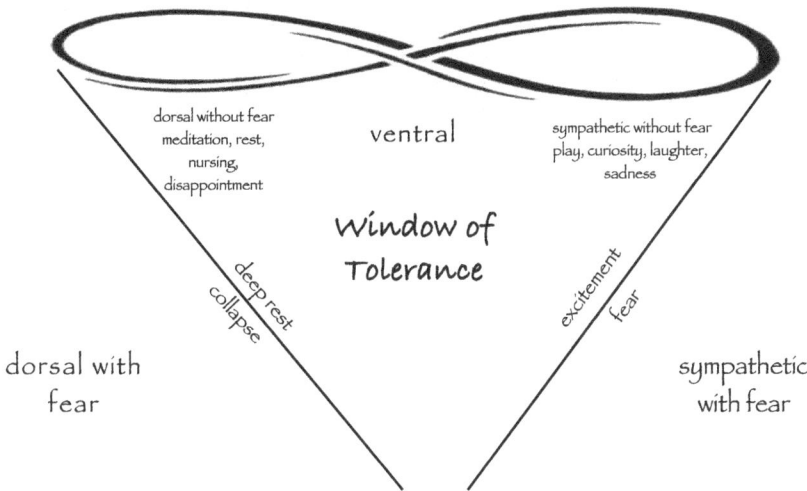

Figure 3.1 Window of tolerance from *The Heart of Trauma: Healing the Embodied Brain in the Context of Relationships* by Bonnie Badenoch.

Source: Copyright © 2018 by Bonnie Badenoch. Used by permission of W. W. Norton & Company, Inc.

You will notice the infinity sign at the top, which captures the experience of our ANS state fluctuating from one moment to the next. The diagonal lines picture how our window of tolerance expands and contracts throughout the day. Our capacity to stay in our ventral state fluctuates depending on the demands on our system. When we are well rested, healthy, and not stressed, our window is likely to be wider than when we are sick, tired, or stressed. On the right side of the diagram is sympathetic activation, and on the left is the dorsal state. On the sympathetic side, when we are inside our window of tolerance, we may feel excitement and engage in play, curiosity, laughter, or even sadness. The sympathetic pathways are under the management of ventral in these states. When there is a neuroception of threat, along with a sense we can do something about the threat, we move outside our window of tolerance into a fight-or-flight response. On the dorsal side, when we feel safe, we can experience deep rest, engage in meditation, breastfeed, and even experience disappointment without collapse. When the neuroception of life threat arrives with a sense of helplessness, we move outside our window of tolerance into dissociation or collapse.

When we are outside our window of tolerance, we are no longer in our social engagement system (ventral state), and our ANS is oriented away from connection and toward survival strategies. In essence, once we adaptively move away from ventral, we are lost to one another. In psychotherapy, the connection between therapist and client is central to the healing process. It is also essential that our clients be in touch with the potentially dysregulating experience of the trauma to be available to a disconfirming experience. How can our clients visit experiences of deep pain and fear with enough access to regulation to heal? This is where the phenomenon of co-regulation comes in.

Let's look at Figure 3.2, which shows how therapists and clients can join through the process of co-regulation.

In this diagram, my client's ANS state is reflected in the inner window of tolerance (inner pair of diagonal lines), and I am the holding person with the wider window of tolerance (outer pair of diagonal lines). Together, these form what we can call a joined window of tolerance. Even though it looks like we are two separate people, we have now become a third entity – the relationship that holds the two of us together. When my client touches on a difficult life experience, the neural net holding the implicit pain and fear

Autonomic Nervous System

Expanding and Contracting Joined Windows of Tolerance

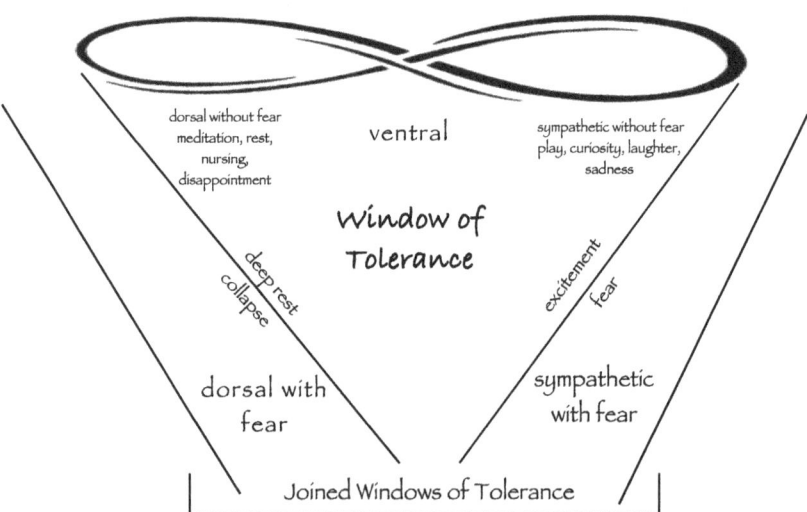

Figure 3.2 Joined windows of tolerance from *The Heart of Trauma: Healing the Embodied Brain in the Context of Relationships* by Bonnie Badenoch.

experienced at the time of that event opens. Because the opening of an implicit memory brings with it the felt sense of what happened at the time, my client's heart may start to beat faster, palms may sweat, belly may tighten in anticipation of harm, and a perception may arise that the situation is not safe. These sensations could easily invite movement into the protective strategy of fight, flight, or dissociation. However, because we have entered a joined relationship, the experience is unfolding in the embrace of my wider ventral capacity. It is difficult to capture this merging of resources in words, but we have all likely experienced it. Because of this, my client can touch on experiences of pain and fear that, alone, would be dysregulating. My offer of a safe ventral presence allows us to stay connected and, together, we can go into the pain and fear of the trauma in the service of healing.

The Autonomic Nervous System's Influence on Well-Being

In much the same way repeated experiences, especially relational ones, create implicit embodied anticipations, our autonomic nervous system is shaped interpersonally (Badenoch, 2018). Early experiences of co-regulation and attunement teach our system that the world is a safe place. Our ventral pathways get a lot of early exercise, so we will likely develop a wide window of tolerance. If our early experiences are more of misattunement, our system may be more oriented toward survival rather than connection, narrowing our window of tolerance. As Deb Dana (2018) tells us, "the autonomic nervous system is 'learning' about the world and being toned toward habits of connection or protection" (p. 5). If what we learn orients us toward sympathetic or dorsal pathways, these become our most easily accessed states. When our ANS neuroceives a threat, either in our external environment or the implicit awakenings inside our brains and bodies, our system adaptively shifts toward strategies aimed at survival. Our mind then observes our state of arousal and looks to explain it based on what is happening in the present moment. It is not uncommon for our left hemisphere to come up with an explanation that justifies how we are responding. Stephen Porges (2015, as cited in Badenoch, 2018) tells us "part of the Polyvagal Theory is that the underlying physiological state functionally drives the personal narrative" (p. 70).

Let's return to my earlier example of visiting the bakery, this time including autonomic responses. I go to the bakery to buy a favorite dessert, and the customer in front of me purchases the last piece. This present-day experience awakens implicitly held pain from my childhood. When this implicitly held memory awakens, it brings with it feelings of frustration, tightness in my body, and thoughts of unfairness. My ANS, in response to what is awakening in my mind and body, senses threat and moves toward sympathetic arousal. I feel like fighting with the man behind the counter. My left hemisphere, with its desire for a settling narrative, evaluates the situation and decides this is the worst bakery ever, offering the conclusion that I should never return. The entire experience likely reinforces my embodied anticipation that I will not be treated fairly in life.

How Neuroscience Informs Sandtray Therapy

As we get a sense for the workings of implicit memory and the autonomic nervous system, we may begin to view our role as therapists a bit differently. Because the neural net holding the embodied part of the trauma must be awake for it to receive a disconfirming experience, our clients are moving away from safety (Badenoch, 2018). If our clients move fully outside their windows of tolerance, the connection between us will be disrupted. When I am able to offer an ample ventral state, it can hold both of us within this joined window of tolerance. In this state, the scene is set for a disconfirming experience, offering that which was needed but not available at the time of the initial wounding. In many cases, just sensing my presence as the implicit memory opens can be disconfirming, because what often makes a difficult experience embed as trauma is the felt sense of being all alone in the pain and fear (Badenoch, 2018). When we distill this discussion down to the essential elements of effective therapy, we find the fundamental need to create safety for our clients, an invitation for neural nets holding implicit pain and fear to open; our offer of a ventral state that can embrace both our nervous systems, and the possibility of offering a disconfirming experience which can pervade the neural net with the felt sense experience of safety.

Sandtray therapy offers a particularly powerful way to provide these essential therapy components. First, engaging with the sandtray orients our clients away from left-hemisphere narratives and toward the wisdom of the body by engaging the senses. Simply touching the sand invites a more embodied state. The symbolic images, along with the natural meditative nature of the process, continues to orient our clients toward right-hemisphere processes. As they relax into the work, their implicit world speaks through the images gathering in the tray. All of this takes place within the safe boundaries of the physical space as it is held by our ventral presence. This creates a depth of safety that is less available when clients verbally relate their personal narrative. In essence, using the sandtray invites the left hemisphere to hand its narrative over to the right hemisphere, where it becomes more fluid and resides in a more open plane of possibilities. As we sit with our clients, respectfully bearing witness to their creation, our brains and nervous systems can settle into deep and safe connection. Our ventral presence can steady our clients' ANS as they venture into uncertain territory. Because the sandtray creation is not bound by the rules and constraints of our clients' daily reality, it offers an opportunity to experience, through the relationships and the movement within the sandtray, disconfirming experiences that may not be available in the outside world.

The Neurobiology of a Sandtray Session

In the following section, I will introduce you to two clients: Max, a fifth-grade boy, who, over a series of sessions, experienced some much-needed care of a younger part of himself; and Carrie, a middle-aged woman with a challenging work environment. We will dissect Carrie's first sandtray to see how the influence of the ANS, implicit memory, and other aspects of neuroscience weave together within the holding environment of a single session.

Max spent his early days in an overcrowded orphanage. His sandtray worlds tended to move and flow as armies did battle and bad guys were defeated. For several sessions in a row, as he gathered good guys and bad guys, he also chose a tiny plastic baby, tossing it into the fray and barely seeming to notice it. The first time he did this, the baby was ignored and trampled by good guys and bad guys alike until I let him know our time together was almost up. Max abruptly paused, searched through the rubble for the tiny baby, and moved it off the battlefield to a relatively safe spot.

As his play progressed over several sessions, I noticed an increase in care being offered to the baby. Sometimes, he would make sure the baby didn't get trampled; other times, he would offer food, and in one of the last sessions before this particular baby stopped appearing in his play, he placed the baby in a small wooden cradle. The cradle in my collection has a blanket that is glued in place. Max needed the baby to be warm and comfortable, so he looked around for a "blanket," ultimately taking a tissue and folding it to just the right size so he could tuck the baby in properly. Max was adopted before he could have formed any explicit memory of his time in the orphanage, and yet the trauma of early neglect was embedded in his system and influenced his present-day relationships. Through his work in the sandtray, along with the interpersonal safety and trust he and I developed over time, Max was able to touch the implicitly held experiences of neglect and offer disconfirming experiences of care. As he played, Max experienced his early trauma from many angles: the neglect, the experience of needing care, the receipt of care, as well as his experience of being the one to provide care and being witnessed and reflected by one who held it all. Outside of his sessions, Max was making progress with his interpersonal difficulties. This is the power of sandtray therapy!

Carrie's Sandtray Journey

The Invitation

I had been working with Carrie for a couple of months when, one day, she walked into my office, took her usual place on the couch and announced, "I think I would like to use the sandtray today." As clients enter my office, they walk past a large collection of figures and a cabinet that holds four sandtrays. Typically, in the first session with a new adult or adolescent client, I briefly describe sandtray therapy and let them know it is available to them should they ever like to try it. I want them to know it is not just for the children I see in my psychotherapy practice. When I introduced Carrie to the sandtray, she politely declined, stating she came to therapy to talk through some difficult dynamics with her manager at work. But Carrie's body told a different story. I had noticed many times, as she walked into my office for her session, Carrie's eyes would go toward the shelves of sandtray figures. Sometimes, her body would pause so she could get a better look. When this happened, I would gently remind her that the sandtray is available to her should she feel drawn to use it. Every time I offered, she declined, and I let her know her response was perfectly fine with me. Each of these interactions communicated to Carrie that she was in charge of her therapy, and using the sandtray would be on her terms if and when she felt ready. Even though I held the opinion that working in the sandtray could be helpful to Carrie, I wanted her to feel safe and not sense that I had any agenda for her to use her therapy time in a particular way.

The presence of the sandtray collection, displayed in a way that is organized and pleasing to the eye, along with any words we may offer, lets our clients know there is a way to speak about the things troubling them without requiring words or analytical processing. From the first time Carrie entered my office, the bookcases holding the sandtray images offered a wordless invitation to her implicit world. Each time she paused for a closer look, it seemed almost as if they were whispering to her. Once Carrie and I built a solid foundation of interpersonal trust, she felt safe enough to accept the invitation. It is important to allow our clients to set the pace and direction of therapy. For some, the attraction to the sandtray will be strong and immediate; for others, it will take a while before they feel comfortable enough; and others will never be drawn to work in this way. For those of us who have deeply studied and personally experienced the power of sandtray therapy, it can be tempting to overencourage our clients to give it a try. However, to maintain safety, it is best to follow our clients' inclinations.

As therapists, it is important to remain mindful of the potential power clients may give us. As we learned from polyvagal theory, connection is a biological imperative (Porges & Phillips, 2016). If a client senses that I have a strong desire for them to work in the sandtray, they may comply in order to stay in connection with me. So how do we know who might be a good candidate for sandtray therapy? I have found it helpful to observe and trust body-based behavioral clues. With Carrie, I had observed the way her body seemed drawn to the sandtray collection. I have had other clients walk swiftly past my shelves without a second look, and it seems unlikely they will choose the sandtray just yet, if ever.

And then there are children, who rarely need any encouragement. I recall meeting Justin for the first time. His parents had told him I could help him with his worry thoughts and that I had a lot of toys. After his mom introduced us in the waiting room, he and I walked back to my office together. Before crossing the threshold, Justin caught sight of my sandtray collection. "Wow! My mom and dad told me you had a lot of toys, but I didn't expect this!" he exclaimed. Before long, and without much in the way of guidance from me, he was selecting figures from the shelves and creating his first sandtray world. Working in the sandtray, like all other relational gestures in therapy, is an offer we make and is best done without any preference as to whether it is accepted now, later, or ever.

The Initiation

As the presence of sandtrays and images whisper an invitation to our clients, their implicit world begins to respond. The moment they decide to accept the invitation, they may feel anxious or excited, have a sense of dread or welcome. All responses can be appreciated as we settle into the safety of the therapeutic relationship and trust our implicit worlds to guide us as the healing journey unfolds. It was no different for Carrie. As we left our seats and moved over to the sandtrays, she let me know she felt a bit nervous about how things might go, but she was excited to give it a try. I reassured her that whatever happened in her first encounter with the sandtray would be just fine, that there is no right or wrong way to do it.

The most important thing I wanted Carrie to know was that she could trust her body to lead the way. We began by having her feel the different sands available (dry and damp). I asked her to tune in to her hands and any other parts of her body that might be speaking to her and simply notice which sand she felt prompted to use. As we move into working with the sandtray, we want clients to orient to the body and away, as much as possible, from any preconceived notions of how to create their sandtray world. In a culture in which left hemisphere–generated thoughts reign, it can require a bit of guidance and permission for our people to move away from cognitions and orient toward their inner world, their bodies, and the behavioral urges that ask them to pick certain images.

Sandtray therapy is primarily a right-hemisphere process. We know from the work of Iain McGilchrist (2009) that our left and right hemispheres operate in two very different and equally important ways. New experiences must first be present in the right hemisphere before they can come into focus in the left. The left hemisphere prefers what is already known, making it a more efficient processor in routine situations. This isn't helpful when we need to orient to what is happening within us in a particular moment. The novelty of each encounter with sandtray images invites the right hemisphere to take the lead, opening the possibility of that which is unknown becoming known. When it comes to problem-solving, McGilchrist tells us the right hemisphere presents us with an array of possible solutions, while the left hemisphere prefers to latch onto a single solution that fits what it already knows. "One way of looking at the difference would be to say that while the left hemisphere's raison d'etre is to narrow things down to a certainty, the right hemisphere's is to open them up into possibility" (McGilchrist, 2012, location 152). From this perspective, it makes sense that we would want to orient therapy toward the right hemisphere. One way of doing this is to engage the body and encourage interoception, or listening inside, which invites wordless implicit memories to arise and manifest themselves in the sandtray, where they can be invited into conscious awareness and explored.

Carrie put her hands in each of the sandtrays and, after a few moments, let me know her hands preferred the dry sand. In order to keep Carrie's right hemisphere in the lead, I avoided giving her any direction about how to proceed beyond encouraging her to look at the images on the shelves and notice where her eyes were drawn and any impulses to touch or pick up something. It is important at this point to avoid calling on left-hemisphere processes by offering a prompt or directive. This can be unsettling for some (therapists as well as clients) because it can be difficult to sit in the mystery of what may emerge. Our left hemisphere craves the certainty of a task to accomplish. We can support our clients at this juncture by breathing with them, offering our ventral presence, and perhaps adding a few words of reassurance. Often, simply letting them know that they don't have to have any understanding of what is unfolding and that there is no wrong way to proceed will do the trick.

The Creation

I watched as Carrie dropped into the process of selecting images from my sandtray collection and placed them on the table beside her tray. After selecting several images, she felt ready to arrange them in the sandtray. She worked silently, and I continued to quietly observe the creation of her world, noticing my own inner sensations and rising curiosity about what was unfolding in front of me. Marco Iacoboni's (2009, 2011) research on mirror neurons and resonance circuits assures me that what I am experiencing may offer a pathway to a deeper shared experience without me having to understand what is appearing before us.

Carrie continued to place the images she selected into the sandtray, sometimes moving them within the world and sometimes making slight adjustments to the placement. After a while, I noticed relaxation in her shoulders and an expression of satisfaction on her face. Her world was complete for now, and she intuitively knew it. She looked up at me and told me she was finished. At this point, I invited her to spend a few moments with her creation and to listen inside for any story the beings in the world or the world itself might be offering. I invited her to share whatever words bubbled up. It is important to note that I did not ask Carrie to analyze her work. That would have called on the prowess of the left hemisphere, and for now,

I wanted her right hemisphere to lead the way. I saw her eyes move around the world as she took in the creation as a whole for the first time.

I, too, gazed at the world in front of us while staying tuned in to my inner experience of it. I was aware that my own implicit world may have been contributing to my experience of Carrie's creation, so I remained open and receptive to what she offered without overlaying my own sense of things. After a few moments, Carrie began to speak. "The woman with glasses is yelling at the woman with her hands over her ears. 'You are so stupid!' she yells. 'When are you going to get things right?' The woman with her hands over her ears is confused. She doesn't know what she has done wrong this time. She doesn't want to hear any more. She just wants the yelling to stop." As Carrie shared, I listened deeply. At times, I repeated her words back to her so she could take them in. Offering this loop of listening and reflection – Carrie speaks, I listen, I repeat her words, she hears them and senses how they feel – invites a deeper, possibly more inclusive story.

As Carrie spoke from her felt sense of the beings in her sandtray world, she tapped into the wisdom of her body and right hemisphere and described it in the form of story or metaphor. When I repeated her words back to her, they were handed to her left hemisphere. This invites a "trying on" of the spoken words and, as often happens, the right hemisphere may offer new bits, either a fine-tuning of what was received or an expansion on the initial experience. I echoed Carrie's words. "She just wants the yelling to stop."

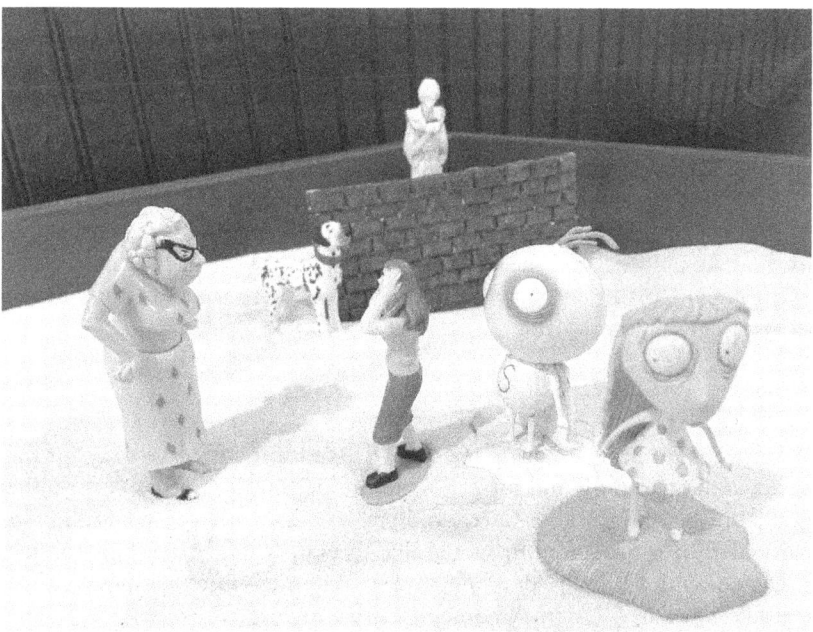

Figure 3.3 Carrie's tray.

Carrie took that in and added, "She is so tired of the yelling. She doesn't know how to make it stop." Carrie went on to describe the being standing behind the woman with her hands on her ears. "This one has a cape and an S on her chest, and she is supposed to be Super Woman, but she isn't Super Woman. She has big eyes with deep circles under them. This is how the woman with her hands on her ears feels on the inside. The one wearing the polka-dot dress has her back turned. She also has big eyes and can see what is happening, but she doesn't want to get involved." Carrie concluded by speaking briefly about a figure dressed in white holding roses who is positioned behind a brick wall. She was unsure what that part of the world was about. There was a dalmatian standing next to the wall. Carrie concluded with, "I don't know why I put the dog in. I just really like dogs." The sharing of the world's story was a beautiful dance between hemispheres and between Carrie and me. As we joined in this way, our brains synced, and my understanding deepened. I tapped into this deep experience and found myself becoming curious about where this world would take us.

To underscore just how much we internalize one another, let's take a brief look at the work of Marco Iacoboni et al. (1999), who discovered the existence of mirror neurons and resonance circuits in humans. While there is still a lot we don't know, it appears mirror neurons help us internalize the intentions as well as the actions of others. They also help us interpret facial expressions and influence our response to what we are observing, supporting successful social interactions (Iacoboni, 2009, 2011). While we may distinguish between self and other, Iacoboni suggests that our neurobiology puts us "within each other" (Iacoboni, 2011, p. 57). This notion is supported by the work of Uri Hasson (2010) on brain-to-brain coupling. His research found that when there is emotionally rich communication, the brain activity in the listener actually begins to mirror the brain activity in the speaker. The higher the comprehension of the listener (based on emotional involvement in the story), the more closely the brain activity matches that of the speaker. When comprehension is highest, the listener's brain activity actually precedes the speaker's. I believe this is what Carrie and I were experiencing, on a neurobiological level, as Carrie spoke and I took in the story of her sandtray world.

Exploration

When Carrie finished sharing the story, I asked if it would be okay for me to ask some questions and for us to explore her creation more deeply. She nodded. I began by asking Carrie if there was anyone in the world she was particularly curious about or would like to understand better. She pointed to the girl with the polka-dot dress, and I asked my favorite question: "What is it like to be her?" After a moment, Carrie responded, "She is stuck. She wants to help, but she is afraid because if she steps in, she will get yelled at, too." I asked a few more questions about the girl in the polka-dot dress and then paused to check in with Carrie to see how she was feeling about us going deeper. Even though Carrie and I had been working together for some time and I trusted her to let me know if something wasn't feeling right, I still wanted to check to make sure what we were doing felt safe and she felt supported. Carrie gave me the green light, and I continued to ask questions designed to deepen her experience of the beings in her sandtray world. There were moments when our exploration went smoothly, and there were times when my questions didn't seem to land. When that happened, I could sense Carrie pulling back, and I did my best to respond in a way that would get us back in connection.

In moments like these, I take comfort in the work of Ed Tronick (1989, 2003), whose research informs us that 33% attuned communication is ideal, and 67% of the time, we will experience a relational rupture which offers an opportunity for repair. This relational dance of getting it wrong and mending it is often, in and of itself, a healing experience, since many of our clients have seldom experienced genuine offers of repair. On this particular day, Carrie and I ventured into some painful territory. She got in touch with the sense of helplessness of the woman with her hands on her ears, along with the sense of overwhelming demands on the one who is supposed to be Super Woman. She could feel the dilemma of the one in the polka-dot dress who wants to help but is frozen with fear. Carrie was also able to sense the woundedness of the woman in glasses who finds fault with everyone and everything.

Going back to our discussion of polyvagal theory, the phenomenon of co-regulation presented an opportunity for Carrie to touch this implicit pain without becoming dysregulated. Her nervous system could lean on mine as I remained in my ventral state. I felt confident that Carrie could deeply feel my presence thanks to our mirror neurons facilitating internalization of one another and our brains coupling as she told her story and I deeply listened and received her. We may have been inhabiting two separate bodies, but in that moment, we became one. Wherever Carrie took us, she knew, on an experiential level, that I was right there with her. This sense of accompaniment is the foundation for deep healing work. To quote Lane Beckes and James Coan (2011), originators of social baseline theory:

> Put simply, individuals in closer relationships experience fewer demands on their own neural resources when solving problems, sustaining vigilance for potential threats, and regulating emotional responses. A growing body of research suggests these and many other processes are indeed distributed across socially interacting brains as people outsource to, or share various tasks with, other individuals. (cf Hutchins, 1991; Wooley et al., 2010; Fitzsimons & Finkel, 2011 as cited in Beckes & Coan, 2011)

Carrie and I also explored the more mysterious part of her sandtray world: the figure with the roses, the wall, and the dog. She experienced the one holding the roses as a resource, but that resource was blocked by the brick wall. Together, we noticed the one holding the roses and the dalmatian share similar coloring, the dog's red collar being reflective of the red roses. Carrie noticed the dog was not stuck behind the wall and sensed he may be able to carry the resource to the woman with her hands on her ears.

Disconfirmation

As Carrie spoke of the dalmatian who was not stuck behind the wall, I sensed the possibility of movement toward a disconfirming experience. As often happens in such moments, Carrie looked at me and asked, "Can I move things around?" I let her know this was her creation and that I fully supported her in doing whatever she felt she needed to do. Carrie moved the dalmatian next to the woman with her hands on her ears. "How does she feel now?" I asked. "Better. A little more supported," Carrie replied. Before our session ended, Carrie rearranged her world (see Figure 3.4) and once again, I saw the familiar settling in her body. "I like it," she said. "This feels better." In her final version of the world, the woman with her hands on her ears has found a way to block the worst of the yelling, which

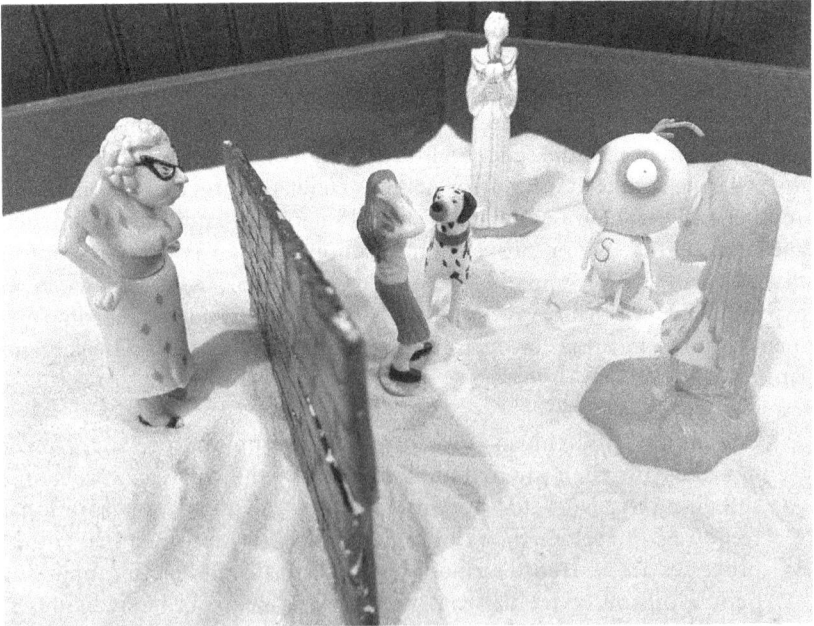

Figure 3.4 The movement in Carrie's tray to block some of the yelling and bring resources closer.

allowed the girl in the polka dot dress to turn inward toward the others. The resource brought by the dog is by her side, and the one with the roses moved a bit closer.

The Healing

When Carrie approached the sandtray shelves, she expected to work on the contentious relationship with her manager. The yelling woman wearing glasses seemed to embody her boss, and she felt like she might be the woman with her hands on her ears. But as Carrie loosened her hold on closely identifying any of the beings in the world, things took a different turn. Implicit memories of being yelled at by an angry father arose alongside her sense of abandonment by her mother, who did not step in to help. The tired one who was supposed to be Super Woman held the helplessness she felt as a child trying to be good enough to stay out of trouble. She also touched into the deep woundedness of a father who both loved and hurt his daughter. Several qualities of sandtray therapy supported Carrie and allowed her to touch these deeply painful experiences without becoming dysregulated. The first was the safety of the therapeutic relationship. We are reminded of the statement "Safety is the treatment" (Porges & Dana, 2018). Working within the metaphor of the beings in her sandtray world also added to Carrie's sense of safety. We were not talking about her mother and her father. We were talking about the girl in the polka-dot dress and the woman who was yelling. In the course of her therapy, Carrie had talked about her mother and father and had described her mother as indifferent. After this sandtray session, she understood that what looked like indifference might really have been fear. This insight was immensely healing for Carrie. Because Carrie's ANS was able to co-regulate with mine, she was able to sit with the implicit pain and fear of her experience as a young child facing a frightening parent. In that moment, traumatic childhood memories were awake and available for modification. Recalling what Badenoch (2018) tells us about healing:

> Memory reconsolidation research has shown that for the felt sense and implicit pattern to change, we need to not only be in touch with the embedded trauma, but simultaneously in the presence of what has been called a disconfirming experience – most often what was needed at the time of the potential trauma but was not available. (p. 13)

As a little girl, when Carrie became the object of her father's rage, she needed safety, protection, and reassurance that she was not alone. In her sandtray world, the woman with her hands on her ears found a way to quiet the yelling, which brought safety, protection, and connection with the one in the polka-dot dress. In my counseling room, Carrie, the adult, was offered a safe experience in which she could touch on traumatic experiences, feeling I was right there with her. The neural nets holding the trauma were wide open and available to be modified by the disconfirming experiences both in the sandtray world and within our therapeutic relationship.

Concluding Thoughts

As you may sense through Carrie's story, entering into the sacred space of sandtray therapy is more an art than a science. Offering the sandtray as a healing tool calls on us to release any agenda or desire to direct the session and, instead, asks us to dedicate ourselves to staying present and co-experiencing, alongside our clients, what is unfolding in each moment. This is no easy task in our current culture, which demands measurable progress toward defined treatment goals and holds the therapist responsible for treatment outcomes. This discussion of the neurobiological processes underlying the healing that is available when we offer the sandtray illuminates the reality that it is actually an art grounded in science. Understanding how sandtray therapy supports healing through a neurobiological lens may help us stay the course and trust our clients to guide us along their unique healing paths.

Sandtray therapy sources the wisdom of the body and right hemisphere, offering an invitation to that which is held implicitly and, therefore, out of conscious awareness, into a healing therapeutic process. Through the use of sand, water, and a collection of images, our inner world can give voice to early experiences, before our brains were sufficiently developed to record explicit memories, as well as experiences that have embedded in our brains and bodies as trauma. All effective therapy must rest on a bedrock of safety (Porges & Dana, 2018), particularly therapies that invite deep work.

Several qualities of sandtray therapy promote safety: the therapeutic distance created by the use of images and metaphor; the inherent permission for clients to proceed at their own pace without direction or intervention from the therapist; the opportunity for clients' nervous systems to co-regulate with the therapist's, allowing the processing of pain and fear that might otherwise be dysregulating; and the felt-sense accompaniment of the therapist by clients, embedding the experience that they are not alone in their healing journey. Thanks to mirror neurons and resonance circuits, along with the phenomenon of brain coupling, therapist and client join to become a third entity as they co-experience the unfolding creation in the sandtray. For both, there is a beautiful dance between brain hemispheres, with the right handing its experience of the sandtray creation to the left, where it may offer words and possibilities back to the right. All of this sets the stage for the possibility of a disconfirming experience, both within the sandtray itself and between therapist and client, that has the capacity to change neural firings in the direction of comfort and well-being.

Over the past few decades, the field of psychotherapy has moved toward empirically supported treatments and evidence-based practice in a bid for credibility (Thomason, 2010). Sadly, this has cast a shadow on therapeutic processes that do not lend themselves to research protocols. Empirically supported treatments must meet rigorous requirements, including proven efficacy in at least two randomized controlled clinical trials. It is essentially impossible to subject sandtray therapy to this type of study because it requires the standardization of treatment procedures in order to ensure all study participants receive treatment in the same way (Castelnuovo, 2010). While there are therapists who use the sandtray in a more directed or prescribed way, which may be more amenable to study, such interventions miss the depth of healing available when the sandtray is offered as an open, agendaless invitation to the client's implicit world. If we think of sandtray therapy as art, sitting in front of the sandtray with a collection of images on hand is like sitting in front of a blank canvas with a vast array of paints and brushes at the ready. Any attempt to impose a standard protocol for what comes next would be like trading the blank canvas for a paint-by-numbers sheet. Sadly, in a summary of empirically supported treatments for adults (Chambless & Ollendick, 2001), there is not a single mention of sandtray therapy, or any other deeply experiential therapy for that matter. Yet we know from neuroscience that our clients benefit when we ground therapy in the body and right hemisphere.

The news, however, is not necessarily all bleak. If we broaden our understanding of what makes a treatment effective beyond randomized controlled trials to outcome studies, we find support for sandtray therapy when it is used within the theoretical framework of psychodynamic psychotherapy. Jonathan Shedler (2010) reviewed multiple meta-analyses, each of which synthesized the outcomes of independent studies looking into the efficacy of psychotherapy. He found that the effectiveness of psychodynamic therapy is more robust than that of other therapies considered to be empirically supported or evidence based. Additionally, unlike those therapies, the data shows that clients who engage in psychodynamic therapies continue to improve after treatment ends. This finding suggests that a psychodynamic approach, which rests on the exploration of material outside of conscious awareness within a safe therapeutic relationship, may be a better choice in the long run. In the case of sandtray therapy, this finding makes perfect sense. Because sandtray offers a way to actually modify wired-in implicitly held pain and fear, it changes the brain. It is my hope for the future that the pendulum will swing away from exclusive support for evidence-based treatments to include scientifically informed processes like sandtray therapy.

Note

1. Gisela Schubach DeDomenico, creator of the sandtray-worldplay method, referred to sandtray figures (commonly called miniatures) as "images" because they are a representation of something that is to come. Once the images enter the sandtray creation, they become "beings" to reflect that they have been enlivened and now hold the essence of what is being projected onto them. I prefer these terms over the more

commonly used "miniature" because there is nothing small about this experience. Also, sandtray images need to be of varying size, so the concept of "miniatures" can be misleading.

References

Badenoch, B. (2011). *The brain-savvy therapist's workbook: A companion to being a brain-wise therapist*. W. W. Norton & Company, Inc.

Badenoch, B. (2018). *The heart of trauma: Healing the embodied brain in the context of relationships*. W. W. Norton & Company, Inc.

Beckes, L., & Coan, J. A. (2011). Social baseline theory: The role of social proximity in emotion and economy of action. *Social and Personality Psychology Compass, 5*(12), 976–988. doi:10.1111/j.1751-9004.2011.00400.x

Castelnuovo, G. (2010). Empirically supported treatments in psychotherapy: Towards an evidence-based or evidence-biased psychology in clinical settings? *Frontiers in Psychology, 1*(27), 1–10. doi:10.3389/fpsyg.2010.00027

Chambless, D. L., & Ollendick, T. H. (2001). Empirically supported psychological interventions: Controversies and evidence. *Annual Review of Psychology, 52*(1), 685–716. doi:10.1146/annurev.psych.52.1.685

Cozolino, L. (2016). *Why therapy works: Using our minds to change our brains*. W. W. Norton & Company, Inc.

Dahlitz, M. (2017). *The psychotherapist's essential guide to the brain*. Dahlitz Media.

Dana, D. A. (2018). *The polyvagal theory in therapy: Engaging the rhythm of regulation*. W. W. Norton & Company, Inc.

Doidge, N. (2007). *The brain that changes itself: Stories of personal triumph from the frontiers of brain science*. Penguin.

Ecker, B., Ticic, R., & Hulley, L. (2012). *Unlocking the emotional brain: Eliminating symptoms at their root using memory reconsolidation*. Routledge.

Geller, S. M. (2018). Therapeutic presence and polyvagal theory: Principles and practices for cultivating effective therapeutic relationships. In S. W. Porges & D. Dana (Eds.), *Clinical applications of the polyvagal theory: The emergence of polyvagal-informed therapies* (pp. 106–126). W. W. Norton & Company, Inc.

Hasson, U. (2010, December). Defend your research: I can make your brain look like mine. *Harvard Business Review*. https://hbr.org/2010/12/defend-your-research-i-can-make-your-brain-look-like-mine

Hebb, D. O. (1949). *The organization of behavior: A neuropsychological theory*. Wiley.

Iacoboni, M. (2009). Imitation, empathy, and mirror neurons. *Annual Review of Psychology, 60*, 653–670. doi:10.1146/annurev.psych.60.110707.163604

Iacoboni, M. (2011). Within each other: Neural mechanisms for empathy in the primate brain. In A. Coplan & P. Goldie (Eds.), *Empathy: Philosophical and psychological perspectives* (pp. 45–57). Oxford University Press.

Iacoboni, M., Woods, R. P., Brass, M., Bekkering, H., Mazziotta, J. C., & Rizzollatti, G. (1999). Cortical mechanisms of human imitation. *Science, 286*(5449), 2526–2528. https://doi.org/10.1126/science.286.5449.2526

McGilchrist, I. (2009). *The master and his emissary: The divided brain and the making of the Western world*. Yale University Press.

McGilchrist, I. (2012). *The divided brain and the search for meaning: Why are we so unhappy?* Yale University Press.

Porges, S. W. (2001). The polyvagal theory: Phylogenetic substrates of a social nervous system. *International Journal of Psychophysiology, 42*, 123–146. https://static1.square space.com/static/5c1d025fb27e390a78569537/t/5ccdfeab104c7b981c2f77c0/1557 003948682/Polyvagal%E2%80%93Theory%E2%80%93substrates.pdf

Porges, S. W. (2004, May 19–24). Neuroception: A subconscious system for detecting threats and safety. *Zero to Three.*

Porges, S. W. (2015). Making the world safe for our children: Down-regulating defense and up-regulating social engagement to 'optimise' the human experience. *Children Australia, 40*(2), 114–123. doi:10.1017/cha.2015.12

Porges, S. W. (2018). Polyvagal theory: A primer. In S. W. Porges & D. Dana (Eds.), *Clinical applications of the polyvagal theory: The emergence of polyvagal-informed therapies* (pp. 50–69). W. W. Norton & Company, Inc.

Porges, S. W., & Dana, D. A. (2018). *Clinical applications of the polyvagal theory: The emergence of polyvagal-informed therapies.* W. W. Norton & Company, Inc.

Porges, S. W., & Phillips, M. (2016). *Connectedness: A biological imperative.* Webinar. http://bestpracticesintherapy.com/silver-month-long-july/

Riener, A. (2011). *Information injection below conscious awareness: Potential of sensory channels.* www.pervasive.jku.at/Research/Publications/_Documents/Automotive%20UI%20 2011%20-%20Information%20injection%20below%20conscious%20awareness%20 CR%20v2.pdf

Roisman, G. I., Padrón, E., Sroufe, A. L., & Egeland, B. (2002). Earned-secure attachment status in retrospect and prospect. *Child Development, 73*(4), 1204–1219.

Shedler, J. (2010). The efficacy of psychodynamic psychotherapy. *American Psychologist, 65*(2), 98–109. doi:10.1037/a0018378

Siegel, D. J. (2020). *The developing mind: How relationships and the brain interact to shape who we are* (3rd ed.). The Guilford Press.

Squire, L. R., Knowlton, B., & Musen, G. (1993). The structure and organization of memory. *Annual Review of Psychology, 44*, 453–495. http://whoville.ucsd.edu/ PDFs/206_Squire_etal_AnnuRevPsych_1993.pdf

Thomason, T. (2010). The trend toward evidence-based practice and the future of psychotherapy. *American Journal of Psychotherapy, 64*(1), 29–38.

Tronick, E. Z. (1989). Emotions and emotional communication in infants. *American Psychologist, 44*, 112–119.

Tronick, E. Z. (2003). *Of course all relationships are unique: How co-creative processes generate unique mother-infant and patient-therapist relationships and change other relationships.* In New Developments in Attachment Theory: Application to Clinical Practice, proceedings of conference at UCLA, Los Angeles, CA.

4 It Is Never Too Late

Healing Trauma Across the Life Span With Sandtray Therapy

Theresa Fraser

Sandtray therapy is often associated with the treatment of children. I believe it can offer deeply healing experiences to all, regardless of age. In this chapter, I will share examples of sandtray journeys taken by individuals across the life span. Developmental tasks identified by Havighurst (1953) will be referenced for each developmental phase.

Much has been learned about development (particularly brain development) since 1958. Most importantly, we now understand that we are not bound to suffer the consequences of difficult life experiences until the end of our days. Thanks to neuroplasticity, experiences of pain and/or fear that have embedded as trauma in our brains and bodies can be healed. As noted in Grayson's chapter in this book, such healing requires the implicit memory of the trauma to be awake and alive in the therapeutic encounter. Sandtray, being body and right hemisphere based, activates implicit neural networks irrespective of our chronological age. Touching the sand initiates a sensory experience that provides physiological soothing when our parasympathetic nervous system is hyper- or hypoaroused. We understand that "engaging with the sandtray orients our clients away from left-hemisphere narratives and toward the wisdom of the body by engaging the senses" (Grayson, chapter 3, p. X). Lowenfeld's quest in the early 1900s "was to communicate with children in a manner that required neither the possession of specific artistic or mechanical skills nor the mastery of language skills" (De Domenico, 1987, p. 9). Her underlying value was that play is a natural adaptive process for each child. This chapter affirms that this adaptive process isn't just for children.

Early Childhood: Forming Concepts and Learning Language to Describe Physical and Social Realities

Garry Landreth shared with the play therapy community that toys can be the words and play can communicate the story (Landreth, 2012). This is particularly relevant in the use of the sandtray with children who are forming concepts and learning language to describe their physical and social realities (Havighurst, 1953). They choose miniatures, sometimes referred to

DOI: 10.4324/9781003055808-5

as beings[1] or images, and place these in the safety of the sandtray container. As the story unfolds, the sandtray therapist witnesses the arrival of each and the interactions of all, as well as the builder's emotional responses. With curiosity, the therapist yearns to learn the physical and social realities both in and outside of the sandtray.

Sabastian was 6 years of age and in the process of being adopted by his maternal grandfather and grandfather's second wife. Sabastian's mother had had him as a young teen. Sabastian was apprehended by DCS at two years of age and placed with grandfather as the closest relative who was approved for kinship care. His grandparents brought him to therapy while the adoption was being finalized. Sabastian's mother had stopped attending visits with Sabastian for more than a year but had recently been initiating contact more often.

Sebastian's grandmother reported that after recent visits with mom, he was clingier and emotionally reactive, having a greater number of meltdowns. He also was experiencing sleep disruptions and crawling into his grandparents' bed each night, which was, in turn, impacting their sleep patterns. Grandmother indicated that she found the sleep interruptions difficult but recognized that Sabastian was seeking connection.

Sabastian and his grandmother came to the play therapy room, where he was immediately drawn to the sandtray. In his first session, he moved the sand around with his little hands, clearly enjoying the feeling of sand flowing through his fingers, as evidenced by the smile that was stuck to his face. In sessions two through four, he used a big bulldozer truck to move the sand from one side of the tray to another. By session five, a being (whom Sabastian described as a little boy) arrived to drive the bulldozer until a big two-headed dragon swooped down and pulled the little boy out of the world. This unexpected action surprised both Grandmother and myself, as it appeared to come from nowhere but was completed with intention.

After these sessions, Sabastian's grandparents let me know that things didn't seem to be changing much at home. However, things began to shift in session six as the story started to deepen. In this session, the little boy was joined in the world by another dragon. This dragon had a large wingspan and was perched on the edge of the sandtray, overlooking all that the bulldozer had accomplished. When the two-headed dragon began to dive, Sabastian paused and asked his grandmother to pick up the other dragon. He then asked her to make sure her dragon hid the little boy. Grandmother's dragon flew up and then down in front of the little boy. The sound of the movement was palpable in the healing space. The majestic wingspan protected the little boy. The two-headed dragon would now only be able to pick him up by sneaking behind him. The little boy was now safe from all that he could see and that which he did not know could hurt him.

Sabastian clapped with glee while his grandmother's eyes filled with tears. She told me later that not only was this the one time he had invited her into his play but also that he now seemed open to her being his protector. Not

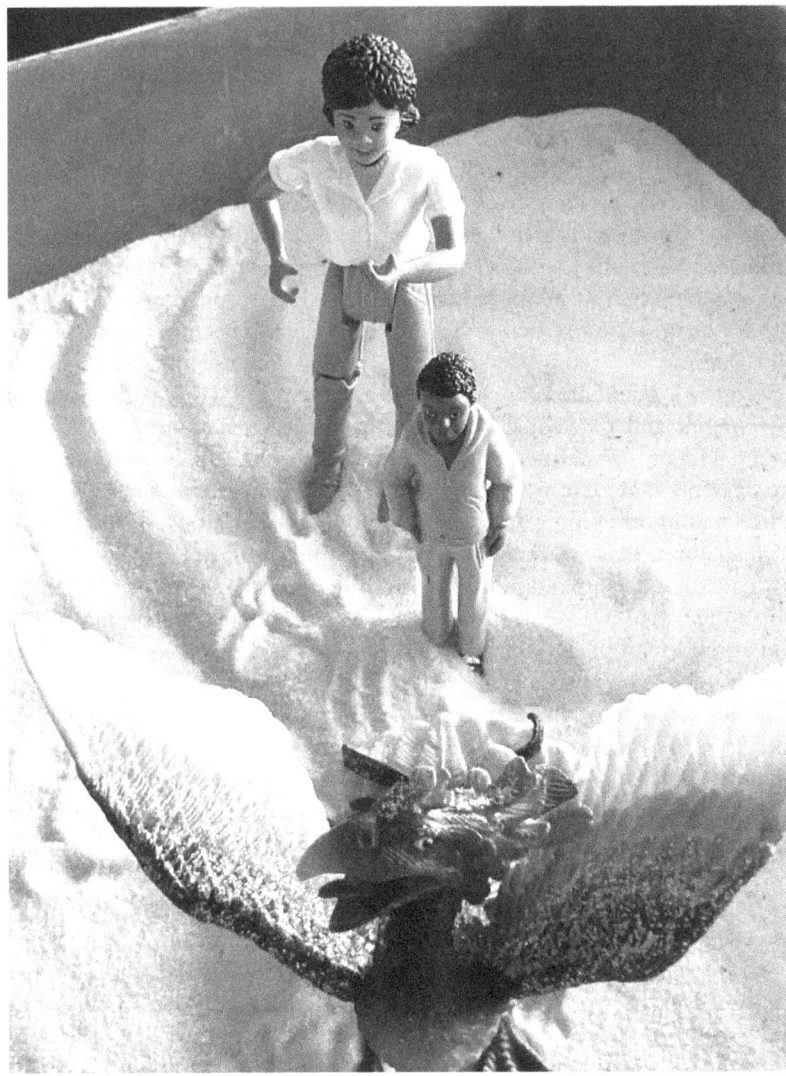

Figure 4.1 Protection.

long after, Sabastian's grandmother reported that Sabastian was no longer climbing into their bed at night. Why was this session so impactful? I believe Sabastian had a powerful disconfirming experience (see Grayson's Chapter 3). The threat of the two-headed dragon was alive in his little body, bringing with it the strong sense of his vulnerability and the history of being snatched away from the bulldozer (where he was in control). In came the second dragon to protect him, which gave him a felt sense of protection as he embodied the little boy in the tray. Sabastian asked his grandmother to operate the protective dragon, and this intensified the play. Sabastian was playing with the themes of safety and protection. After this session, he permitted his caregivers to protect him both in and out of sessions. His sandtrays demonstrated that he was using the miniatures to describe the physical reality of living with his grandparents and the social reality of his developing parent/child relationship with Grandmother.

Middle Childhood: Developing Conscience, Morality, and a Scale of Values

When I met Raymond, he was an 11-year-old boy who was a ward of the province. He was in his third foster placement and had been assessed as having Asperger's syndrome. His foster mom reported that he was often argumentative with peers and authority figures. He had little contact with his biological family except for occasional visits with his paternal grand-mother, who lived nearby in senior housing. Raymond certainly seemed to be struggling with the developmental tasks of middle childhood: developing conscience, morality, and a scale of values (Havighurst, 1953).

We can look to Raymond's nervous system for clues about the origin of his difficulties. When our autonomic nervous system has a neuroception of threat, we move toward the adaptive survival strategy of fight or flight. Raymond was being suspended more often from school due to meltdowns after interacting with peers (fight). He also was leaving school without per-mission when frustrated with teachers or his educational assistant (flight). Luckily, he would always return to his foster home. While his foster mother experienced frustration with Raymond's inability to join with her emotion-ally, she was grateful that he experienced their home as a safe refuge. Might it be possible for Raymond to increase his felt sense of safety within rela-tionships? He was referred to therapy in the hope that, together, we could create experiences of safety within the therapeutic relationship that could then generalize to the larger world.

Raymond was drawn to the sandtray and particularly happy that he "didn't have to talk," because he had not enjoyed previous experiences with verbal therapy. When Raymond was invited to choose images (miniatures), he was not happy that there were symbols that "cross lovers" have in their churches. Raymond was raised in a faith that didn't believe in religious symbols, so he refused to remain in the sandtray space if there were any cru-cifixes on the shelves. I offered a basket with a lid in which he could place the two crucifixes so they could be contained out of sight. As he did this, he informed me that the cross is a lie because the Bible actually states that Jesus died on a stake.

His ability to contain the crucifixes brought a smile to Raymond's face. In this first session, he spent the whole time carefully looking over all the images and even suggested that I reorganize what shelves "things" were placed on. Once I let him know that these "things" were kept on specific shelves so others could find them easily, he stopped mumbling about how he didn't like the setup.

At the start of his second session, Raymond shared that he knew exactly what he wanted to build this time. He intentionally moved from shelf to shelf, collecting images in a basket. His sandtray world was a scene devoid of human figures. Animal families showed up with a fence that divided wild from domestic. Vegetation provided shade to the lions, who looked like they were gathering by a water hole. He carefully placed everything and, once done, sat down triumphantly exhaling a deep breath of satisfaction and wearing a huge smile. Raymond didn't want to tell me the story of this world. He felt it was clear that anyone looking at the world could see what it was about. He did manage to share that if he gave this world a title, he would call it *"comfortable,"* after which he left as quickly as he had arrived. This sandtray was a wonderful example that the therapist does not need to know what the builder's process is for healing to occur. Raymond was working out his inner conflicts while I witnessed the story.

Raymond continued to come for weekly sessions, saying little but creating worlds that had boundaries and fences and animal families living by the "rules that everyone should know." Domestic animals could never visit the wild and vice versa. By session 12, he was open to me asking some questions about his creations. He shared with me that the day would come when someone would break a rule, and then we would all see what would happen. That day came in session 14. Raymond picked up a black kitten and moved it ever so slowly toward a leopard. As predicted, the leopard pounced and killed the kitten. Raymond repeatedly stated that the kitten should have known and then that the kitten and its mother should have known. He periodically glanced up to see if I was watching and check for my reactions to the unfolding events. He reflected that the mother should be the one to clean up all the blood, as the death was ultimately her fault because she didn't protect her kitten.

Session 15 was cancelled because Raymond was ill, and the following week, he asked if anyone had played with the kitten. I told him that all images are available to anyone who visits the playroom. He easily found the kitten and the kitten's mother, telling me I was right about keeping the organization of the figures consistent, remarking that it is nice to know where things were on the shelves. The world he created this week was different from what had shown up before. No fences were added; instead, there were mama animals and baby animals. As he built, Raymond talked about how he had been thinking that mothers usually protect their babies and teach them the rules.

Raymond continued to attend therapy, and as time went on, he began to identify times when he experienced frustration, most often centred around following rules. He also began to share his understanding that he approached situations differently than others due to his Asperger's diagnosis. Raymond

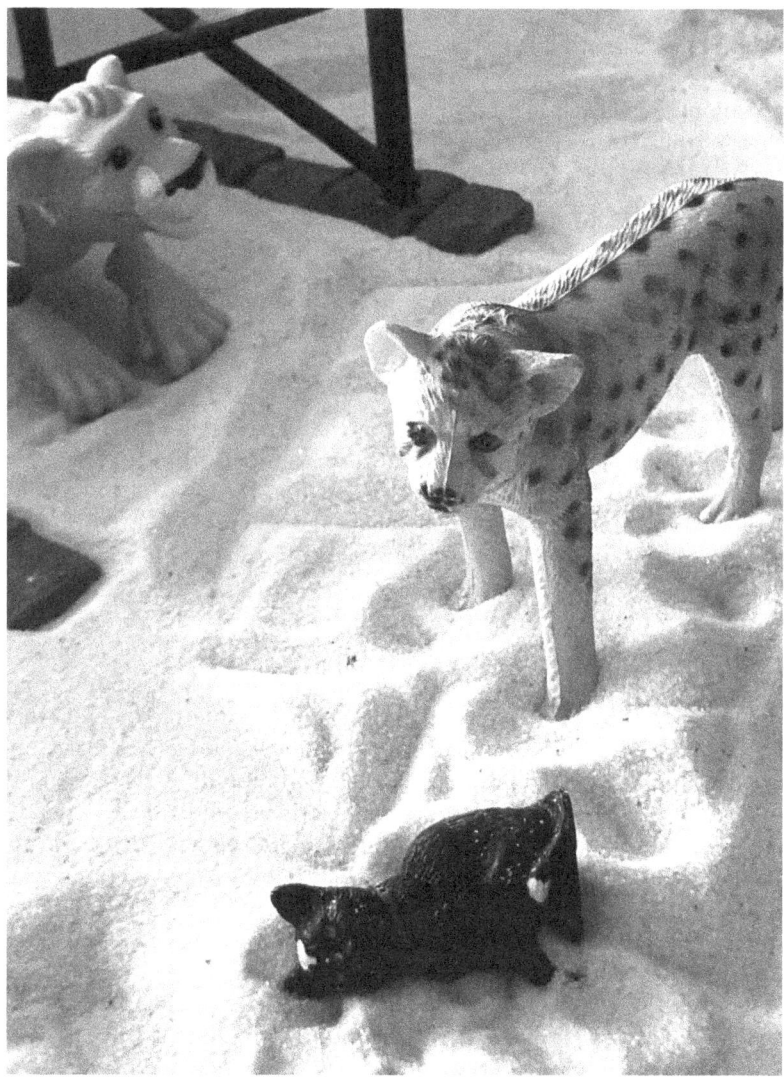

Figure 4.2 Lack of protection.

could identify that his previous meltdowns were often a result of others not responding to his expectations or requiring him to be flexible. He added that this happened most often between him and his mother when he lived with her. He was learning to breathe deeply when he felt conflicted and shared that this was a skill his foster mom had taught him.

In time, his sense of morality and conscience became less rigid. Raymond was working through this middle-childhood task by wrestling with his development of conscience, morality, and values. His foster mother reported that his meltdowns at school and episodes of running away had decreased. He also began to ask her when he needed something. This was new in their relationship, and for the first time, she felt both needed and heard by Raymond. They were experiencing connection.

Raymond taught me that I didn't need to have the builder verbally share the story while I witnessed the sacred process.

Adolescence: Achieving a Masculine or Feminine Social Role

Shaun came to therapy seeking treatment for gender dysphoria. This is one of the 11 developmental tasks of adolescence that Havighurst identified and the one most challenging for Shaun. Shaun was named Shauna at birth and said he began to recognize that he was Shaun at approximately 8 years of age. His parents referred to him as their tomboy, and Shaun became more and more withdrawn from peers as they continued to play with "girl toys." At age 11, Shaun told his parents that he would prefer to be called Shaun and intended to transition to high school as a male student. Shaun's parents were supportive of their child expressing his gender identity and wanted him to get the necessary supports to transition when the time was right. They attended his first therapy session and let me know that once Shaun began to present to the world authentically, extended family members became rejecting. In that session, we discussed the need for a referral letter for hormone blockers that would be a first step before Shaun could access masculinizing hormones as an adult. In cases such as these, it is the therapist's responsibility to document a long-lasting and intense pattern of gender nonconformity or gender dysphoria, gender dysphoria that began or worsened at the start of puberty, [and to] address any psychological, medical or social problems that could interfere with treatment as well as informed consent (World Professional Association for Transgender Health, 2001). (BC Trans Health, 2020)

Even though Shaun's parents were consenting to treatment and said they intend to support their child through his transition, it was still my responsibility to provide them with psychoeducation in addition to my support. I explained all this to Shaun and his parents and let them know that while there are many therapists who will issue a referral letter after a few sessions, I work a little differently and have found that using the sandtray can be helpful.

I didn't give Shaun any guidance about the type of world to build but rather invited him to use any images in the playroom to create a world in the sand. In his first tray, Shaun created a scene in which children (he later identified as peers) were shopping, dancing, and having pajama parties. Shaun placed one figure in the far end of the world, where he could see all that was going on in "girl world." This figure was hiding behind a barrier, disconnected from other beings in the world. In subsequent worlds, this figure began to come out of the hidden area and eventually morphed from a small female figure into a tall basketball player. Initially, Shaun talked about the identity struggles that the basketball player experienced and identified how isolating it felt to have to pretend when acting as the little girl. Shaun also disclosed that no one knew that the little girl had tried to die before she felt strong enough to share who she was. Shaun added that if the girl's parents hadn't listened or been supportive, there would likely be a coffin in the world.

Shaun's sandtray worlds clearly communicated his need for hormone blockers. With no medical or mental wellness issues that would interfere with treatment, I felt confident in providing the referral after four sandtray sessions and a parent psychoeducation session. I invited Shaun's parents to return for a hormone recommendation when Shaun approached adulthood. Providing hormone replacement therapy letters is not a gatekeeping process for a WPATH therapist. However, witnessing Shaun's sandtrays affirmed the importance that he needed hormones to achieve a masculine role.

Young Adulthood – Learning to Live With a Marriage Partner

At age 24, Chantel married her first love right after completing an undergraduate degree in criminology. She and her wife moved to another part of Canada, where Chantel got a job at a youth custody centre. When she arrived at my office, she was not necessarily seeking a therapist trained in play therapy or expressive arts but was happy to find someone who could bill her benefits package and was also trained in EMDR. She had heard that EMDR could quickly address the symptoms she was experiencing, which she attributed to her work with violent youth.

Chantel was immediately drawn to the sandtray and inquired if adults usually came to play. I assured her that many adults work in the sandtray. Some use only the sand, and others also take advantage of other available interventions that integrate with the sandtray. Following her desire to try the sandtray, I invited Chantel to follow her heart and pick a few miniatures to place in the sand. She became visibly upset, started to cry, and told me she had never cried in therapy before and didn't understand why simply touching the sand struck her in such a powerful way. I asked if she could sense being in the sandtray world from the perspective of the three beings she had placed there. She couldn't. Chantel told me she felt as if their words were stuck in her throat. She spent the session weeping while touching the sand and stroking the head of one of the beings.

Chantel returned later that week and settled on the comfortable couch. She related that she had been dreaming of the three beings since her last session, and she now knew what they had wanted to say but couldn't. We sat in silence, and for a while she held one of the beings cupped between both of her hands. Periodically, she used Kleenex to wipe her tears. After a while, she approached the sandtray, placing the one in her hands, retrieving the other two, and adding them to the world. She completed the tray by adding a deciduous tree and a building.

I took my place across from her, and together, we gazed at the world until she began to speak. She pointed to the one she had held in her hands and said that this one has been telling the others how scared he feels when people yell or swear at him. Another of the beings stated that he feels the negative energy around him in his body and, at times, wants to throw up. With these words she drew a circle in the sand around him, noting that this would protect him. The third one had a voice that was different from the others. This one told the others to stop being so sensitive and to ignore the negative voices and energy. At first, Chantel described it as a strong presence that wanted to support the scared one, but then she acknowledged that although this strong one appeared supportive, it was making the scared one feel less safe. The strong one yelled and bullied to get his point across. Chantel then moved the strong one toward the home and stated that this one usually stayed in this part of the world, watching what was going on everywhere else. Chantel pondered her creation and told me that she felt better now that words could be spoken.

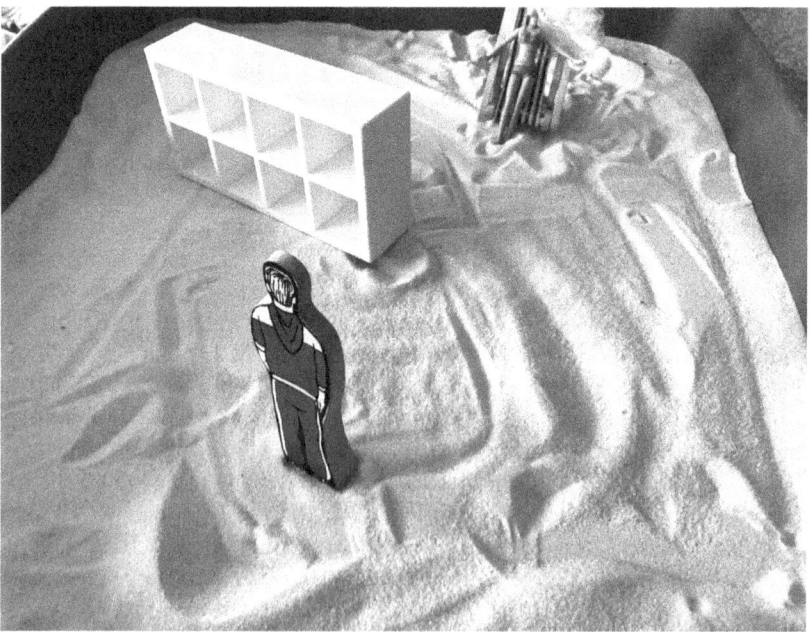

Figure 4.3 Hiding.

Chantel returned a week later. This time, she placed the building in the centre of one sandtray and then asked if she could use another tray. In the second sandtray, she shifted and moved sand methodically, creating pathways all around the world. In these pathways, she added shells, beads, gems, and some blue material she identified as rain. She placed angels in each corner and a bridge in the centre. Once done, Chantel looked up and said that this was the world of peace and support and that it felt starkly different from the world with the building she had labeled as "home." She wanted to explore the "home" world first.

When we travelled in the "home" world, Chantel's body was stiff and her words intentionally chosen. She told me that the scared one lived in the home with the strong one. The strong one sounded supportive but was often critical about the scared one's reactions to negative energy and questioned why he had to feel scared in the first place. I asked Chantel if there were any other beings who could join the scared one so he didn't have to be alone with the strong one and might feel less scared. Chantel said she had spent a lot of time wondering about that possibility but felt that the scared one needed to spend more time in the other world instead. In time, she hoped the strong one would choose to join the scared one there.

I met with Chantel again a few weeks later, and she told me that she was including more self-care practices in her day-to-day routine. She was sleeping more, drinking alcohol less, and walking daily. She shared that her wife had finally found employment, a life stressor that had not been previously disclosed. Chantel smiled easily and seemed calm and confident. She said she felt better than she had in a long time and promised to set up a subsequent appointment in a few months. The unique aspect of Chantel's process was that Chantel identified one reason for coming to therapy. However, she didn't need to share that she also was learning how to live with her marriage partner. This relationship was under great stress as a result of moving, new employment for her, and lack of employment for her wife. They were finding their way as a couple together, and Chantel was ensuring that she was making her health needs a priority. The conversations she shared in the sandtray were the beginning of her journey to find personal healing in the sandtray.

Middle Adulthood: Accepting and Adjusting to the Physiologic Changes of Middle Age

Sharon was a cancer survivor who had undergone a double mastectomy, chemo, and radiation to treat her cancer. As we settled in to get to know one another, she told me that she had found middle age (specifically menopause) an adjustment. However, her cancer treatments had added to the difficulty of adjusting to the physiological changes of middle age. She was struggling to accept this older, scarred version of herself. I had provided play therapy for a friend's granddaughter, and, knowing of my work, her friend suggested

Sharon come to talk with me about her experiences and the process of coming to grips with her changed body, which included the loss of her hair. Sharon sobbed as she related what she had gone through. It was a surprise to her that losing her hair would be more upsetting than losing her breasts. Her upcoming reconstructive surgery would, to some degree, restore her breasts, but baldness was an obvious sign of her cancer. She wore head scarves because she didn't like strangers prodding. She poignantly stated that talking about it made her feel that it had far too much power in her life.

After using lots of Kleenex, she asked me how this "sandtray thing" worked. I invited her to choose images that spoke to her and place them in the sandtray. She started by choosing sculptures that depicted family relationships and placed them along the outside edges of my wooden tray. Next, she chose a cartoonish warrior and a piece of coral I had found washed up on the beach in the Bahamas many years before. The coral looked very much like a brain, and children often labelled it so. Sharon placed the warrior on top of the coral in the middle of the tray. She didn't talk or identify any of the images chosen; instead, she built methodically while taking deep breaths. One would think she had done this before, because her eyes remained steadfastly on the world instead of making eye contact with me.

After a time, Sharon looked up and stated that the warrior was not welcome in this world. He was familiar to her because he kept showing up in her head. It seemed to me that, like the children before her, Sharon was experiencing the coral as a brain. She sat back, looked at me, and asked, "How do I get rid of him?" I wondered who he represented. Could he be someone in her life? Could he be someone else? Could he be the cancer? This wasn't clear in my mind. I needed to refocus and remind myself that the most important thing I could do in that moment was to follow Sharon's lead. I didn't need to know specifics about the warrior to be with Sharon and her question.

I responded with more questions. Is there anyone else in the world who could help with this task? Did others want him gone also? Could they voice their thoughts or speak to this being on her behalf? Sharon stood up and physically moved around the tray, talking about the others, who were sons, daughters, siblings and friends. After she introduced them to me, I invited them to speak to the one who was taking up more space than was welcome.

Sharon was quiet at first as she sensed the responses of the other beings in the world. When she did speak, she told me that they recognized how much time the warrior was stealing. He wasn't a good warrior; instead, he represented doubt, sadness, and feelings of vulnerability and impotence. He was the culmination of negativity and fear. He had robbed Sharon of hope. With one flash of the wrist, Sharon leaned over and toppled the warrior off of the brain. He landed facedown in the sand. Sharon sat looking at the sandtray, displaying little emotion but looking physically tired if not defeated. She then spoke, stating that this made the others happy, but the brain was now lonely. She asked if it would be okay for another being to

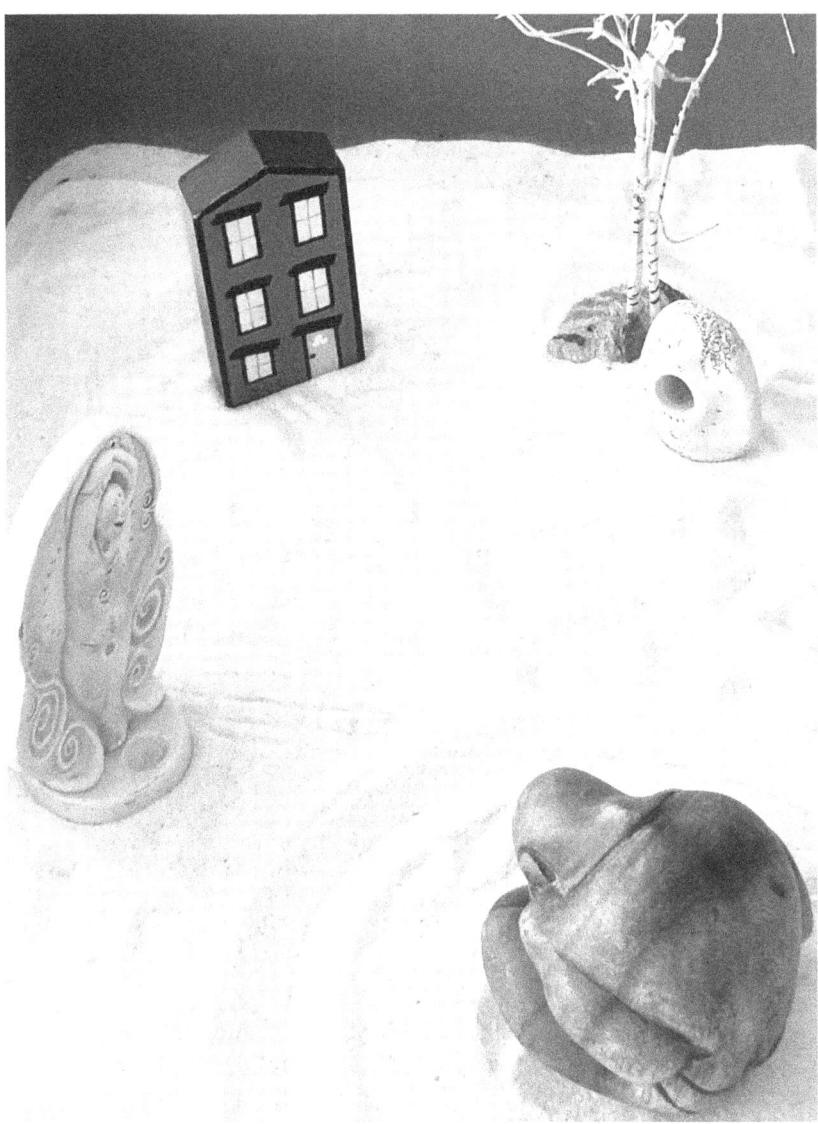

Figure 4.4 Creating safety.

join the world. She slowly surveyed the shelves and eventually found a little stone with the word "hope" inscribed on it. The stone took its place on the brain. Sharon then moved the family members closer to the brain, where they formed a circle. I invited her to take a photo, saying she might want a photo of this version of the world versus the warrior. We sat together in

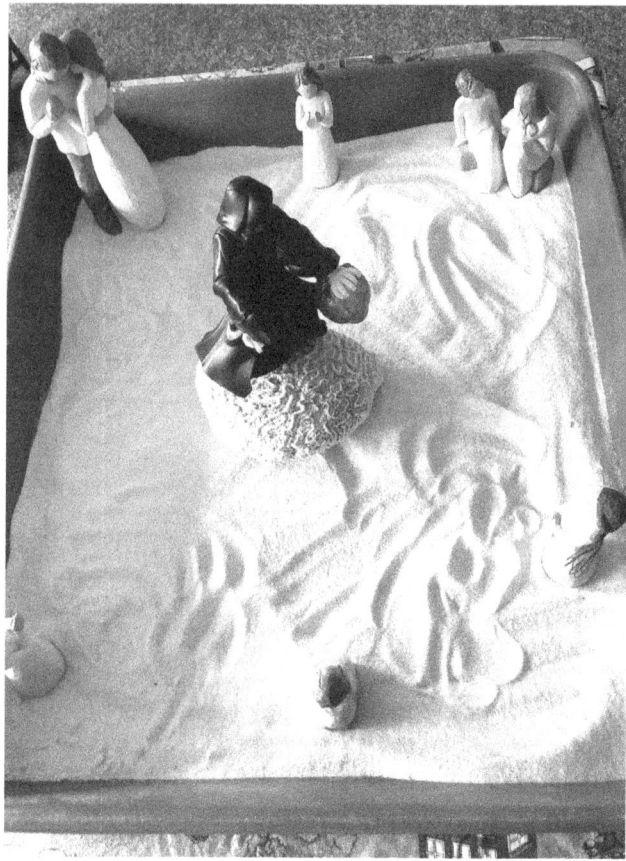

Figure 4.5 Robbing hope.

silence for a while, gazing at her world. After a few moments, Sharon spoke of her realization that she was disconnected from loved ones. Throughout her treatment, she had accepted help from family and friends. They purchased groceries and drove her to appointments, but emotionally, she had distanced herself. She did not want to talk about the cancer or other things like possible death or disconnection from loved ones. Instead, these dark thoughts took up residence in her thoughts and dreams. Now, except for breast reconstruction, she was done with treatments. She realized she was finally in a place to embrace hope and connection again. She took pictures of the world with her cell phone, and treatment ended after only a few sessions.

Later Maturity – Adjusting to the Death of a Spouse

Fred arrived in my office stating that he had researched my background as well as sandtray. Fred had been a high school teacher with a full career teaching biology and geography. Knowing that I, too, was a teacher, he was optimistic we would be a good fit. In our first session, he told me he and his wife had always planned on retiring in Florida, but she had died five years prior, and he was now more interested in retiring somewhere else but wasn't sure where that might be.

Fred spent a good bit of time looking at the images on the shelves. He didn't talk at all but instead hmmmed periodically. After about 10 minutes, he sat down at the sandtray and placed images in the tray one at a time. In the centre of the sandtray was a female figure, and he announced that this was his wife. I reflected that this is *the* wife and Fred nodded. He then placed a boat alongside the wife, pointing towards a bridge with a dolphin swimming in water. He used shells to border the world and placed many trees close to another corner. There was an area that looked dark, with wood pieces and black plastic material bundled up in little pieces. One corner lay barren until a book was placed there.

When Fred finished placing the images he had selected, I invited him to silently gaze at the world and see if he felt that anything needed to be added or changed. He jumped up and picked a golden retriever dog and placed it beside the book. Fred then looked carefully around the world and took me on a tour, beginning with the corner with trees. This part of the world felt peaceful, and the wife in the middle could move here or into the water to relax and listen to the birds that would visit the trees every spring. Fred then talked about the dolphin who followed the boat around. Every year, the boat would visit this world and reunite with the dolphin, who was waiting. The boat sometimes went to the dark corner but was in danger of getting stuck in the garbage. The garbage didn't get bigger or smaller but was omnipresent. Fred then touched the sand in front of the book while the dog looked onward. He let out a sigh and said that this spot was one that was a quiet place for the husband. He noted that the husband couldn't be seen in this world because he had left a long time ago. It was too hard to stay in this world because the wife was so lovely and nice to be around. Fred ended the session, thanking me but not booking a second session.

About a month later, Fred phoned and again thanked me for my wise counsel. My experience of my time with Fred was one of witnessing his sandtray and not of providing any counsel at all. He told me that upon leaving the session, he realized that even though he was close to retirement, he did not want to make any big decisions about moving for a while. He wanted to renovate his current home to the way he wanted it, including a quiet place for reading. He also got a dog. His wife had been allergic, so they never owned a dog. He had grown up with a golden retriever and decided to get another. He was enjoying walking the dog daily. He spoke of his loneliness, as he and his wife had never had children, and how he appreciated the company of his new canine companion. Fred also recognized that although his wife had died five years ago, he still had not grieved her the way he needed to, so he was giving himself permission to tell stories about her and go through old photos. We ended our phone call with Fred letting me know he might return for another session sometime in the future.

Fred came back to the sandtray room six months later. He was in good health and continued to walk his dog daily. He told me that he still had days where he would pick up the phone to call his wife. Sometimes, he would spray his bedroom with her perfume and hadn't dated since she died. He admitted to being pretty lonely with no wife and no children. Recently, he had joined a 50-plus social group and signed up for a French course, as he hoped to travel to France in a year or two. Early retirement had given him the opportunity to do things he never had time to do before except during the summer months. Fred found his initial experience with the sandtray to be beneficial and, this time, he wanted to do another tray and dedicate it to his Ruth. He wanted to show her how he was coping with her loss, as he felt that she was always with him and worried about him. He also wanted her to know that he missed her but felt like he had hope for the future.

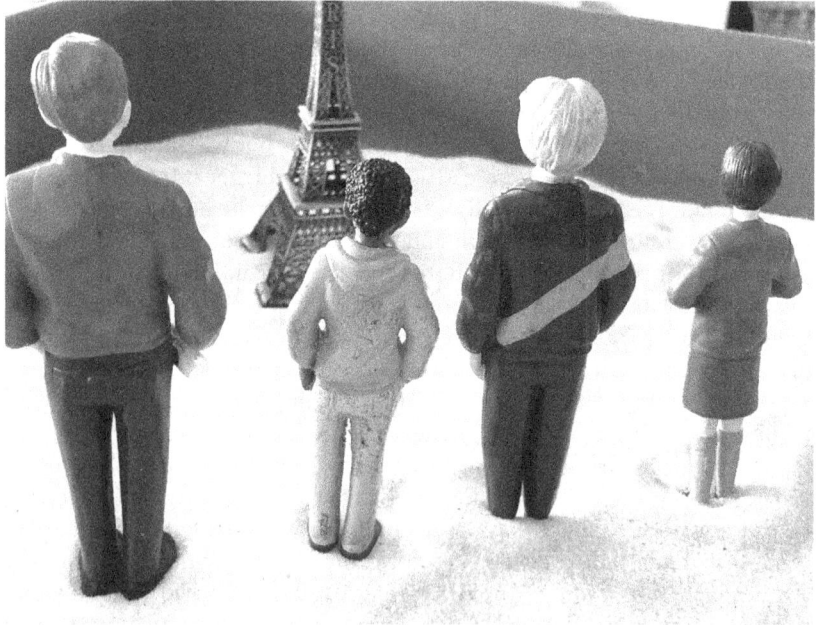

Figure 4.6 The Future.

This tray was difficult to witness given that I was also grieving personal losses at that time. As a therapist, it can be hard to hold this very sacred space and not let your emotions overrun the precious gift of being a witness. I held my tears as they welled up for Fred. He picked the special being that was placed in the middle of the tray. A dog and a book were placed in the centre. The dark place that had been in Fred's previous tray did not manifest in this world. A boat and a dolphin were placed near the middle. As I watched him wipe a tear, he pulled a structure from his pocket, and I noticed that it was a little metal Eiffel Tower. Last but not least, he chose a female image and two children from my shelves as well as a male figure. He placed all of these close together and seemingly walking in the same direction. They faced the special being in the center. Fred put his hands in his lap and smiled. He said he had a title for this world, and he called it *Future*.

When we toured the world, we travelled to the water area and visited the Eiffel Tower in France. He introduced me to the man, the man's girlfriend, and her grandchildren. He then said that he wanted to tell the special one how he felt and pulled a pre-written letter from another pocket. I will not share the details of this letter here due to confidentiality, but it is important to note that it was a tearjerker. Fred told the special one what he had been doing since he retired and described his hopes for the next year. He then placed the letter in the sand, asked to take a photo, and, as he had previously, thanked me for my time and left.

Across the Life Span

These sandtray journeys were organized under the developmental stages identified by Dr. Robert J. Havighurst, who was an American scientist and expert on human development and aging. He identified tasks that humans process in six stages from "infancy and early childhood" to "later maturity." Havighurst believed that each human has three sources of experience that inform our growth and development. These experiences are physical maturation, as seen in Sabastian, Shaun and Sharon's stories, personal values as demonstrated in Chantel's and Fred's stories, and tasks that get accomplished as a result of societal pressures (expectations). This was Raymond's story.

Our role as witness permits us to observe and feel these worlds. They connect feelings, memories, and experiences in a powerful way for the builder (whatever their age) and therapist as the witness. Each of these vignettes illustrate that the sandtray can be a powerful tool to use therapeutically across the life span. "We all ache to be heard and held in the reality of our experience, without judgement or any impulse toward fixing" (Badenoch, 2018, p. 13). The sandtray therapist who trusts the process and holds the belief that the builder (whatever their age) intuitively knows what the journey needs to be will honor a right-brained process of connecting thoughts, feelings, and experiences. It is a challenge at times, as we can experience self-doubt about our role. It is during these times that we need to remind ourselves and each other that the builder knows the way.

Note

1. In the practice of sandtray-worldplay, it is customary to refer to sandtray figures as either images or beings. The use of the term "being" reflects the sentient nature of the image once it is enlivened by the world creator.

References

Badenoch, B. (2018). *The heart of trauma: Healing the embodied brain in the context of relationships*. W. W. Norton & Company, Inc.

De Domenico, G. (1987). *Sand tray world play: A comprehensive guide to the use of sand tray in psychotherapeutic and transformational settings*. Vision Question into Virtual Reality.

Havighurst, R. (1953). *Developmental tasks and education*. Longman's Green.

Landreth, G. L. (2012). *Play therapy: The art of the relationship* (3rd ed.). Routledge.

World Professional Association. (2001). *Standards of care for the health of transsexual, transgender, and gender nonconforming people 7th edition*. https://www.wpath.org/media/cms/Documents/SOC%20v7/SOC%20V7_English.pdf

Part 2

Stories of Healing in the Sandtray

5 Troubled Waters

Navigating Difficult Life Transitions

Rita Grayson

Life is a series of transitions, beginning with our departure from the womb and ending with our death. Some transitions are expected and fairly predictable, such as beginning and ending life's role as a student. Other transitions may be hoped for but less predictable, like getting married or becoming a parent. The most difficult transitions are those that seemingly come out of nowhere: an accident, illness, or the death of a loved one. What every transition brings with it, whether joyous or painful, is the stress associated with change.

In 1967, the research of two psychiatrists, Dr. Thomas Holmes and Dr. Richard Rahe, resulted in what we now refer to as the Holmes and Rahe Stress Scale. Their research sought to determine if there was a connection between difficult life events and physical illness. Five thousand patient records were reviewed, and 43 life events were identified and assigned points depending on the degree of life upheaval associated with the event (Noone, 2017). The life experiences ranged from the death of a spouse and divorce as the most stressful to major holidays and minor violations of the law, such as getting a traffic ticket, as the least stressful (Holmes & Rahe, 1967). To use the scale, one simply identifies which of the 43 events have occurred during the past year and adds up the associated points. A link was found between a high score on the Holmes and Rahe Stress Scale and the likelihood of a stress-related illness arising in the next 2 years (Noone, 2017).

How can we, as therapists, help our clients navigate these stressful life transitions? It is one matter when a client arrives with a problem that can be solved or a symptom that can be relieved. But when it comes to big life changes, like a loved one's death, the ending of a marriage, the onset of a serious illness, or even the birth of a child, there is generally nothing to be done. Therapy becomes more about being with what is and accompanying our clients on the journey as they navigate the twists and turns before them. In these cases, perhaps the most important thing we can offer is our willingness to suffer with them so they don't have to go it alone (Badenoch, 2018a). What follows is the story of a middle-aged woman who, through her use of the sandtray, uncovered the source of a nagging sense of discontent, only to realize the path to relief would ask her to turn her life upside down.

DOI: 10.4324/9781003055808-7

Orienting to the Journey

Monique came to therapy seeking help for a vague sense of dissatisfaction with her life that had been with her for some time. She found it confusing because, from the outside, her life looked ideal. Monique had been married to her husband for 25 years, and their three children were thriving. Her oldest had recently graduated from college and was enjoying his first career position, her middle child was doing well at the state university, and her youngest was a senior in high school who had recently been accepted into the college of her dreams. Monique held a senior-level management position in a large corporation, a job she professed to love. They lived in a nice home, drove nice cars, took interesting vacations each year, and were financially stable. And yet, in her quieter moments, Monique felt there was something missing.

When I first encountered Monique in my waiting room, I was immediately drawn to her. She greeted me with a warm smile and a firm handshake and made easy conversation as we walked back to my office. When she caught sight of my sandtray collection, she exclaimed, "Wow! That's a lot of stuff!" I chuckled, silently relieved that she had given me the opportunity to let her know I am not, in fact, a hoarder as some might assume! I briefly described sandtray therapy and let her know it was available to her if she would like to give it a try. Jokingly, she asked if I had a crystal ball in my collection. "I feel like I need someone to peer into a crystal ball and tell me why I'm not satisfied with this great life I have." I told her I did not have a crystal ball or any special powers to see into the future but suggested working in the sandtray might actually be preferable, as it would allow her inner world to communicate about her sense of dissatisfaction.

As we settled into our initial session, Monique shared a bit about her life. She is the youngest of four children; her parents are still alive and married to each other. She grew up in a fairly rural setting with easy access to grandparents and cousins. Her siblings are now scattered around the country, but they generally see one another over the holidays. She met her husband in college and described the marriage as a solid partnership. There were no obvious traumas other than a car accident (no serious injuries) in her 20s and an emergency appendectomy in her 40s. Monique was looking forward to her 50th birthday in a few months. She wondered out loud if it could be this upcoming milestone birthday or the prospect of an empty nest causing her unease. I assured her those might be good places for us to start, and we would see where the journey took us.

Bonnie Badenoch (2018a) likens the role of therapist to that of a Sherpa. The Sherpa provides expertise needed about the terrain, weather, necessary supplies, and other challenges the journey might hold. But it is the traveler who initiates the trek and identifies the desired destination. As Sherpas, we bring our vast experience and expertise in a support role, offering guidance and supplies as needed. The client, as Trekker, determines how much to push, how much to rest, and whether to even venture out of the tent on any given day. In keeping with this theme of client as traveler, Monique was experiencing wanderlust but did not yet have a sense of where she wanted to go. It was time to explore some possible destinations.

After a couple of sessions talking and generally getting comfortable with one another, Monique was ready to venture into the sandtray. The early sessions of a therapeutic engagement are often about building interpersonal trust and safety, which is the essential foundation for healing (Badenoch, 2018b). Just as the Trekker must be confident the Sherpa has the capacity to navigate whatever lies ahead, our clients must know, through their experience with us, that we can calmly and respectfully hold them throughout their therapy journey.

Monique's first few sandtrays touched on the bittersweet nature of preparing to send her youngest daughter off to college. This was not particularly new territory for Monique, as two of her children had already left home. But this one seemed different in a way that was difficult to define. We held the experience together, curious about why this one felt unusual beyond what might be expected with the youngest child. Monique and her husband had often talked about the freedom that would come when their day-to-day parenting duties ended. There was talk of downsizing and early retirement, all things Monique looked forward to.

It was roughly her third or fourth sandtray session when something new showed up. In the upper corner of her world was a miniature dried steer skull, complete with horns. Next to it lay some driftwood and a scrap of tanned leather. She spoke of the other aspects of the world, notably skipping over this desert-like corner. When Monique finished telling the story of her world, I gently inquired about the skull, driftwood, and cowhide. It was then the tears started to flow. For several minutes, we sat in silence, connected in that wordless space that often arises in a sandtray session. After a time, in a quiet voice that belied the conviction of her words, Monique said, "That is my marriage."

Leaning on the work of Iain McGilchrist (2009), we can appreciate the qualitative differences of narratives originating in the left hemisphere as compared to those coming from the right hemisphere.[1] In general, left-hemisphere processing is more analytical, logical, linear, and literal. The left hemisphere can produce a narrative of our experiences that has the settling quality of "making sense" given the facts of the situation (Badenoch, 2011). Viewed from a left-hemisphere perspective, Monique had difficulty finding fault with her current state of affairs. She and her husband worked together like a well-oiled machine. The house and yard were kept up, bills were paid on time, healthy meals were cooked, and the children were attended to. What is missing from a left-hemisphere accounting is the felt-sense quality of relationships.

The right hemisphere provides us with a more holistic view of the world, along with a sense of the emotional, relational, and bodily held responses

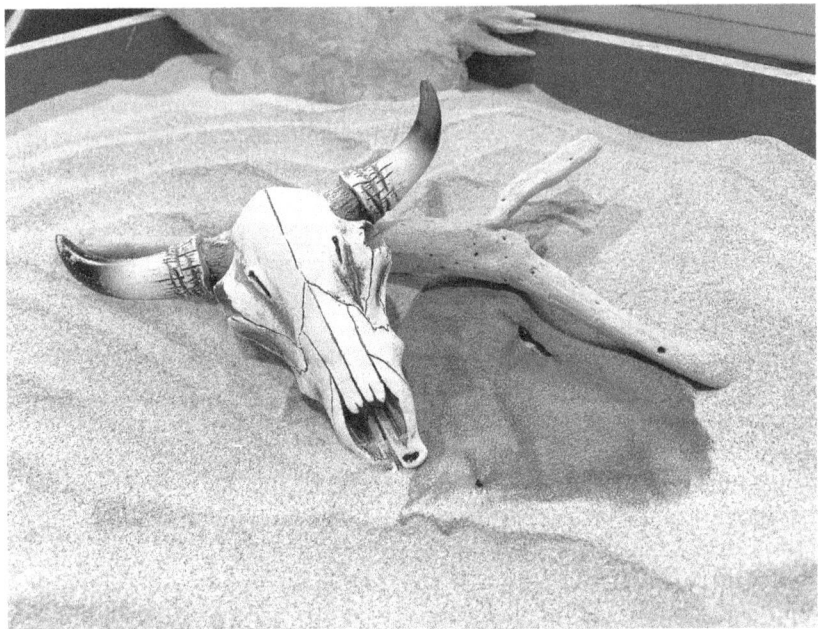

Figure 5.1 Monique confronts the desert quality of her marriage.

to our lived experience (Badenoch, 2011). Sandtray offers the possibility of grounding therapy in the right hemisphere, as it invites the body, rather than left hemisphere–generated thoughts, to guide the process. Monique's left-hemisphere assessment of her life followed the foregone conclusion she had nothing to complain about. However, the unease that inhabited her body told a different story. Honoring that whisper from within, she bravely sought a Sherpa who might be able to offer some guidance about how to start her journey. That guidance came in the form of an invitation to engage with sand, water, a library of symbolic images, and the containment of a tray. Monique accepted the invitation, allowing the story of what she thought was true to quiet, making room for her inner wisdom, held in her body and right hemisphere, to speak.

It is no easy matter to sit with the agony of another, as Monique and I did the day she faced the desert-like quality of her marriage. She was at a crossroads. Would she retreat into the relative safety of the left-hemisphere story that her marriage was not that bad, or would she move into the desert to gain deeper understanding? I was also acutely aware of the challenge in front of me as Monique's Sherpa. We were at the threshold of very tender territory that would, in all likelihood, touch my own experience with divorce. With this thought, the kind face of my clinical consultant came to mind, and I felt my system settle with the knowledge that I, too, would have support and accompaniment with any personal responses I might experience related to Monique's journey.

On the Path

Over the next several months, Monique continued to create sandtray worlds, and she began talking with her husband about her loneliness and desire for more connection in their relationship. She would arrive to some sessions knowing she needed to express herself via the sandtray and would immediately begin creating. In other sessions, she needed to talk. We spoke mainly of fear and grief. Her fear that she was making a mistake, her fear that she would end up alone, fears about navigating the day-to-day without a partner to lend a hand. We sat with her grief. The potential loss of the future she and her husband had envisioned for so many years. The loss of this man who was, at one time, so dear to her. The possible loss of the social life that included their married friends. Together, we sat with her sense of failure. We listened to the echoes of her faith tradition that deemed divorce to be a sin. Sometimes, there was anger. The "How could he?" and "How dare he? and "Why didn't he?" questions would arise, and we would sit with them, mutually understanding the answers were irrelevant but understanding that giving voice to them was essential. During this time, the conversations with her husband continued, but the connection they once shared remained elusive.

Over this period of time, I noticed a trend in Monique's sandtrays. The desert was still there, but resources and opposing experiences began to appear. She began to divide her trays with a river running diagonally from one corner to its opposite. One side remained dry and lifeless, while the other side began to show signs of new life and possibilities. Sometimes, there were sharks in the water, making the passage away from the desert seem too dangerous to attempt. But eventually, boats appeared in the river offering the possibility of safe passage.

Outside of her sandtrays, Monique's narrative also began to change. Initially, she talked about her marriage in terms of how it could be worse: no one was cheating; no one was an addict; no one was physically abusive. The degree of isolation and loneliness was dismissed because it was not as intolerable as other worst-case scenarios. Initially, I attributed these kinds of statements to Monique's justifiable fear of striking out on her own as a woman in her 50s. But as I got to know Monique better, I came to realize that, on a deep, implicit level, Monique did not feel she deserved better when it came to relationships. This made sense given what Monique had shared about her early relational life.

I noticed my divergent responses to this new realization; on the one hand, I felt a sadness for the woman beside me who had accepted disconnection as the relational norm for so long, but I also felt a spark of hope at the arrival of an emerging sense of being worthy of love.

As more nourishing possibilities began to emerge in Monique's sandtrays, I noticed that statements of "It could be worse" were gradually replaced by "I want a shot at something better," and eventually "I deserve to be with someone who really loves me."

We might wonder what brought about this change. I credit two parallel processes, one in the sandtray and one in the relationship Monique and I had forged. As Monique began to put new, possible experiences (love, acceptance, satisfaction) into her sandtrays, she was able to experience them with her whole self. In this act of embodied experiencing, what might begin as a notion of what could happen transforms into a felt-sense experience of that possibility actually happening. Monique's creation of a river in her sandtray made room for something other than life in a desert. Populating this new area with trees and other living creatures allowed her to experience what life might feel like outside the desert. In the sandtray sessions in which Monique added boats and physically moved those boats away from the desert, she could feel that movement in her body and know, experientially, that she had the power to create her own destiny, even if it meant navigating shark-infested waters. Equally importantly, she experienced me, right there with her, which embedded an experience of accompaniment, leading to the felt-sense awareness she would not have to navigate these difficult passages alone.

The cultivation of a safe and supportive therapeutic relationship is just as important as being skilled in facilitating a sandtray journey, if not more so. There are a few neurobiological principles at work here. Iain McGilchrist (2009) tells us that how we attend to our people actually changes them. If I were to see Monique as weak and insecure, I can say with some certainty that her therapy would have taken a different course. If I saw her as incapable of change, I would likely have supported her evaluation that her lonely marriage was "good enough."

This brings us to another challenge of being a therapist. Had I not resolved my own uncertainties about my marriage (regardless of whether I decided to stay married or not), I do not believe I could have held her struggles with any clarity and would likely have taken the natural course of coloring her experiences with mine. This underscores the need for all of us who do this healing work to have our own Sherpas, our own support for the inevitable co-suffering that comes when we enter the wilderness with our clients. Fortunately, in Monique's case, I found her to be completely capable, and I had reached sufficient resolution about my own marriage to enable me to receive her with as little perceptual bias as possible. Conversations with my consultant about this case were reassuring that I was seeing things as clearly as possible given the reality that we cannot help but see things through our own idiosyncratic lens.

A second principle from neurobiology worth noting comes from the work of Stephen Porges on co-regulation (Dana, 2018). Porges tells us there are three branches of the autonomic nervous system (ANS), and they are hierarchical in nature. In mammals, the preferred state is called ventral vagal parasympathetic, also referred to simply as our ventral state. Porges calls this our social engagement system, because in this state, we experience connection with one another. When our ANS senses a threat in our internal or external environment, we move out of this ventral state and into a state more oriented toward survival than toward relationship. Co-regulation is simply the phenomenon of one nervous system shifting to match the condition of a nearby nervous system. Because ventral is the preferred state, it is more likely that the nervous system in a state of alarm will co-regulate with the one in a ventral state, restoring any felt sense of connection that may have been lost.

This becomes important when intense emotion arises during therapy. When Monique first became aware of the connection between the desert in her tray and her marriage, her pain was palpable. At this juncture, there was a possibility of her nervous system adaptively moving into sympathetic arousal, which would prompt a fight-or-flight response aimed at protecting her from the pain of what was arising in that moment. But in order to fully absorb the impact of what was presenting itself in her sandtray, it was important for Monique to remain as present as possible.

As Sherpa, my job in that moment was to stay in my ventral state, offering her nervous system an opportunity to co-regulate with mine. If I did so, she would not feel alone in her pain and would be more likely to integrate this new information into the developing narrative of her life.

Beckes and Coan (2011) offer us two ideas from their research in the area of social baseline theory. The first is that emotional information is an important component of good judgment and decision-making, and second, the perception of being accompanied through challenging circumstances can reduce the level of distress experienced. As Monique sat in the painful realization that her sense of unease was coming from marital dissatisfaction, she needed to remain present with this emerging experience so she could exercise good judgment about her future. My ability to stay in my ventral state offered a reassuring sense of safety and connection with the deep knowing that whatever twists and turns her journey would take, we would face them together.

As Monique's sandtray journey progressed, she became more and more comfortable with the notion that she deserved more relational goodness than what was available in her marriage. She worried about living on her own, and she questioned the impact of divorce on her children, but she began to believe it was okay to prioritize her own happiness. At the same time, her husband was beginning to acknowledge his own dissatisfaction. Together, they made the decision to go their separate ways. For both, the vision of being in their empty nest together was simply too empty. The road to this decision had certainly been an agonizing one for Monique. What began as a felt sense that something wasn't quite right turned into a major life transition.

Years later, Monique would tell me she couldn't have done it without me. I used to respond to statements like these by reflecting to the client that they did all the hard work. But given the supportive knowledge of interpersonal neurobiology, I now see the truth in that statement. Neurobiologically, we were never meant to go it alone.

Reaching the Point of no Return

On every trek, you reach a point at which the degree of difficulty is equal whether you decide to turn around and go back or forge ahead to your destination. For Monique, this moment came with the decision to divorce. With her determination to forge ahead, Monique's therapy journey took yet another turn. Some of her sessions were dominated by the needs of the day: what and how to tell the kids; when to put the house on the market. But Monique did not leave the sandtray behind, as she had found it indispensable to her journey thus far.

We began to see sandtray worlds emerge that we would later categorize as either "vision trays" or "hell trays." In the beginning, they appeared equally, but over time, the hell trays faded in favor of the vision trays. Monique's vision trays were variations of a common theme. They always contained two houses, one formal and one informal, perhaps even whimsical. There was typically a river separating the land in the front of the tray as well as the

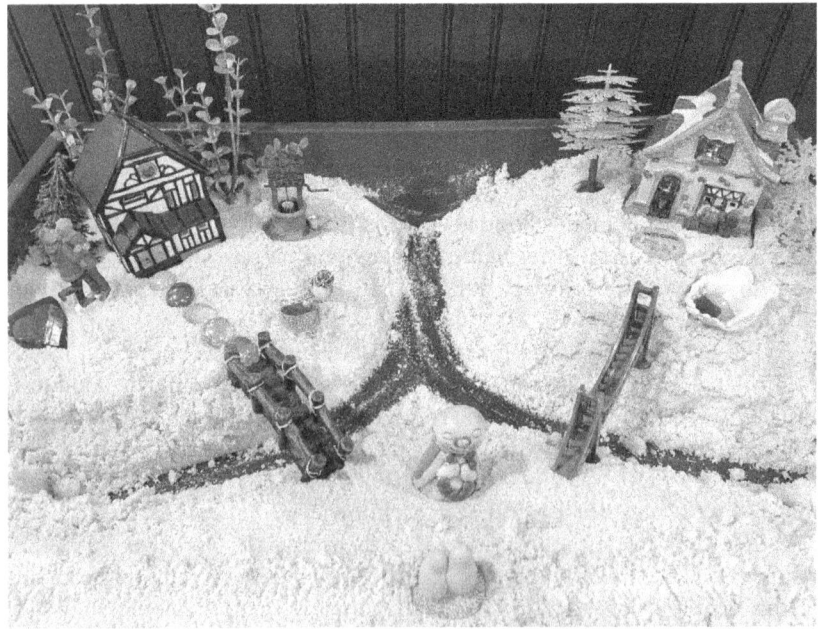

Figure 5.2 Monique's vision tray.

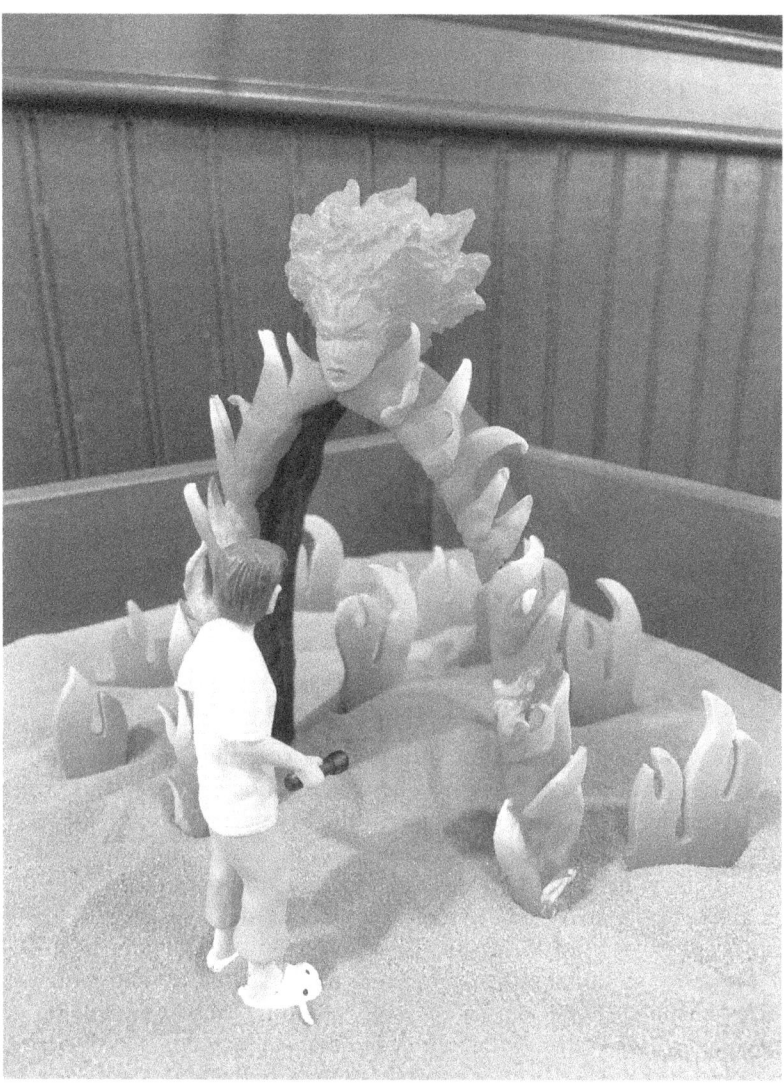

Figure 5.3 Monique's Hell tray.

two houses. Bridges allowed easy access to and from the different parts of the world. Without fail, near the whimsical house was a loving couple, a heart stone, and a wishing well, among other things.

Monique's "hell trays" took on different looks, depending on which chamber of hell she found herself in on any given day. Sometimes, there was destruction by fire, sometimes a tornado, sometimes a deep pit that was nearly impossible to escape. Often, there was the figure of a woman holding a flashlight. This became an important theme for Monique as she expressed determination to examine every aspect of her divorce experience, pleasant and unpleasant alike, in order to learn as much as possible in the hope of avoiding similar pitfalls in future relationships. She likened her divorce journey to a visit to hell and was determined to explore all the nooks and crannies of each chamber so there would be no compelling reason to go back for a second look!

Over time, we began to notice a new experience arising in Monique's vision trays. A sense of the spiritual found expression in the form of feathers, flowers, stones, shells, and other natural items. Often, this part of the world would be illuminated by candles. Occasionally, there would be a meditating figure. Verbally, Monique shared her awakening interest in connecting with the Divine. Her husband identified as an atheist, and Monique's own spiritual beliefs were not deeply rooted. For the course of their marriage, they lived without any outward expression of a spiritual belief or practice. The suffering Monique experienced as she moved through her divorce, along with the freedom she now felt to find her own path, opened space for Monique to resume the spiritual exploration that began as a young child but was dampened, first by formal religious education and later by partnering with a man who strongly dismissed the existence of a greater power.

Marking the Transition

One day, Monique came to her session with a startling request. "Will you facilitate a family sandtray session designed honor our transition brought on by the divorce?" She must have read the bewildered look on my face, as I had never encountered such a request before. She continued, "We have ceremonies to honor a marriage and ceremonies to grieve the loss of a loved one. Why can't we have a ceremony to acknowledge a divorce?" The logic of her request did not escape me. How could I say no? Divorce is generally a private affair, so we settled on an extended sandtray session that would include Monique, her soon-to-be ex-husband, and their three children. Her extended family was not local, but had grandparents, aunts, and uncles been available, it may have been supportive to include them. I wasn't quite sure about the mechanics of the session, but I was solid in my sense of where we might begin and where I hoped we might end (understanding that the ending was ultimately up to Monique and her family). The family would come to me in the throes of a divorce that was rocking their worlds, individually as well as collectively. My hope was that, together, we could create a vision of life after the divorce dust settled.

When Monique's family entered my office, they were greeted by my sandtray collection, five rectangular trays, one for each member, as well as the large round tray I use for ceremonies. Monique opened the session by reiterating why she asked for this gathering and showing her appreciation that her request was honored. She spoke of her hope that all family members would find the experience helpful and supportive. While Monique's family members had never worked in the sandtray, they were not strangers to the process, as Monique had told them about her work in the sand. With a brief introduction to the process, I invited each member to create a sandtray world, encouraging them to let go of any preconceived notions about what it might be about but instead to allow their eyes to find the images on the shelves they felt drawn to and their hands to arrange the selected ones in the tray however it felt right to them. I let everyone know that they could continue creating their individual worlds until they felt "just right" and that they might notice a settling in their bodies when their creation was complete.

I sat and watched as each person created a world, noticing the deep gratitude in my heart for these humans who, as their lives were being upended by divorce, were still willing to come together as a family. When all the individual worlds were complete, I offered each family member an opportunity to share their world with the others.

Monique's husband went first. His world included a spiral, and he walked us along the path that began with life before Monique and included meeting and marrying her, the birth of their children, career transitions he encountered along the way, and ended with the figure of a shepherd-like man holding a lantern in front of him to illuminate the path (not unlike Monique's woman with the flashlight). He spoke of the joys as well as the struggles along the path and ended with uncertainty, mixed with hope, for the future.

The youngest child shared next. Her world showed five spokes connected to the center, where there was a large tree in full leaf. At the end of each spoke was an image that represented a family member. She described her experience of each, ending with the observation that even though each family member had their own life, they could all gather in the center under the tree and appreciate its shelter.

The oldest child's world had more to do with his newly launched career. One corner held the disruption of the divorce, and he expressed his desire for the turmoil to go away so he could concentrate his energies on creating a solid foundation for his future as an independent adult. There was some concern that if things did not go well for his mom, he would have to step in as "the man of the family," a role he was not prepared to assume.

The middle child's sandtray world was divided in two. One side contained college life, while the other showed family life. There was no bridge connecting the two. On the shore of college life and facing family life was a worried-looking figure. This family member spoke about his difficulty being away at college with everything happening at home. He expressed concern that his parents were "glossing over" things when they spoke on the phone to keep him from worrying.

Monique shared her sandtray last. I smiled as I gazed upon the now-familiar vision tray. She had placed a house in each upper corner separated by rivers with bridges connecting them. The "shore" in the front of the tray held three distinct areas, one for each child. In the center was a large heart-shaped stone with five people standing around it. Small stepping stones connected each area of the world to the center, not unlike her daughter's world. She acknowledged the difficulty of the present situation but assured her family that, while this was the end of a marriage, this was not the end of their family. She told them of the commitment she and their father shared to remain comfortable in each other's presence, so the children would not have to choose sides when it came to big life events like graduations, marriages, and grandchildren.

It was time to bring the independent worlds together into a family world. I invited each person to select parts of their individual worlds that felt most significant and bring them to the round sandtray. Monique's husband brought the man holding the lantern, the youngest child brought her beautiful tree, the oldest brought the disruption he wanted to go away, the middle child brought the worried one, and Monique brought her bridges and stepping stones. Each family member placed their selections in the round tray.[2] Once this initial sharing and placement was complete, I invited family members to bring whatever else moved them into the circular tray. I let them know they were free to choose anything from their individual worlds or the sandtray collection, but items from another person's tray could be used only with specific permission.

I watched as this family world transformed. Comfort was brought to areas of distress, possibilities brought to areas of uncertainty, connections brought to areas of isolation. In the end, the middle child, who had voiced concern about being too far away while his family struggled, found several long strands of Mardi Gras beads. He began to weave them throughout the tray, sharing strands with his siblings so they could join in. I observed Monique and her husband in this moment and could feel the love, pride, and delight they shared in the family they had created. As we ended, I invited family members to comment. The youngest daughter summed it up for all of them, saying, "The family only dies if you kill it."

A few months after that session, the marital home sold, and Monique and her now ex-husband moved into separate homes and separate lives. The move took her farther from my office, and she came less and less often. I was not concerned, as I knew Monique had navigated this difficult life transition well. I also knew she carried me within her, as a resource she could access, whether we were physically present with one another or not.

Thanks to the work of Marco Iacaboni (2011) on mirror neurons and resonance circuits, we are coming to understand the process of co-internalization. I am alive in Monique as she is equally alive in me. Calling one another to mind brings with it the felt sense of care, warmth, and support we shared in our time together. In this way, those who have nourished us along the way continue to be a resource we can call on when needed.

Discovering New Territory

Monique would pop back in for a session here and there, particularly as she began to consider dating. On one such occasion, Monique recounted the events of the Thanksgiving holiday that had recently passed. She and her daughter had decided to run in the local 5K Turkey Trot, after which they met up with her other sons at the home of her ex-husband for a Thanksgiving feast. In that session, Monique also shared that she had met a man who seemed quite interesting and was clearly smitten with her. We talked about the excitement that sat alongside the fear as she wondered if she was ready to love again. Fast-forward a couple of years, and I heard from Monique again, this time by email. She and her new man were still going strong. Her children and her ex-husband were doing well. They continued to get together as a family to celebrate birthdays, graduations, and other momentous occasions. At the end of the email, she asked if I remembered her vision trays. They immediately sprang to life in my mind as I read her closing comment: "It all came true! The two houses, the kids going back and forth effortlessly, right down to that kissing couple I always put next to my house. Do you remember when I asked if you had a crystal ball? I guess I created my own in the sandtray. Thank you for sticking with me."

I can honestly say the pleasure was all mine. Every day, I am grateful for the privilege of walking a part of life's journey with the courageous people who come my way. And I am deeply grateful to be able to offer them the deep healing that can arise in the course of a sandtray journey.

Concluding Comments

In one of the many conversations Monique and I shared over the course of her therapy, she expressed a sentiment shared with her husband, "We may not have been able to sustain a good marriage, but we can have a good divorce." She went on to explain their definition of a good divorce as one with minimal fighting, one that put the well-being of the children at the center, one that preserved funds by talking through things rather than having lawyers speak for them, and one in which, once it was all over, they would be comfortable in one another's presence.

I believe we can all agree that navigating the difficult waters of divorce with such grace is the exception rather than the rule. The anger, resentment, and interpersonal injury that lead couples to divorce often drives a desire to blame and punish one another.

I am curious about the reason things went differently for Monique. While I would like to credit her powerful work in the sandtray, I am sure it is more complex than that. The work of Simonič and Klobučar (2017) reminds us that the presence of help and support through the divorce process exerts more influence on the eventual outcome than the intensity of the stress experienced along the way. But how did her sandtray journey contribute to the relatively peaceful unwinding of a 25-year marriage? First, I believe it provided clarity for Monique. When she approached her husband about her dissatisfaction with their relationship, she was able to be clear about what was missing and what she needed from him. Those conversations centered on the qualities of the relationship itself and not the qualities of the people involved. Second, through her sandtray work, Monique understood she needed to rediscover herself as an individual before she could make a mindful decision about whether or not to stay married. This took time, slowing down the process enough to give both of them time to do some soul-searching. Monique bravely shared the personal insights from her sandtray journey with her husband which, in all likelihood, invited him into similar exploration.

Third, Monique created a vision for herself and her family that carried them through the divorce process and supported them in the years that followed as they created a new normal for their family. Monique's vision was not simply an intellectual idea. It was sourced from her deepest knowing, created by her own hands, and repeated over and over until it was in her bones. This vision became so deeply embedded in her that it was literally unthinkable that things would take a different route.

But perhaps most important of all was the contribution of Monique's husband. Had he been revengeful and determined to punish Monique, all the vision trays in the world could not have altered this couple's course. But he was not those things. It is Monique's opinion that, as she shared her struggles in their marriage and owned her part in them, her husband got in touch with his own dissatisfaction with his life and began to imagine a future for himself where he was free of the obligations he felt as Monique's husband.

Even in cases where the journey is more painful and a happy ending seems elusive, working in the sandtray can provide clarity, vision, and the opportunity to rediscover and redefine oneself as an individual, which are key elements for anyone going through a divorce. The greatest comfort you can offer is the unwavering accompaniment of a Sherpa who knows the destination is achievable and will be there every step along the way.

From the Therapist's Perspective

I often feel conflicted when clients show up with stories and life challenges that are similar to those I have faced in my own life. On the one hand, I think "Who better than someone who has been there, done that?" On the other hand, I know I am heading into territory where I will be challenged to see my clients as clearly as possible and not make any assumptions that my experiences are similar to theirs. This was particularly true with Monique.

When we first met, I had been divorced for only a few years. I might not have taken her on as a client, but when we first spoke, neither one of us had any idea her journey would lead to divorce. There were many times in her process that we would land in territory that was personally familiar to me. In these moments, I noticed my own urge to offer guidance or reassurance, and I had to remind myself that neither one of us had any idea how this would go for Monique. I was also aware of the moments I wanted Monique to move more quickly through her pain, as it was touching my own pain. At these times, I was particularly grateful for my clinical consultant, who was and continues to be an indispensable resource to me.

When I chose therapy as my profession, I assumed my job would be to help people. They would come to me with problems, I would apply my knowledge and skill, and their problems would go away. It was early in my career when I learned it doesn't always go that way. Through my study of interpersonal neurobiology, I have come to understand more deeply that my role is to create a safe relationship for the people who come to me and be as fully present with them as humanly possible. Certainly, my knowledge and skill come into play, but only in response to what is unfolding moment by moment in the therapy session. Sometimes what is called for is not the application of a particular therapeutic technique but rather the willingness to co-suffer. Monique and I did a fair amount of co-suffering. In those times, it was my number-one priority to let her know we were in this together. I often wanted to fix things for her, which of course was impossible, and I often had to remind myself that I was easing her pain simply by accompanying her on the journey. Sometimes it is when we think we are doing the least that we are helping the most.

As is true with just about every sandtray journey I have ever witnessed, trusting the process is key. Oftentimes, when working with a client, we can't draw a straight line between what is unfolding in the sand and what is happening in their lives. It may take many sandtrays over many sessions before subtle but immensely important changes appear. Over the course of my time with Monique, I had to trust her inner world to guide the pacing and direction of her journey. This is one challenge of sandtray therapy I seem to have mastered after many years. Throughout Monique's journey, I was able to trust the process because of my own personal experience with the sandtray. Deep and intimate knowledge and experience with the terrain, coupled with strength and courage, is what makes a Sherpa a Sherpa.

Notes

1. For the sake of simplicity, we refer to left-hemisphere and right-hemisphere processes, although the actual mechanisms are more complex. More accurately, we could refer to left- and right-mode processing, as some of what we attribute to the left hemisphere takes place in the right and vice versa.
2. I purposefully chose a circular tray for the ceremonial ending of Monique's family session. The circle can symbolize wholeness, which felt important to underscore. The

divorce would end the marriage but not alter the composition of the family, which would remain whole regardless of perception. In general, I do not recommend working in circular sandtrays unless the client so chooses. I prefer them for ceremonies or other times when the act of bringing individual parts into the whole is important.

References

Badenoch, B. (2011). *The brain-savvy therapist's workbook: A companion to being a brain-wise therapist*. W. W. Norton & Company, Inc.

Badenoch, B. (2018a). *The heart of trauma: Healing the embodied brain in the context of relationships*. W. W. Norton & Company, Inc.

Badenoch, B. (2018b). Safety is the treatment. In S. Porges et al. (Eds.), *Clinical applications of polyvagal theory: The emergence of polyvagal-informed therapies*. W. W. Norton & Company, Inc.

Beckes, L., & Coan, J. A. (2011). Social baseline theory: The role of social proximity in emotion and economy of action. *Social and Personality Psychology Compass, 5*, 976–988. doi:10.1111/j.1751-9004.2011.00400.x

Dana, D. (2018). *The polyvagal theory in therapy: Engaging the rhythm of regulation*. W. W. Norton & Company.

Holmes, T. H., & Rahe, R. H. (1967). The social readjustment rating scale. *Journal of Psychosomatic Research, 11*, 213–218. doi:10.1016/0022-3999(67)90010-4

Iacaboni, M. (2011). Within each other: Neural mechanisms for empathy in the primate brain. In A. Coplan & P. Goldie (Eds.), *Empathy: Philosophical and psychological perspectives* (pp. 45–57). Oxford University Press.

McGilchrist, I. (2009). *The master and his emissary: The divided brain and the making of the western world*. Yale University Press.

Noone, P. A. (2017). The Holmes-Rahe stress inventory. *Occupational Medicine, 67*, 581–582. doi:10.1093/occmed/kqx099

Simonič, B., & Rijavec Klobučar, N. (2017). Attachment perspective on marital dissolution and relational family therapy. *Journal of Divorce & Remarriage, 58*(3), 161–174. doi:10.1080/10502556.2017.1300015

6 Lost and Found

Reuniting With Self: Tales of the Wandering Psyche

Sean P. Jennings and Aimee L. Jennings

Tales of the Wandering Psyche

By the turn of the millennium, graduate school was over and 'real life' had officially started. Sean had opened his private practice under his master's-level license while completing his residency in pursuit of a doctoral license. Aimee had just left a community mental health agency to work with a private grant funded school-based counseling program. Significant changes abound, and sure enough, the momentous shift came when Aimee felt a "pull" toward sandtray. She arrived home one day with a flyer about Theresa A. Kestly of the Sand Tray Training Institute of New Mexico. The advert was for a series of trainings over five days. It was the first time Theresa came to Florida. Sean was a bit hesitant, and money was tight, but Aimee pointed out a couple of things: she was going no matter what; her work was paying for the hotel and her part of the trainings; and the trainings were held at an oceanfront hotel, where Sean could surf in the mornings, evenings, and lunch breaks. It was settled, we were going! At this point, we both had been play therapists for 6 years and were traditionally trained using sandtray – more like "sandbox" – in the playroom with children. Neither of us had ever considered using sandtray with adolescents or adults, picking a sandtray off the floor and putting it on a table, nor keeping our hands out of the sandtray. We had not yet even heard the names of Lowenfeld and Kalff! Before the cognitive knowledge, before the deep passion and respect for the powerful modality of sandtray came the *experience*.

Our Experience

Our experiences during those initial 5 days of training were very consuming. Dora Kalff (2003) described sandplay as "a Western form of meditation," and our absorption into the process was just that: very mindful and meditative. We were able to share our insights and knowledge with each other, furthering our relationship. Our passion, respect, and love of sandtray started in those early days and have exponentially grown over the years. Having experienced the power of sandtray personally and with clients, we

DOI: 10.4324/9781003055808-8

became committed to continuing our training. During the journey, we have gone through many stages of connection, disconnection, and reconnection to different elements of the process, ourselves, and each other. Both of us love the incredible balance sandtray offers between the experientially rich *knowing* and the cognitive knowledge derived through dialoguing between the conscious and the unconscious. Sean's mind jumped to integration of sandtray with clinical and developmental theories and the similarities shared with Rorschach principles and the synthesis with many other psychological modalities. Aimee's focus aimed towards integrating the energetic experience and the intuitive powers involved in healing. Let's refer to them as the "head and heart" approaches. We honor both, and though we have our own leanings we explore and develop both approaches within ourselves. We will differ at times in how we see sandtray, though it is through the interaction of differences that we reach new insights and integration, leading to synthesis. Having taught sandtray workshops together, for 10 years we have found it helpful to harmonize our voices in an effort to convey concepts to a diverse audience. Theresa A. Kestly (personal communication, May 5, 2020) said it is "essential to have a personal and meaningful experience" with sandtray in order to fully facilitate the witness role. Dan Siegel (2010) discussed "explaining" is a left hemisphere–dominant process, while "describing" is a whole-brain activity, as it requires the experientially rich right hemisphere to integrate with the wordsmithing language centers of the left hemisphere. Hopefully, we have begun a description and not an explanation of our personal and meaningful connection to sandtray, for it is our approach to share ourselves in order for those learning to connect and ignite the parts of self that relate.

We are tasked with writing about client experiences of disconnection on intrapersonal and interpersonal levels and the use of sandtray in reconnection. We have decided to use an amalgamation of clients into specific examples illustrating the differing ideas put forth in the chapter. We have recreated real sandtrays using similar but not the same miniatures, as well as various sand colors and tray shapes different from the original, unless the exact miniature or sand or tray was significant to illustrating the concept. Our goal was simple: if one of the clients we merged into the stories were to see the pictures and read the text, they might say "that is me and that is not me" to the degree that we all recognize ourselves in others and still feel uniquely us. The process to decide using composite stories or specific individuals' stories went as follows:

Aimee: I am not sure how I feel about using specific clients as examples. I am torn.

Sean: I am as well. On one hand, I want to convey the specific reconnection experience in its pure powerful form, but at the same time, I feel weird and protective of the original experience. I do not want to violate the sanctity of the protected space.

Aimee: Exactly! On one hand, I want the authentic energy to be present, but it also feels hard to put that out there – even with consent. For me, it feels like my needs are coming before the client's, even though the sessions (for many cases the actual therapy) have been over for a long time.

Sean: Well, I agree, but let's go deeper. We both love when books and articles have specific case examples and we benefit from those, so why would we not do it? We discuss specific cases in our workshops. Is this that different?

Aimee: Yes and no. No, it is for educational purposes, and we have consent, so it is not really different in theory. But yes, it feels different *energetically*. In our workshops, we begin with confidentiality and recognizing everyone's growing edge will come out to play. We are part of that sharing process by sharing our experiences in a sacred space. It is not the same with a book, in black and white and without presence.

Sean: Yes! That is the conflict I was having as well. It is missing the intimacy and the immediacy, which contribute to the parallel process. The parallel process where participants are revealing intimate details of themselves and we are revealing intimate details of our work and process. The energetic exchange is missing! By using a specific builder's[1] story, we gain the power of the process in its natural form but also incur an uncomfortable disclosure, and by using blended examples without a singularly identifiable builder, we maintain comfort but also encounter some amount of synthetic experience. So for us, we are deciding to construct examples using recreated sandtrays with blended backgrounds to be presented as a single person for continuity and readability purposes.

Aimee: Yes, sounds like a good integration. We get to (hopefully) capture the authentic process and feel comfortable in the disclosure. I love when others use case studies, but I agree we are not at a level where we can comfortably do that yet, so this feels like a good solution.

We demonstrate our process as we believe our interactions and processing of material through "heart and head" help us identify differences, similarities, and hopefully integration – within self, between each other, and for the clients' benefit. When thinking about connection-disconnection-reconnection and Tronick's (2007) language of connection-rupture-repair, Hegel's dialectics came to mind as a frame to understand the clients' work as well as our parallel process in understanding what manifests through the use of the sandtray. For those unfamiliar, a common example of a Hegelian dialectic would be Being – Nothingness – Becoming (Maybee, 2020), where the concept of Being naturally leads to the concept of Nothingness, and then they are combined into the unified concept of Becoming. Becoming implies both Being and Nothing; you can become a being and you can become nothing. In Maybee's (2020) detailed definition of Hegel's dialectics, she deftly delineates the dialectic does not have to be thesis-antithesis-synthesis, as it can be concept-different concept-next concept (through development or unity). This seems to be useful as a method to explore the process and understanding of sandtray experiences. Maybee (2020) further states the dialectic does not have to be triadic, which frees us up to explore ideas and other sides of the idea and, hopefully, develop an integration, synthesis, or unity. The very experience of Hegel's dialectic coming to mind as frame for discussing reconnection and unity experiences may have been synchronous unto itself. Hegel's philosophy was partially influenced by Plato's concept of the Forms (Maybee, 2020), which are universal knowledge and ideas that exist in a different realm than the world. Jung (1990, p. 75) partially based his concepts of the collective unconscious and archetypes on Plato's Forms as well. Thus, a chapter that aims to explore connection-disconnection-reconnection in sandtray using a method of inquiry (Hegel) influenced by the same source (Plato) that influenced Jung's theory, and subsequently sandplay therapy, may have its own serendipity! It is therefore our hope that the ideas and manner in which we express them are inclusive to all sand therapy practitioners.

Case 1

Cheryl presented as a 5-year-old female in Kindergarten with selective mutism. She did not talk to adults and would occasionally whisper to peers in class. Both her parents were in substance use recovery and had been divorced for 3 years prior to counseling. During the course of counseling, her father married his girlfriend. Cheryl's mother struggled in recovery and has some emotional stability issues but worked hard at containing herself. Her mother had significant attachment issues she was addressing in her own counseling. The parents had shared custody, and Cheryl talked readily at both homes and in session. She reported positive relationships with both parents and her stepmother. She enjoyed art and communicated mostly through drawing and sandtray. Cheryl presented as very intuitive, highly sensitive, and emotionally attuned to others and reported her best relationships were with her animals. Her mother referred to her as an indigo child. She often took care of others' emotions, especially her mother's.

Cheryl's first world is depicted in Figure 6.1 (A). She approached the first world by carefully scanning the miniatures, particularly the animals. She was intentional in her approach. She discovered a camel that is very flexible. She took the camel and bent the legs up and carefully laid the camel on the sand in the bottom right corner of the tray (Figure 6.1 (B)). She then proceeded to vigorously dump pretty much everything she could onto the camel until the tray was filled. She repeated this process for several sandtrays.

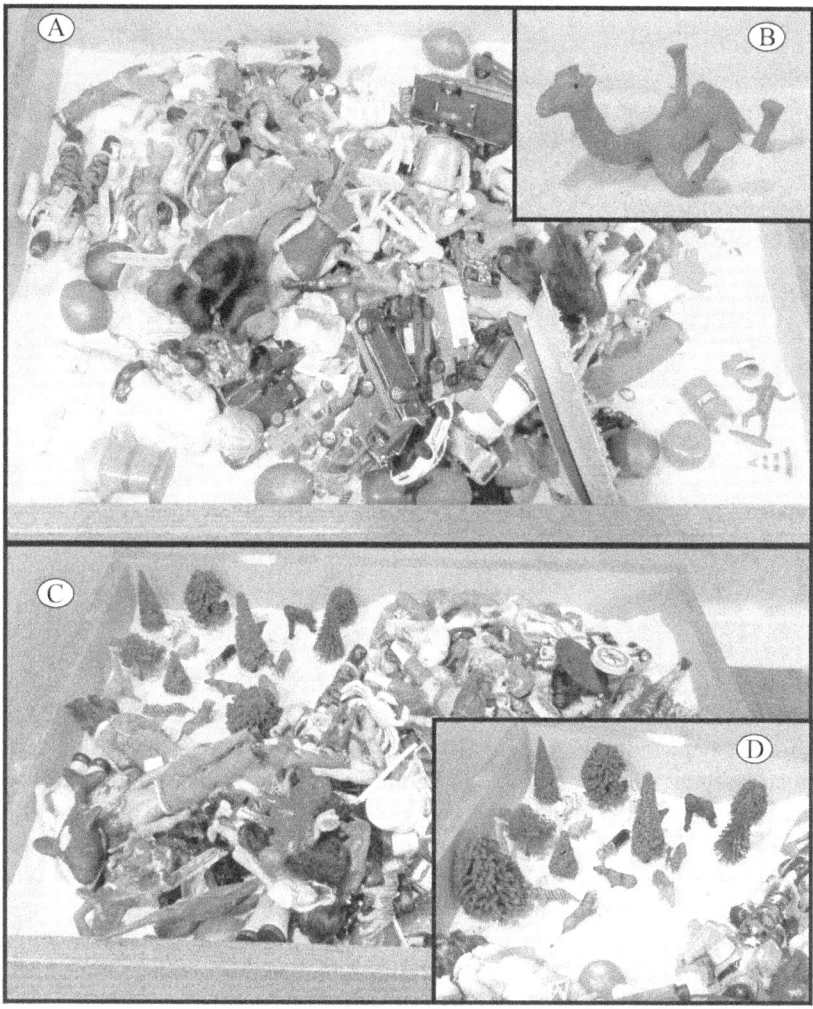

Figure 6.1 A – First tray; B – Close-up of the camel figure; C – Second tray; D – Close-up of small clearing in second tray.

Figure 6.1 (C & D) show the first tray where an area of the tray was not filled by dumping and, in fact, had a small scene of animals in a treed area. She continued to build sandtrays in this fashion. She picked the camel every time, and each time she bent the legs up, placed it in the bottom right corner, and dumped miniatures on top of the camel. Over time, the area of organization would become bigger, and the area of dumping on top of the camel became smaller and contained.

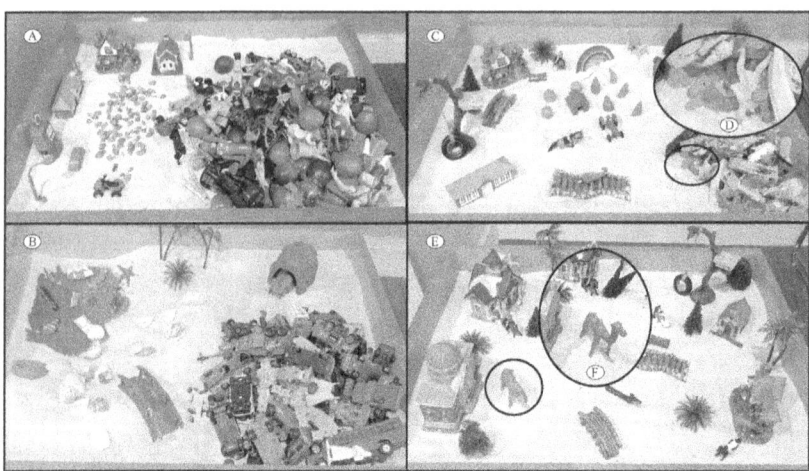

Figure 6.2 A – Third example of increased containment; B – Fourth example; C –
Fifth example; D – Closeup of camel and actually seeing the head in fifth
example; E – Camel is free and visiting people; F – Close-up of camel out
and about.

Figure 6.2 has more examples and demonstrates Cheryl's process. Figure 6.2 (A) is the third example and took place quite a bit into counseling. The tray depicted in Figure 6.2 (B) is representative of more than half a year in counseling. The last example in Figure 6.2 (E & F) depicts one of her last sandtrays prior to termination. Figure 6.2 (E) is the complete world, and (F) is a close-up of the camel. By the end the camel was out and walking around to the school, after-school program, church, and neighborhood. Cheryl was talking to adults and had made friends and had a best friend.

One way to conceptualize Cheryl's case is to understand she was completely overwhelmed and flooded emotionally. She was inundated with her own anxieties and, as a highly sensitive child, was inundated with everyone else's emotions. Her different parts were out of balance, lacked harmony and leadership. Her internalized mother and fear of her mother relapsing or having depression/anxiety while she was at school, her anxious self about school and social relationships, her desirous self who wants to make friends and connect with others, her animal-loving self who wants to just be with animals, etc., were at odds with each other and were demanding her focus with equal intensity. Through the sandtray process, she was able to externalize the flooded experience and slowly untangle what was tangled, creating boundaries to contain the different parts, developing harmony between competing areas, and eventually, leadership emerged.

This is not based on interpretation but rather the edification of Cheryl's own description into the language of internal family systems. As Cheryl created the small contained areas, she would call them different names like "my animals love" and "learning me" or other phrases that gave the distinct connotation she was referring to inner experiences. At the beginning, her presentation was reflective of the internal chaos of tangled selves, and by the end, the internal organization was evident by her reported behavior at home and school and displayed in the sandtray.

Processing of Case 1

Sean: Describe the disconnections.

Aimee: Cheryl was disconnected from her naturally intuitive and highly sensitive self. Her anxiety, manifested into selective mutism, further disconnected her from others. In the disconnected state, her fear of abandonment propelled her deeper into the safe sanctuary of animal relationships, which disconnected her from her desire for human relationships. She would experience nurturance and the ability to nurture with animals and thus felt connected and safe, but that part of her was blocking her from accessing the needed energy to overcome the fear of exploring the social world.

Sean: What was the rupture?

Aimee: As best as I can surmise, there was attachment disruption due to the parental relationship during the clear-cut attachment phase and the parents struggling in early recovery. Though her mother worked very hard at containing herself, Cheryl was so clearly aware and in tune with her mother she just was a conduit for her mother's emotional experience, which she had no defenses against or ability to understand. One might say she was overly connected to her mother, entangled, and thus unable to connect with self or others. Her own anxiety prevented her from accessing her natural growth parts, her growing edge.

Sean: What was the dumping like?

Aimee: That was shocking, not cognitively shocking like "I can't believe someone would do that" but energetically shocking like lightning bolts of anxiety were coursing through my body. I say energetically, because just saying emotionally would leave out the very physical sensations of the emotional experience. My body felt the dumping. It was not because of the force with which Cheryl was dumping things, because she was so purposeful the dumping was "controlled chaos." She was controlling the dumping to communicate how important it was so I could fully understand "this is important," as opposed to showing the chaos by dumping in an uncontrolled manner. The analogous behavior in her day to day life would be her anxiety manifested into overcontrolled speech, selective mutism.

Sean: Talk a bit more about the explanation around using the term "energetically."

Aimee: Some people have an immediate reaction, like "that is not scientific" or "that is more of that crazy pseudopsychology babble." Yet it is used every day in description when people talk about "there is so much excitement in the air" or at sporting events, "the crowd is electric." The exclusion of collective colloquial phrases for experiences by scientists for the sake of legitimizing science sounds like a move for superiority to cover a sense of inferiority, very Adlerian. I love science and the scientific method, but there is also natural knowledge. Natural knowledge is scientifically unproven information not meant to be confused with "naïve" knowledge (that which one knows based only on their individual subjective experience) but rather data of collective experiences in recurring patterns across cultures and time not by chance alone. I am not saying there should not be scientific inquiry or that we should readily buy into everything, but there does need to be room for the art with the science. I just get frustrated.

Sean: Then let's play a little bit with the Hegelian dialectic for this issue of using "energetically." We know there are experiences of physical sensations, and we know there are emotional and motivational experiences. We know the human body requires energy (food) to run and thus expends energy. We know having physical sensations will expend energy, and we know emotional experiences require and expend energy. Thus, a Helgelian dialectic could be sensation experiences discharge energy – emotional experiences discharge energy – energetic discharge. The energetic discharge would be the supraordinate concept holding both sensation and emotion energy consumption. Panksepp (1998) discusses the energostatic theory related to monitoring energy balance; thus we know there are changes in the brain regarding energy supply changes. Would it be feasible to believe mirror neurons may perceive such changes in others? Well, before we go too far beyond the data, how about we argue you can sense another person's energy expenditure when in close enough proximity? People get "heated" or "cool off"; psychodrama therapists have talked about warming up and cooling down clients for close to a century. So, we know you can sense another person's energetic discharge and there are established therapeutic techniques designed to recognize and regulate a client's energetic discharge. Another quick dialectic would be warming up – cooling down – energetic adjustment. Using the terminology "energetically holding, energetically containing, or energetically adjusting" sounds pretty reasonable with the current science, and a content analysis may indicate language reflects natural knowledge.

Aimee: I like that integration of science and natural knowledge. I think it fits nicely with how sandtray itself is such a wonderful modality for integration.

Sean: How did repair occur?

Aimee: Well, now I am going to say "through energetic adjustment"! My holding space for Cheryl allowed her to explore her parts of self and allowed for her innate healing process to begin putting the pieces together. I believe my ability to contain my own anxiety as I energetically felt her anxiety helped the co-regulation process. We can think about it through the lens of Porges's (2011) polyvagal theory and the application of the window of tolerance by Badenoch (2008) and Dana (2018). The co-regulation container allowed her to repeatedly "pop" into the sympathetic and come back to the ventral parasympathetic, eventually allowing her to remain in the ventral parasympathetic and thus "*sit*" with her experiences longer to recognize and connect with other parts of herself.

Sean: What is an intervention you did that you liked?

Aimee: I have to go with how we dialogued with different parts and introduced coping skills to help shield the incoming emotions of others. Cheryl would work in the sandtray and work on a part of herself. We would do other play-therapy activities outside the sandtray, where I am directive, and when she would introduce the part she just worked on in the sandtray, I would introduce more direct methods for skill development. Then she would go back and work more in the sand to discover more of herself.

Sean: How did Cheryl's play practice personally impact you? What did you learn/connect with self, relationship, and life?

Aimee: It was such an incredible and honoring experience for me. At the time I saw Cheryl, I was just getting my sandtray legs under me. I am not talking about how long that took! I intuitively knew what she needed and felt confident and fully trusted the process. It was through our work that I received a huge boost of confidence and competence. It was just one of those cases where everything came together for the betterment of the client, and it was how it needed to happen. I consider what I said a connection to spirit. When I get disconnected from spirit, a rupture, I need to do repair work in the form of self-care in nature. Through repair and reconnection with spirit, I am able to be effective in helping others, thus balancing my needs with clients' needs.

Case 2

Jackson first came to therapy when he was 12 years old. His parents were both recovering substance users, and his father had recently begun drinking again after 19 years of sobriety. His drinking was episodic and generally kept away from Jackson. Jackson had not seen his father intoxicated, as his mother went to great lengths to minimize his exposure, but at the same time, Jackson was aware his father was drinking again. Jackson's father would drink on business day-trips. His father had been an outstanding athlete in high school and would have been a professional baseball player had it not been for his early substance use. Jackson's father was often asked to coach Little League, and he turned down head coaching spots but would always help out with skill building. Jackson only played baseball in order to be with his father. Jackson was brought in initially to just check in with how he was coping with the shift in the family, as Jackson's parents were in therapy.

Figure 6.3(A) depicts Jackson's first sandtray world. He discussed "baseball dad" as the area with the baseball players and beer bottles and cans all around. He also referred to a leprechaun in the same area as his uncle. His maternal uncle had also relapsed. Jackson reported it was sad but that he and his friends could not see any of it. He described the Harry Potter characters as he and his best friends and added "there are more than three of us, and

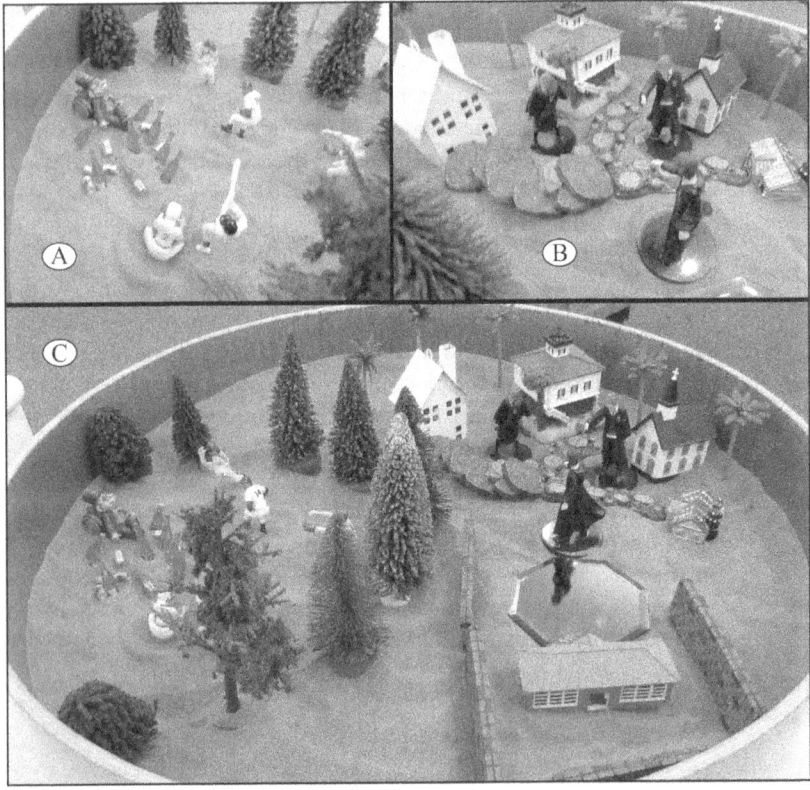

Figure 6.3 A – Uncle and Baseball Dad; B – Friends; C – The first tray.

we are all boys." Jackson's support system outside of his mother consisted of four best friends. The other four children went to the same private school together, and Jackson went to public school. Jackson reported he had friends at school, but they were "school friends" and that his real friends were his best friends in the neighborhood. He indicated he did not have a strong desire to make friends at school because he did not need them, he had his neighborhood friends and that was all he needed.

I informed his parents he seemed to be coping well and had a solid support system, and that unless they saw something concerning, he did not need therapy.

A couple of months after Jackson made his first sandtray, his father had come home on a Saturday seriously drunk and was making a scene on the front lawn. This was the first time Jackson was witness to his father's behavior when intoxicated, and his mother quickly called one of the four friends' parents and asked if they could take Jackson for the night. They of course agreed, and Jackson was whisked out of the house for a sleepover. His father had been escorted off the front lawn by a police officer and was required to leave the house. After Jackson returned home from the sleepover, he talked with his mother and told her he was feeling pretty sad about everything. He decided he would go hang out with his friends. He called one of his best friends and was told they were no longer allowed to be friends with him because of his father. When Jackson called the other three friends, he discovered they all said the same thing. All the parents were very upset that their children had been exposed to hearing about the behavior and wanted nothing to do with Jackson and his family. Jackson felt betrayed, rejected, and abandoned. He immediately came in for therapy. Please see Figure 6.4, as this is the world he built immediately following the incident.

Figure 6.4(A) shows the whole tray. There is a wizard that is controlling things and has put a spell on everyone. The boy fell into the well, and none of his friends can see him; he is hurt and needs help. The shark cannot cross the wall and is keeping the boy trapped on his part of the world if the boy "even gets out of the well." The friends cannot see the boy because they "turned their backs" away from him. Jackson identified he felt horrible and just wanted his friends back. He talked about his hurt feelings and his anxiety about not having friends.

Following the incident with his father and his best friends, Jackson suddenly became the target of bullies at school. Figure 6.5 depicts a world about his experience being bullied. Jackson is very clear and labels miniatures with specific bullies' names. There are children that are not being bullied, and they are also not helping Jackson. Jackson reported he felt very alone and that he could not count on anyone.

Middle school was rough for Jackson, but he slowly went from the peer status "rejected – withdrawn" to "controversial." Jackson was developing new friends, and slowly, the bullying ended. He finally found the close friends he was looking for when he joined the theatre club. Figure 6.6 (A–C)

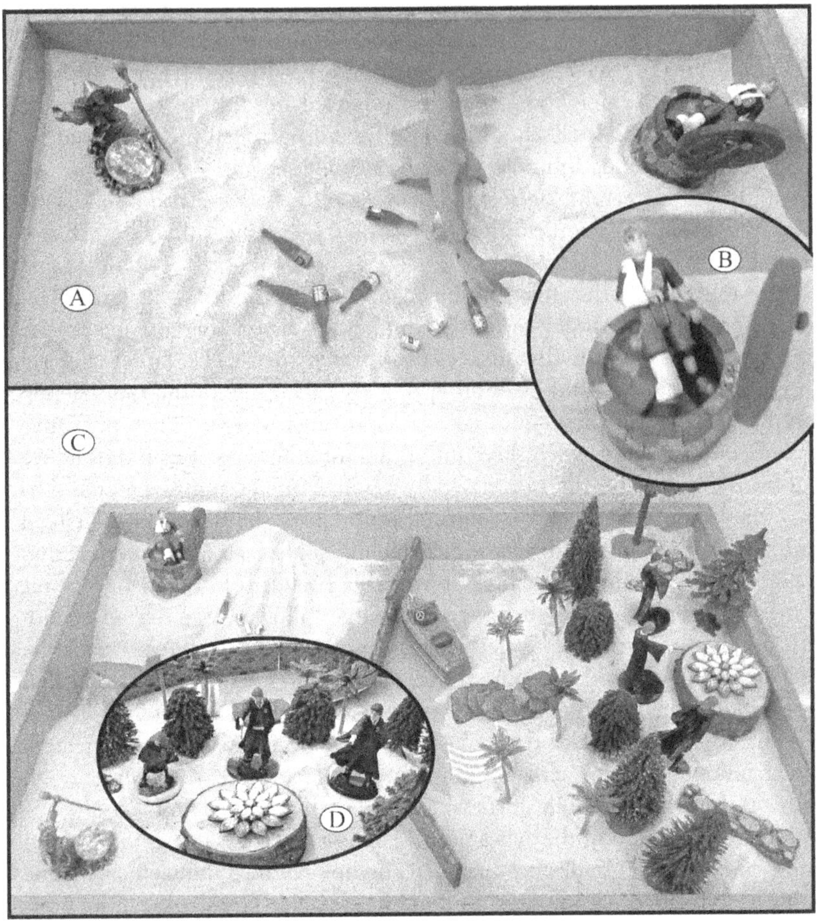

Figure 6.4 A – Tray following best friend betrayal; B – The wizard and the boy in the well; C – Boy in the well; D – The friends with back toward boy in well.

depicts his journey to meeting his "tribe" as he referred to his new friends. Jackson terminated therapy, went on to high school, and then after graduating high school, he decided to go to college abroad. Figure 6.6 (D-H) is a sandtray Jackson built when he came back for a session to say goodbye before he left to start a life in a different country. Figure 6.6 (D) shows how he first methodically groomed the sand. Figure 6.6 (E) is the world. Figure 6.6 (F & G) depict two different angles on the "Buddha Garden" he built for his mother, who is represented by the leaf miniature. He discussed using the brick walls he used to use in worlds as barriers and now was using them as part of the walkway because he sees everything that happened as

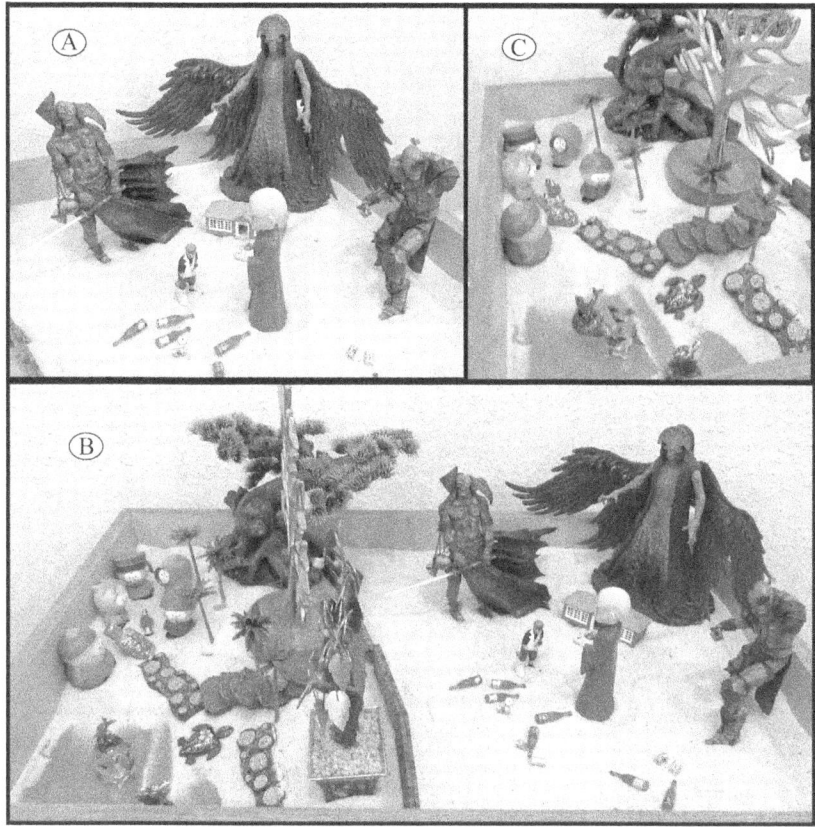

Figure 6.5 A – The bullies; B – Bullies on one side and other kids on the other; C – Kids not being bullied.

how he got to where he is now, and he does not feel upset by it. In figure 6.6 (H), he said he believes he has wisdom and that through his gained understandings, he is comfortable with being alone, as represented by the figure in the wooden cone-like miniature. Jackson said, "he is alone but people can come in and he can go out to them."

Processing Case 2

Aimee: Describe the disconnections.

Sean: Well, Jackson was clearly disconnected from his peers and his best friends. He was disconnected from his father. On an intrapersonal level, he was disconnected from his confidence, and as soon as he lost his confidence, he severely spiraled, and with the hits his self-esteem

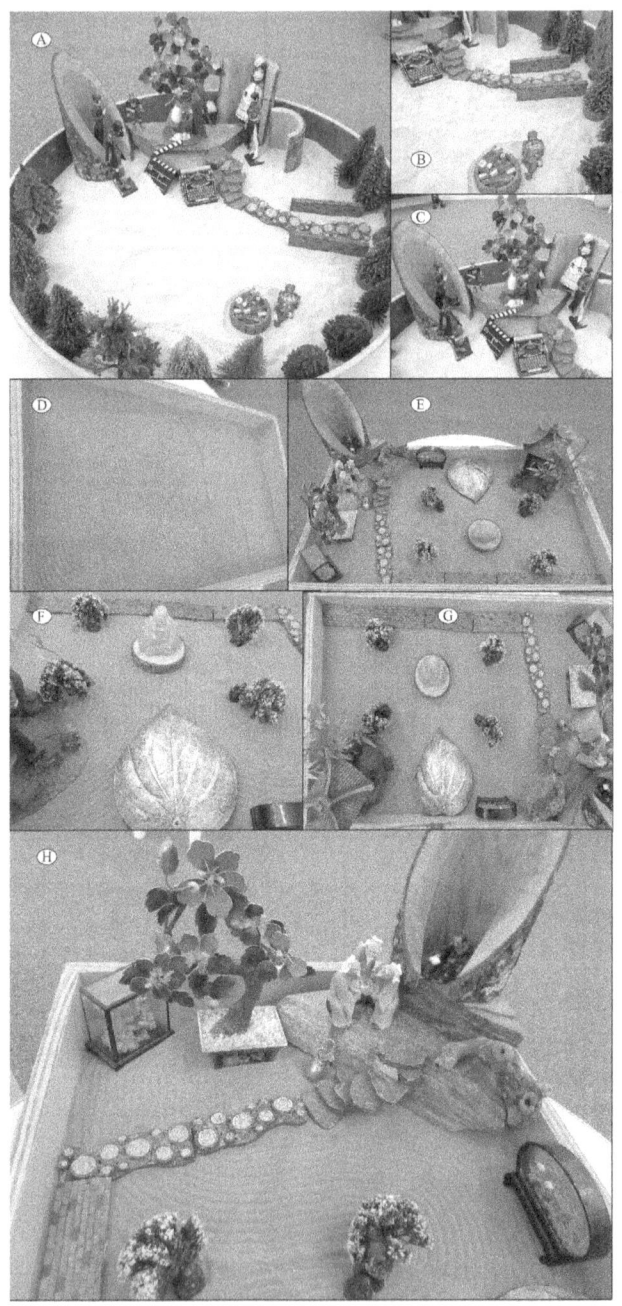

Figure 6.6 A – Jackson finds his tribe, the stage; B – The pathway to the stage and his uncle; C – The stage; D – The sand before Jackson built the goodbye tray; E – The goodbye tray; F – The Buddha garden; G – The Buddha garden from above; H – Wisdom and comfort.

and self-concept took, he immediately became a victim to bullies. The low self-esteem and poor self-concept were like blood in the water to bullies; they could energetically smell his vulnerability. These disconnections can be viewed through family systems, internal family systems, object relations, cognitive behavior theory. However a person conceptualizes the disconnections, it remains that Jackson was in pain and isolated within himself and from others. Thinking of Jaak Panksepp's (1998) seven innate motivational circuits, it would seem being disconnected from self and others contributed to the activation of his rage, separation-distress, and fear circuitry, and those dominated his affective experiences, most notably the distress and fear, which may have contributed to the bidirectional dynamic between him and the children who bullied him.

Aimee: What was the rupture?

Sean: The initial rupture was his father's relapse, but the big event was losing the friends. That was huge right as middle school was starting.

Aimee: What emotionally did you pick up on while holding space?

Sean: That is a good question! Initially, the first tray and interactions were great, and holding space felt really easy. He was so verbal and attuned to his emotions; it was really cool. When he came in after the friend incident, holding space was still pretty straightforward. At one point in the therapy, I started to feel some somatic pain in my left side. I was not sure why, but I queried about his left side, and he reported one of the bullies had thrown him in a locker, and he hurt his left leg. I think it was such a great example of paying attention to our bodies and the information they hold, which inform us for our builders. Emotionally, I could feel the sadness and not that much anger – some but not as much as I would have had if I were him.

Aimee: How did repair occur? Was there a bridge or gateway?

Sean: I think he started to reconnect with himself once he was able to let go of the victim role. Once he reconnected with himself, he rapidly was able to reconnect with others. The major task was getting him to let go of the victim role. I think the bridge was his father. He loved his father and was able to use boundaries with his dad. At some point, it was noted he was not as kind towards himself as he was towards his father. Hegel indicated the moment one concept is defined, then the opposing concept will immediately come into being. So the moment self-rejection was present, then self-acceptance must be at least a thought. Sometimes, it takes a while to find those concepts, but if we hold space and allow the client to drop into the world, they will find it faster than I can find it!

Aimee: Talk more from the "heart" approach. How does that fit in with all of this?

Sean: I think holding the free and protected space allowed Jackson to explore the environment and genuinely *"sit"* with the internal experiences being projected into the sandtray world. I truly believe the nondirective approach and focusing my energy on holding space and creating the warm, caring environment really allowed him to drop into the world and reconnect with parts of himself he had not been in touch with for a while because it was not safe. I think by not holding any interpretation, it allowed the unconscious field to be open for emotional connection without an underlying presumption of knowing. I could feel him wanting me to "fix" his father because I was still seeing is dad in therapy for a while.

Aimee: Discuss an intervention(s) you did that you liked.

Sean: I liked the suggestion to join theatre! At one point, he was stuck as to how to meet people and was doing a lot of "yes . . . but . . . no it won't work" responses to suggestions and ideas. When it came to socialization idea, he was having difficulty engaging in mutual brainstorming, not unlike polyvagal "freeze." Not the full "freeze" but the early entry into the dorsal parasympathetic with him feeling a powerless victim state and lacking energy to engage, particularly when it came to the fear stimulus of the relational context of peers. I believed we distracted with adolescent humor, which pulled him back into ventral parasympathetic, and utilizing middle school stereotypical thinking, I said something along the lines that theatre kids accept everyone and are totally nonjudgmental, and he latched onto the lack-of-judgement concept. He said he would join theatre. We practiced "the secret of middle school" by using some homemade techniques like "the air of confidence" and "faking it 'til you make it."

Aimee: Was there an intervention that was problematic?

Sean: There were a couple of things. One was to have his father rubber band a picture of the family (Jackson and his mother) to the outside of his wallet. The thought was if you want to drink, you will have to go through your family. It did not have the desired effect, as it did not slow his father's drinking down at all. Since Jackson knew about this intervention, and he knew his father was still drinking, the message he gained was "my dad doesn't love me enough to stop drinking." Another intervention was a method to deal with bullies. Not only did it not work, but he got in trouble with the school, got made fun of by the bullies, and he got put in the "friend zone"[2] with a person he liked. That was not great!

Aimee: How has this client or clients impacted you, and what have you learned/connected with *self, relationship,* and *life*?

Sean: I gained so much it is amazing. It was processing this case in this way that I stumbled upon the disconnection/reconnection to community. When the best-friend debacle occurred, remember, home was tense and school was not the main source of support; the neighborhood was the safest and thus connection to community.

When the best friends dumped him all at once, he was basically rejected/shunned by the community. His mother did well by not telling the other parents off, because that would not help, but it was clear the feeling of being ousted by the community was present. When Jackson started to come out of his victim stance and take on choices, he had just decided to study a very hard language to learn. It is also the language that is spoken in the country to which he moved. The language helped his self-confidence at that time, but it also gave him a foreign culture/community to become a part. I think his rupture with his complacent neighborhood community became disrupted, and after healing enough, he became curious and explored his environment, looking to join another community. If his best friends did not shun him, perhaps his connection to that community would have kept him in the Central Florida area for the rest of his life. I think he healed in such a way that he did not run away from any feelings of rejection or hurt by the community. Instead he gained confidence by developing best friends at school, which became his "next community." I think he then felt confident enough to explore his environment further, move to a foreign country, go to college where he would study completely in his second language, and become assimilated into that culture, which became his "current community." So, I reconnected with that "explorer" inner part of myself.

Summary

We have enjoyed learning by writing this chapter together, and we hope you have learned something as well. It would be a bonus if you had some fun while doing it! As Theresa Kestly (2014, p. 62) helps us remember there are the three Rs to integration of play (recognize, rely on, and reinforce), we think there are three Rs to the synthesis/integration/unity process of the Hegelian dialectic process we demonstrated in processing sandtrays: *rationale – reverse – refinement*. The *rationale* is the first position or understanding, the *reverse* is taking another direction, exploring our first understanding by taking an intentionally different direction, and that will hopefully lead to *refinement*, the integration of differing ideas. We will leave you with some dialectics for you to think about and play with; perhaps you will come up with different integration concepts: connect – disconnect = collocate; rupture – repair = healing; conscious – unconscious = being; aware – unaware = information; cognition (head) – emotion (heart) = human . . . enjoy!

Notes

1. We use the term "builder" for the person constructing the world and "witness" for the person observing/aiding in the processing of the world. For many readers, the

builder is known as the client and the witness as the therapist. Similar to how the change from "patient" to "client" connotates a redistribution of power within the therapeutic relationship, for us, the change from client/therapist to builder/witness connotates the role shift in expertise. The builder is the expert, and the witness becomes the student/receiver of manifested knowledge.

2. The "friend zone" is a generational colloquial term referring to when one person is romantically interested in another person, but the feeling is not reciprocated. The person of interest does not directly reject the person but rather continues to lead the person to believe there is a "chance" in order to continue to get their needs met through friendship.

References

Badenoch, B. (2008). *Being a brain-wise therapist: A practical guide to interpersonal neurobiology*. W. W. Norton & Company, Inc.

Dana, D. (2018). *The polyvagal theory in therapy: Engaging the rhythm of regulation*. W. W. Norton & Company, Inc.

Jung, C. G. (1990). *The archetypes and the collective unconscious* (R. F. C. Hull Trans., 2nd ed.). Princeton University Press. (Original work published in 1959).

Kalff, D. M. (2003). *Sandplay: A psychotherapeutic approach to the psyche* (E. R. Verlag Trans.). Temenos Press. (Original work published in 1980).

Kestly, T. A. (2014). *The interpersoanl neurobiology of play: Brain-building interventions for emotional well-being*. W. W. Norton & Company, Inc.

Maybee, J. E. (2020). Hegel's Dialectics. In E. N. Zalta (Ed.), *The Stanford encyclopedia of philosophy* (Winter 2020 ed.). https://plato.stanford.edu/archives/win2020/entries/hegel-dialectics/

Panksepp, J. (1998). *Affective neuroscience: The foundations of human and animal emotions*. Oxford University Press.

Porges, S. W. (2011). *The polyvagal theory: Neurophysiological foundations of emotions, attachment, communication, self-regulation*. W. W. Norton & Company, Inc.

Siegel, D. J. (2010). *Mindsight: The new science of personal transformation*. Bantam Books.

Tronick, E. Z. (2007). *The neurobehavioral and social-emotional development of infants and children*. W. W. Norton & Company, Inc.

7 Through the Eyes of a Child

Sandtray Therapy With Children

Caron J. Leader

Amy didn't tell me much about why I have to talk to someone, but I think it's 'cos I get mad all the time and don't listen. She and Paul say I don't listen sometimes and the last family I was with got mad at me when I didn't listen too. I have been to a place like this before but not in a really long time. I didn't want to come, yelled at her and hid in my room. Every time I go talk to someone, I get in trouble and have to move to another place. I am scared and mad. Amy is sitting next to me and we are waiting on a couch with other people I don't know. There is a lady on the phone talking and when we came in and she didn't even look at me. She talked to Amy and then told us to sit and wait. Amy gave me her phone and I am trying to play but my brain won't let me. There is a fish tank behind me, so I turn around and look at it. Oh, there is Nemo and I see Dorie too!

I think someone is coming over to us! She is kind of old and white like Amy but has curly hair like me. She is smiling and says hi to me first. She says her name is Mallory and puts her hand out to me. I freeze and don't know what to do and just sit there looking away. It seems like Amy already knows her. She asks us if we want to go to her office. I don't want to go but I don't think I can say no. I say nothing and look out the window. We go past the lady on the phone, past a hallway and down another hallway past some rooms with people in them and around a corner. I feel dizzy. I see some weird stuff in one room but we go by too fast so I can't see what's in there. The lady takes us into a big yellow room. She talks to me first. She says a bunch of stuff, but I don't really hear the words. I am sitting as still as I can and looking straight ahead trying not to blink. I can see there is some weird stuff in here too.

Finally, she asks me if it would be okay if Amy left and we played for a while. Play? Play what? I don't play with old people like her and have never played in one of these places! She does seem kind of nice, but I don't really want to! I feel scared again. I still don't think I can say no so I slowly nod my head up and down. Amy leaves and we sit for a while. I feel frozen waiting for her to do something but am moving my eyes around the room. She is quiet for few minutes looking around the room with me. She asks me about what I see, and I point to some small dolls. She says I can pick them up if I want to and I go get them.

Then she says I can pick up other stuff if I want and she will show me the playroom in a few minutes but first she needs to say something very important to me and asks if I can listen carefully. My eyes get really wide and I sit up thinking she is going

DOI: 10.4324/9781003055808-9

to tell me I have to go back to the last family! I am so scared that I hold my breath. I didn't like them at all! She says she knows I had to talk to a lot of grown-ups since I was really little and when I moved in with Amy and Paul. She says she understands if that was scary for me and made me worry. She asks me if I know what scary and worry mean, and I shake my head yes. She says anybody would feel that way if they moved a lot. Then she says she is a helper kind of grown-up. She said her job is just to help me and not to decide if I have to move. She says she is Amy and Paul's helper too and Amy brought me here so she could help all of us! She tells me she is not here to talk about what I am doing wrong and is not going to take me away from my brother, Amy, or Paul. It is like she is reading my brain! Then she said she is not the same kind of helper like a mother, a teacher or a coach and wants to help me feel better but first she just wants to get to know me.

She says one of the ways she gets to know kids like me is by playing with them. She asks me if I have any questions and I slowly nod no but I am not so sure. Then she asks if I am ready to see her playroom. I nod yes but this time I actually want to nod yes. I don't feel as scared. We get up and leave the yellow room going back out the way we came in, I think. Then there is that room with all the weird stuff. We are going in there! She asks me to go in first and I move slowly into the room but then suddenly I stop, and my eyes go very wide as I look at all the stuff. I can't believe what I am seeing! There are shelves on each wall with all kinds of little toys! I see dolls, cars, trees, furniture, little people, play food, all kinds of animals and a bunch of Disney princesses! And in the corner, there are masks and dress-up clothes too. In the middle of the room, there is a round table just the right size for me.

She asks me if I'd like to sit down. As I get closer to the table, I see a big blue box filled with orange sand. I have never seen orange sand! I can't stop looking around at all the stuff. I touch the edge of the table and the lady asks if I want to touch the sand. I step back a bit, surprised. Touch it only if you want to, she says. I stick one finger out and touch the orange sand just on the top. I have played with sand a few times but never this much of it and never orange and never with a lady at a place like this. I can't believe how it feels. She says I can sit if I want to or stay standing. Then she says I can put both hands in the box and move the sand around. I want to do that but for some reason I get scared again and don't move. She says it is okay if I don't want to. She also says she has other colors of sand if I don't like the orange color, but I don't hear what she is saying anymore because suddenly, I have both of my hands in the sand and am moving it through my fingers. It feels so soft and kind of cold. I can't stop moving my hands in this orange sand. I can hear the helper lady say some stuff, but it is so hard to listen. I do catch her saying I can make the sand into mountains, get it wet or move it around to see more of the blue tray, which I do and see blue on the bottom.

She says this is sandtray and that we are going to be playing in this room a lot if I like it and I will get to pick out any of the toys on the shelves too. She says if I want I can put the toys in the tray and play with them. She calls this building a world and I think that sounds kind of fun. I don't feel as scared and sit down. I look at the helper lady and she smiles. I ask her if I can go pick out something now and *she says sure. I go right to the shelf where all the play food is and grab all kinds of yummy food!*

Working With Children

This vignette is a fictional version of how a child might feel when being introduced to a therapist and sandtray. A child's apprehension and concern when visiting a therapist's office for the first time can only be imagined from our adult perspective. However, it is likely a time of anxiety and uncertainty for many children and can easily be disorienting. When a child with a history of difficult life experiences enters a therapist's office and is expected to talk, they are being set up for a failed therapeutic experience. It is unrealistic to think a child can verbalize their experience. Many well-meaning therapists see children without specialized training. The reality is if therapists are working with children who have trauma, attachment disorders, severe behavioral and/or emotional problems, it is essential they develop a skill set based in solid mental health theory and therapeutic models that are effective for children.

Anna Gomez (2013), child therapist and author, discusses the level of expertise and how vital it is for child therapists to obtain advanced training before working with children with complex developmental trauma. Just as important as determining a specific training path is a therapist's individual process work. A therapist must understand their own early childhood experiences that could hamper their clinical interventions. She states clinicians that do not do their own healing work will have difficulty attuning adequately to their clients and might themselves become activated when working with children. Finally, a child therapist must understand cognitive development to offer children a way to process their experiences in a safe, comfortable, and appropriate manner.

Play therapy serves as an invaluable therapeutic tool when working with children. A child's play is an important part of how neuronal connections are formed, especially surrounding social engagement (Gomez, 2013). However, playtime can be nonexistent for some children, as their caregivers' ability to play might be limited for many reasons. Lucky for the child therapist, play is a child's natural means of expression. Using toys, dress-up, art, and movement, coupled with creativity and spontaneity, a therapist can support children to become comfortable with play. If given the opportunity, a child will use play to safely negotiate inner conflicts, emotions, and positive and negative experiences, build and/or test relationships, and express their inner and outer world.

Sand is one of the many mediums used in play therapy. Most children really love it and, with little instruction, jump right in. Gisela Schubach De Domenico, a pioneer in sandtray therapy, discusses the value of sandtray-worldplay (her method of sand tray therapy) with children as she highlights the barriers some clients present with when they walk through a therapist's door. Many adults have difficulty with cognitive processing as well as expressing their emotions and experiences. This is more so the case with children, "whose intellectual, emotional and language development is insufficiently complete and cannot present the complexity of their psychological experiences" (De Domenico, 1995, p. 3).

Because sandtray offers a child an opportunity to fully use their senses as they create something tangible, it can also lend more creative options to the therapist as they expand a child's therapeutic experience. The multidimensional, archetypal, symbolic world of sandtray allows a child to play, imagine, explore, work out, and test all manner of inner and outer expressions. All experiences of life can show up in the tray as De Domenico's phenomenological background emphasizes. The therapist's work is to provide a supportive, open, and present witnessing so a child is allowed to create or recreate whatever manifestations of conscious or unconscious elements come out in the sand (De Domenico, 1995).

Each sandtray session centers around building a sacred world, one with images that depict the child's psyche as they are allowed to freely create and integrate their being into the here and now. As De Domenico so elegantly describes, "It evokes the archetype of the creator, the undifferentiated Self in the process of becoming" (De Domenico, 1995, p. 5). The attuned and present sandtray therapist is witness to a great unfolding of a builder's being as they work through experiences that have delayed their integration and move into wholeness.

Improved self-awareness, emotional regulation, and integration of maladaptive information are key goals of therapy. Only when a therapist is present and attuned can this vital work take place and produce desired outcomes. For true treatment success with children, proper attunement is essential. If therapists are not attuned when working with children, they could be repeating attachment wounds or activating children negatively. Of course, even the best therapists are unable to attune and be present every moment, but if therapists are not trained in child-specific methods and/or have little understanding of attachment disorders, trauma, or child neurodevelopment, attuned presence will be even more challenging.

The attuned child therapist uses their training and skill to complete a thorough assessment of a child's full experience in order to determine the best therapeutic course for treatment. Sandtray is not for everyone, and treatment planning involves obtaining a client history that includes a full caregiver interview. Gomez (2013) suggests the child therapist must assess the caregivers' attachment style, trauma history, ability to play, ability to self-regulate, and their strengths and resources and discover what the care giver considers their child's problem areas. All this involves paying careful attention during the interview, as caregivers often do not provide this information freely as they are focused on their child's negative behaviors and could be activated themselves as they start the therapeutic process. A proper assessment will take more than one session, and therapists must help guide the process and support caregivers as they learn about their clients (Gomez, 2013).

Working With Jackie and Her Family

Jackie's case highlights difficulties, pitfalls, and missteps along with successes. It is a case that, as of this writing, has not successfully been discharged. Jackie's parents gladly granted me permission to share their experiences in the hope it would help other clinicians and parents facing similar challenges. This case touches the core of our human need for connection and understanding, as well as our resiliency and capacity to change.

Jackie is a 9-year-old biracial girl who was adopted when she was 4 years old. Her adoptive parents, Pam and Leonard, were referred to me due to difficulties they were having with communication, acting-out behavior, discipline, and difficulty bonding. In a brief conversation with the referring therapist, I learned of Jackie's complicated early traumatic experiences, difficulties with the foster care placement of one of her older sisters, and the adoption of her younger brother prior to Jackie's placement.

Beginning to work with a family with experiences like Jackie's and her parents is never easy. It is hard to vicariously witness the full range of human experiences and how the grim side of these manifest in mental and behavioral problems. It can be even harder to witness the impact that adult life struggles and tragedies have on children. Taking in the pain and suffering Jackie's parents shared and their need to find a way to connect with and understand their daughter, made for some initial unease, and I felt pressure to find quick solutions and provide relief for this family. However, relying on my training and knowledge versus the immediate emotional tug allowed me to form a solid treatment plan that included the use of sandtray. Remembering that, first and foremost, a connected and safe relationship with Jackie and her parents was paramount, I focused on attuning and listening carefully as treatment began. I knew the best result would come if I withstood the pressure to move too fast, follow the parents' emotional pace, or allow sympathy for their suffering to drive treatment.

The task of gathering a thorough history began with the chaotic backdrop of difficult emotions, vague memories, and limited reports that were culled out in bits and pieces during the first few sessions. This task was made even more difficult as the story of Jackie's adoption unfolded. Jackie's mother, Pam, reported they began with fostering Jackie's older sister and younger brother, who were 7 years old and 4 months old at the time. Pam had less than 12 hours' notice to prepare for the arrival of her son, which is often the case with emergency placements. Jackie's sister came next, ultimately leaving within four months, and Jackie arrived soon after. These were hectic and frightening times for Pam and Leonard, and the initial information they learned about Jackie when she arrived was swept away into the trauma vortex. Jackie's parents always intended to adopt after they could not conceive and wanted to take in siblings, but despite positive intentions and foster training, they were not prepared to manage the severe emotional and behavioral issues their foster children presented.

During these first sessions, Pam often became tearful as she described her experiences during those early days. She told about Jackie's sister and her episodes of rage that led to self-harm, her waking up screaming in terror, how she could not be soothed, leaving the family in a state of utter panic. After 4 months of trying, Pam and Leonard could not continue, and with great remorse, they requested that Jackie's sister be removed. She was transitioned to a group-home facility, where she remains to this day.

Before Pam and Leonard could even settle from this experience, child protective services began encouraging them to take in 4-year-old Jackie to foster and ultimately adopt. Both parents were reluctant after the experience with her older sister but felt pressure to keep Jackie and her brother together. Pam and Leonard agreed Jackie did not have the severity of issues her older sister exhibited, but they described her as extremely difficult.

In my first phone contact with Pam, I discussed my assessment process, telling her I would need both mother and father to attend at least three sessions so I could get a solid history and provide psychoeducation about complex trauma and attachment issues and discuss our treatment plan. I warned her that it might result in my referring them to a therapist trained in a specific attachment disorder treatment method and gave them the option to start with this type of therapy instead. They elected to begin treatment with me, as there is no local therapist trained in the suggested attachment therapy, and they trusted their referral source.

Once the assessment phase began, it became clear that Pam and Leonard needed to share the trauma they experienced while fostering Jackie's older sister. It seemed as if Jackie's sister was still living with them, and perhaps much of their distress about her was projected onto Jackie. However, they were able to communicate their concerns about Jackie, which included her aggressiveness, defiance, and poor boundaries. They also felt she was very loud and disruptive, and Pam worried about her capacity to bond with them. Both parents wanted help in educating her about being adopted.

My persistence, patience, and listening for clues of Jackie's history, her potential treatment targets, and issues of attachment allowed a picture of her early life to slowly come into view. Jackie not only witnessed her biological father's death when she was 18 months old, but reportedly, her biological mother demanded Jackie hide this fact from police. According to Pam and Leonard, Jackie's mother had been involved with child protective services for some time, and her oldest girls had been removed multiple times. Once Jackie came along, this was the norm, and a permanent separation process for these children had been started.

While it is not certain that Jackie was sexually abused, it was reported that her oldest sister sexually abused her second-oldest sister. Jackie demonstrated inappropriate touching and masturbation per her previous foster parents.

Both parents were severely neglectful and emotionally absent, leaving the care of the children to her oldest sister. It is unclear how many times Jackie was removed from her parents' home, how many foster families she lived with, or how much of the time she lived with her maternal grandmother and how positive this relationship was for her. As the pieces of this puzzle formed, it became clear Jackie's early life was filled with insecure attachment and complex trauma.

Jackie arrived at the second session, even though I had not completed the assessment phase with her parents. But here she was with Pam, both of them looking at me expectantly with bright smiles. Jackie was ready to play! I shifted focus to building rapport with Jackie and grabbing what background history I could. Just like in the vignette at the beginning of this chapter, in this first meeting with Jackie, it was important to let her know my role in her life and that I was not going to be like a mother or a teacher or make decisions that would affect her staying with her parents. I also briefly introduced her to the sandtray room, and then we set about to play a game.

Jackie chose Candy Land, and we sat on the floor together to play. There were no expectations, no rush, no pressure as the play took place. I didn't ask any questions about her background, as it felt important to allow space for Jackie to feel comfortable and get to know me. The game was fun, and Jackie clearly wanted to win but was not mean spirited as she made strategic moves to grab the victory. She was observant and inquisitive; looking around the office and asking questions about things in the therapy room. She did not share much but was not overly guarded either and seemed to genuinely enjoy our time together. She agreed to come back, and I felt the therapeutic relationship was off to a good start.

Jackie showed up again for the third session, this time with her father, and I had to quickly switch gears. As is common, our treatment plans have to be adjusted when client needs show up differently than expected. I decided to use this session to introduce Jackie to sandtray and started by providing a more detailed tour and description of sandtray. I described the different types of sand textures and colors along with the various trays then talked about the miniatures and described the building process.

I told Jackie to use whatever color sand and size tray she pleased and to pick some miniatures or none at all. De Domenico (1992) calls this type of sandtray session "free and spontaneous" play. "The builder can work uninhibited by directions, instructions or interventions while the therapist silently witnesses the play until completed" (De Domenico, 1992, p. 11). Once the play is done, the client may speak about their creation and the therapist may ask probing questions to deepen the experience for the client (De Domenico, 1995).

Like many children, Jackie went right to work without much prompting, instinctively knowing this sand and tray were meant for play. She chose pink sand and began by moving the sand around, making a flower-type pattern.

Then she collected some miniatures, picking several people: two infants; two girls; two adult dolls; furniture; and a car. She talked as she worked, saying these people were moving into their new house. She carefully built a bedroom for the babies and one for the girls, a kitchen with a large bounty of food, and put the adults' room in the middle. She said the adults were sleeping, and the children could do whatever they wanted. Jackie said the girls needed to give the babies food, saying they needed all the healthy food. She had the girls tuck in the babies, kissing them good night. Jackie moved the girls to the car, saying they were too young to drive but were going to try to do it anyway.

Jackie often looked up while building, seeking eye contact. I don't know if she was making sure I was attentive or if she was seeking reassurance that she was doing a good job. It felt important to give her my undivided attention while she worked. It seemed equally important to note her pace and match the rhythm of her breath and movements, not in a rote or invasive manner, but rather to aid in attunement and connection. Jackie's building was thoughtful and purposeful as she carefully created the scene.

Referred to as the "questioning phase" in sandtray-worldplay (De Domenico, 1995), this next part of the process allows the therapist to shift positions and see the sandtray world from the vantage point of the builder.[1] I asked Jackie's permission, which she eagerly gave, and I moved beside her

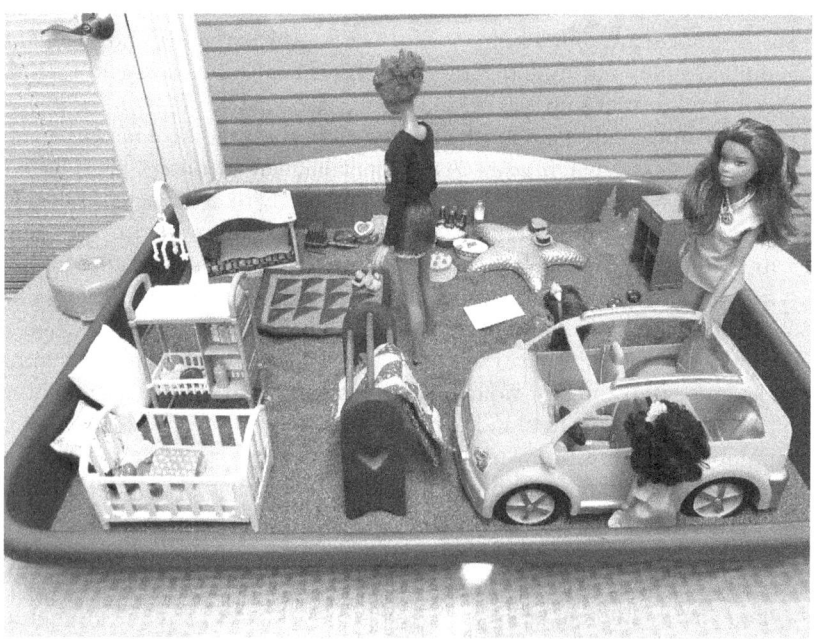

Figure 7.1 Jackie's first tray.

to view the creation. Jackie explained that she was in the tray and was both one of the babies and one of the little girls. She said the other baby was her twin brother, Luke. She shared information about the children's bedrooms and gave elaborate details about the importance of the healthy food, saying they liked having the food, and adding that she liked feeding the babies best. Jackie said the adults are always sleeping in this world and did not even know the girls got into the car. She said she liked this tray very much and felt safe when the babies were being fed and tucked in.

Suddenly, Jackie had jumped forward several sessions in her treatment plan before I had a chance to assess her level of affect tolerance and emotional regulation, much less help her build these skills. In this third session, she was starting to work with her unmet needs. It is recommended this type of work be introduced to a child after providing psychoeducation through play about emotions, physical sensations, and thoughts, then do work to install skills and build strengths that can assist when processing difficult experiences (Gomez, 2013). It appeared Jackie was able to tolerate what she built and focused on what felt good after it was completed, especially when the babies were being nurtured with food and soothed with their bedtime ritual.

As you may have gathered, the assessment phase was not going according to my plan. The session preparation, training protocols, and history taking were being thwarted by the family's life circumstances and Jackie's unmet needs. This is often the case when working with children. We attempt to follow treatment plans, but often, clients show up wanting and needing to go a different direction. Therapy is an organic process, and we must make space for what shows up and adjust the treatment protocol rather than allowing the protocol to dictate.

This first sandtray session provided useful information. It was clear Jackie had a lot of strengths and resiliency. She was able to be in touch with her unmet needs without dysregulation. However, she saw herself as two different ages, one being the same age as her younger brother. Here were clues about her difficulty regulating her emotions, how she might be confused regarding her role in the family, and why she might regress when her needs were not met.

Jackie and Pam came together to the next two sessions, so I decided to use the time for psychoeducation. While I believe it is important to provide both parents with information on attachment and complex developmental trauma, it became clear that Leonard's 12-hour workdays would make it difficult for him to join us. It was also obvious that Pam was feeling more of the caregiver stress. She needed to talk about her experience with Jackie's older sister and continued to voice fears about not being as close to Jackie as she was to Luke. Both parents maintained Jackie was too loud, overly impulsive and aggressive, excessively needy for her age, and would not do what they asked. Pam worried that Jackie was potentially dangerous to her brother, as she did not seem to understand their age differences. In addition, as is often the case, Pam had her own family-of-origin trauma that was being touched by her struggles in parenting Jackie. Pam and Leonard needed support and education.

Daniel Siegel (2014) has written extensively about the importance of understanding children's security of attachment to their caregivers and suggests that connection and attunement can be improved with mindfulness, flexibility, and playfulness. I decided to use Siegel's framework with Jackie's parents and recommended his book, *Parenting From the Inside Out*, to help Pam and Leonard better understand Jackie's developmental challenges. In session, I reviewed the importance of early brain development, and we worked on positive redirecting. In a session where Jackie chose to play Candy Land, I asked Pam to only observe and resist any urge to intervene or comment. Jackie's desire to win resulted in occasionally and gleefully knocking down my pawn. She angled for the higher number when the spinner landed on the line, saying that was her rule. Whenever she was about to do something mischievous or make a winning move, Jackie would make eye contact with her mother and me. I gave her room to be competitive, and we agreed her spinner rule would prevail. If Jackie pushed a boundary too far, I gently and playfully stood up for my character. I used every opportunity to encourage positive behavior, keeping the atmosphere jovial and light. Somehow, I won the round of play but offered for Jackie to go first in the next round to ease her disappointment. She took the loss like a champ and agreed to a rematch.

I invited Pam to join us with the instruction to simply play and leave me to redirect Jackie if needed. The dynamic immediately changed as Jackie became protective of her mother, clearly wanting her to win. Jackie challenged my moves and only made eye contact with me when she tested a limit. She told her mother how to play, taking a parental role. I maintained the same steadiness, gently and playfully redirecting Jackie when needed and encouraging both she and her mom when they helped each other. I kept consistent boundaries, using Jackie's spinner rule even when it did not favor her or her mother. This round ended with Jackie taking the win, and we celebrated her victory. Jackie ended the play by comforting her mother, reassuring her she would win next time.

When Pam and I processed the play session, Pam shared concerns about Jackie's willful desire to win, along with her willingness to use aggression to do so. She had observed similar behaviors at home and worried that Jackie lacked empathy. Pam also noted Jackie's protectiveness toward her, saying she often has to correct her from parenting her brother. She commented on how I kept things playful and consistent, not getting upset or angry but gently challenging Jackie when she tried to change the rules. She saw Jackie mirror me and respond positively when encouraged. Pam was able to see how this allowed space for fun and avoided arguments or tantrums. Watching me play with Jackie made Pam wonder about her own relationship to play, observing that she does not spend much time playing with her children and curious about whether her own parents played with her as a child. Pam described herself as quick to anger, jumping to negative conclusions, and handing Jackie punitive consequences. I suggested a homework assignment for both parents to play with the children, together and alone, using the tools of mirroring, redirecting, allowing space for appropriate competition, and encouraging positive behaviors versus highlighting negative ones. They agreed to this experiment to see how play might change things at home.

Despite the start of treatment not going according to plan, Jackie's parents reported improvement. They were reading Siegel's book, better understood the importance of consistent discipline, reduced using yelling as a consequence, began using redirection, and added play into their routines. They told me Jackie was less aggressive, but they were still concerned she was hyperactive, unable to focus, and too clingy and upset at bedtime. Pam revealed Jackie's doctor had previously diagnosed attention deficit hyperactivity disorder and had recently switched to a new medication, leaving Pam feeling unsure about Jackie being on medication. I suggested they pursue psychological testing and a medication evaluation to confirm the diagnosis. In an attempt to underscore our progress, I highlighted Jackie's interest in therapy and her ability to be redirected during sessions as good indicators she was moving in a positive direction and was invested in the process.

Unbeknownst to me at the time, these positive observations caused a breach in my attunement with Pam. She let me know she needed a break from therapy. I gave her the requested space, and eventually, she contacted me to schedule time to discuss what happened. Pam courageously shared that my comments about Jackie's ability to be redirected in session felt like I was saying she was unable to redirect Jackie well, which meant she was inept. She said she felt unheard when I suggested a medication evaluation, because she did not want Jackie on medication. Pam tearfully and vulnerably shared that her mother made her take antidepressants when she was young, and she now feels dependent on them.

Pam's reactions were very surprising, as I felt our previous session had ended well. I was at a therapeutic choice point: I could defend my well-intended comments or apologize for the misstep. I was truly sorry Pam felt criticized and knew what was needed most was a repair of the relationship rupture. Given the information she shared about her own childhood, it was imperative she felt validated and experienced our relationship as one in which disruptions could be repaired. I apologized and commended Pam for her courage to discuss her experience with me. She was tearful and clearly overwhelmed but agreed to move forward with Jackie's individual and family sessions.

Jackie's next session started with a brief update from Pam, who reported improvement and said she was not sure if it was because Jackie was changing or if it was because she was calmer. Jackie was anxious to build another sandtray "just like her first one." She requested to see the photo of her first tray, took a look, and said, "I want to use that orange sand today." She slowly chose the same miniature figures, dressing them with care. Then she picked out a buffet of food and set up the children's bedrooms. As before, she often looked up at me for encouragement. When she finished building her world, she told me it was her birthday, and the mother doll was getting her party ready. After preparing food and drink, she had the adult doll bring out the goodies. She acted out the party, with one girl clapping and jumping up and down as the cake was presented. I asked if the clapping girl wanted the others to sing to her, and Jackie nodded yes, eyes riveted on the scene. I sang "Happy Birthday" as the doll blew out the candles and everyone ate cake. The birthday girl tidied up, tucked the rest of the children in bed, read them a story, then kissed them goodnight as the adult doll slept.

Jackie was very excited about this tray and said everyone loved the cake and, like with the first tray, she felt happy and safe. Because she used positive emotional states when describing these moments, I chose to enhance them by asking Jackie to find them in her body and choose miniatures to help remember the feelings. She excitedly picked some miniatures, and we embodied them. This technique allows the builder to take on the characteristics of the miniature, acting out in real time how they might feel and what they are doing. Embodiment facilitates a deepening of the builder's experience that is then shared with the therapist, enhancing positive connection (De Domenico, 1995).

This session felt intense to me and seemed to reflect Jackie's continued processing of her unmet needs. Like in the first tray, she painstakingly

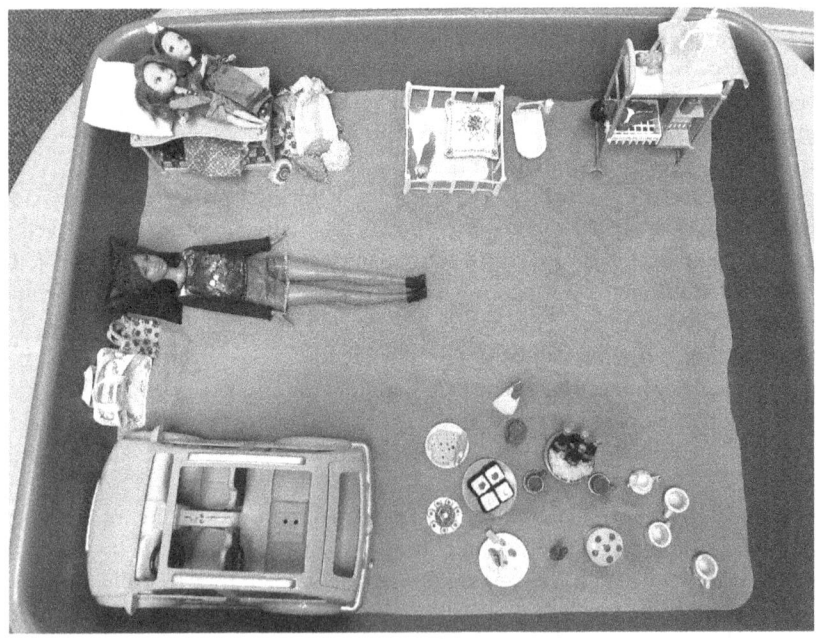

Figure 7.2 Jackie's second tray.

chose each miniature, especially mulling over her food choices. She was so methodical during her miniature collecting time that the hour was slipping away. Knowing the time spent choosing miniatures was just as important as building her tray, I stayed present and attuned as she selected figures, providing help when requested. The building phase was swift, as she quickly placed her chosen figures and planned her birthday party. Once complete, Jackie showed the tray to Pam, sharing the details of her special party. Pam listened attentively, and it was clear there was positive connection and attunement happening between the two.

For Jackie's next session, I wanted to focus on resource development using a directed sandtray approach, where "the therapist assigns a topic, an experience, or an interaction to be worked on during the session" (De Domenico, 1992, p. 11). I asked Jackie to choose miniatures that made her feel good, happy, and safe. She collected several and placed them in the tray one at a time. I asked her about each, questioning the type of emotion it invoked, where she felt it in her body, and how it might feel in the tray. When possible, we embodied them. Jackie chose nine items and took her time as she shared each one. She struggled a bit to connect physical sensations with emotions but excitedly announced where she felt the sensations once she knew. For example, she chose a unicorn and a rainbow, deciding these two were a pair and came together. She said they made her feel happy and described a tingling sensation throughout her whole body.

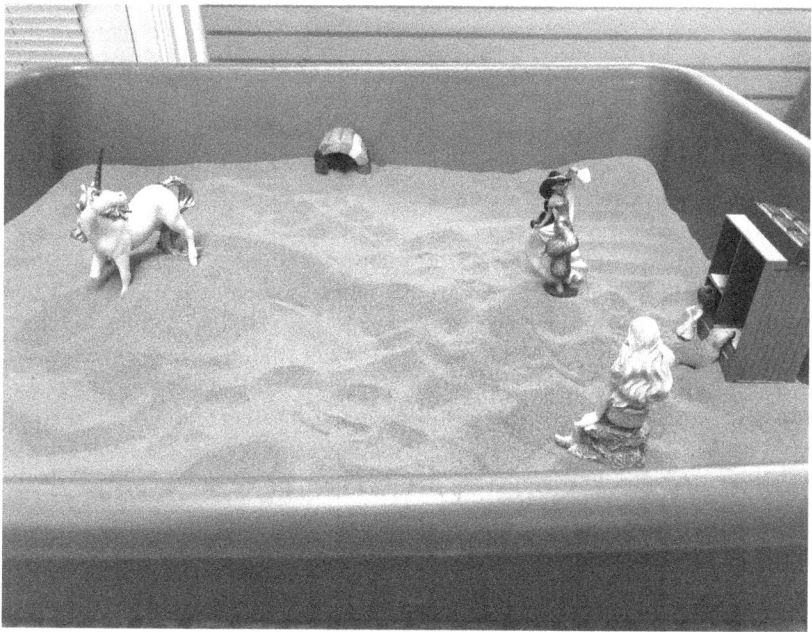

Figure 7.3 Jackie building a resource tray.

We continued this work in the next session, ensuring each miniature was thoroughly experienced as they were enhanced and embodied.

Some may find this work time-consuming and not worthwhile. However, a slow pace and careful processing of positive emotional states is important for a child with little modeling of positive emotional regulation. We referenced Jackie's work in this tray in many future sessions. It became a resource for her when she experienced difficult emotional states. She drew pictures of them so she could take them home to look at and feel. Jackie never seemed bored during these strength-building sessions. In particular, she really enjoyed acting out the characters with me, finding it quite humorous.

As of this writing, Jackie's parents are seeing improvements: her aggressiveness is lower; she tolerates redirection; tantrums have stopped; and she is better able to self-soothe. They still struggle with clinginess at bedtime, some defiance, and seemingly random moments of upset that are likely triggered by her painful past. Pam and Leonard still question which behaviors are typical for a child her age and which are related to trauma. Like all parents, they get irritated and lose patience, but they are able to repair attunement breaches. They now understand more about attachment styles, complex developmental trauma, and how Jackie's behaviors have been shaped by her unfortunate early life experiences. They continue to have individual sessions and are engaged in family therapy with Jackie. Committed to Jackie's individual work, Pam and Leonard are eager to see Jackie progress, grow, and become an independent, secure girl. Jackie and I have established a strong therapeutic relationship, and we both look forward to sessions. Due to the COVID-19 pandemic, we have switched to a virtual platform, but the resources, targets, and work she did in her sandtray sessions are still being used, creating new challenges and opportunities for us all.

At the beginning of treatment, I was unsure of Jackie's prognosis given her difficult life experiences and the challenges I had to navigate early in treatment. However, her resiliency, along with her parents' determination, have produced a very different outcome. Jackie is thriving and connected and is now experiencing typical developmental issues. Pam and Leonard have given her a chance to experience secure attachment as they support her, adjusting and growing right alongside her. She has family members who are present when she succeeds and when she fails, helping her negotiate the difficulties of life. They are an incredible and courageous family, finding their way toward successfully integrating their difficult life experiences so they can live a healthy and happy life. For me, I feel privileged and inspired by witnessing their trials and joys in this process.

Note

1. In sandtray-worldplay, the one who creates the sandtray world is often referred to as the builder, and the therapist is referred to as the witness.

References

De Domenico, G. (1992). A psychotherapeutic technique for individuals, couples and families. In *Sandtray world play: A comprehensive guide to the use of the sandtray in psychotherapeutic and transformational settings*. Vision Quest Images.

De Domenico, G. (1995). *Sandtray world play: A comprehensive guide to the use of the sandtray in psychotherapeutic and transformational settings*. Vision Quest Images.

Gomez, A. (2013). *EMDR therapy and adjunct approaches with children*. Springer Publishing Company.

Siegel, D., & Hartzell, M. (2014). *Parenting from the inside out: How a deeper self-understanding can help you raise children who thrive*. Tarcher and Pedigree. (Original work published in 2004).

8 Who Am I?

The Journey of Self-Discovery

Rosalind Heiko

The most precious gift we can give girls is the liberty not only to listen to the greater voice of themselves but to act on it. This is the simplest kind of freedom and the most sacred sort of empowerment. (Simmons, 2009, p. 253)

Let Us Meet Mist

It became quite clear that even a "klutz" like me (meaning a very clumsy person in Yiddish) could appreciate the sinuous grace and beauty of a client who herself was an aspiring 12-year-old dancer. I first met Mist, my client's name for herself, in the waiting room of my office. She was surrounded by her family. At my greeting, she rose fluidly from her chair, her hair pulled back tightly in a bun at the back of her head, dressed for dance practice. She was prepared (although I didn't quite realize that fact at the time) to begin her healing work as she did everything, with her whole and very fierce heart. In my recollection, she was always moving delicately, either bending over to reach for something on a shelf in the sand room, elegantly arranging her feet in one of the ballet positions, or speaking with fluid hands. It was a delight to work with her, and I came to admire her quiet strength alongside an intense focus she brought to bear on her dancing, her work, her relationships, her conversation.

What Mist Had to Face

Mist rose by leaps and bounds to the pinnacle of achievement in her class of competitive dancers while maintaining academic excellence. She demanded perfection from herself in performance and in her relationships. She could not understand why she was so agitated and frightened most of the time. She knew she had mastered confidence, commitment, and resilience in her technique and chosen discipline. Her mother, who had been critically ill, had made remarkable medical progress in the last half year since undergoing several traumatizing hospitalizations and having to be resuscitated at several critical junctures. Her younger siblings appeared to have moved on after

DOI: 10.4324/9781003055808-10

expressing uncomplicated grief over the medical trauma. This eluded Mist. She continually asked herself why she could not stop going over and over what had happened to her mother. Why could she not quit pulling out her eyelashes, eyebrows, and even the hair at her hairline? She could tell it drove her mother "crazy," but she could not help herself.

Mist was the oldest of four children, with Latinx ancestry. Her mother, as well as her father, proved to be strong allies as the therapeutic process was underway. They initially sought treatment for eyelash pulling (trichotillomania), within the context of a presentation of overall anxiety and agitation in her daily life. Her mom was initially fixated on Mist's hair pulling.

Mist's work focused on three aspects: the trauma experienced through her mother's medical challenges and near-death experiences; her need for a healthy reconnection with her parents; and a focus on reestablishing her path of self-identity through a combination of talk therapy, dreamwork, and sandplay. Mist was able to speak about being "angry and sad" about her mother's "heart holes" from the first time I met her. Her mother confided in me at the initial parent session that her daughter's eyelash and hair pulling was an incredibly painful reminder of the stress and agitation her daughter was experiencing, likening the experience to hearing "nails on a chalkboard." She constantly reminded her daughter to "stop!" It was difficult for Mist's mom to allow Mist to control her own response to the clinical hypnosis protocol for trichotillomania. She felt the need to direct her daughter's actions and point out when her daughter began to "pull." This ran counter to how the protocol was administered and diminished its effectiveness.

Mist struggled mightily with "failing" to immediately conquer her eyelash and eyebrow pulling. She blamed herself for not being strong enough to stop immediately. Mist conscientiously reported on her lack of progress (using fidgets, breathing and distraction techniques) for the first several months of therapy. In fact, I actually avoided speaking directly about pulling unless Mist brought it up. I knew it was imperative to provide a sheltered and nonjudgmental container for Mist to explore her emotional reactions and make her own decisions about handling the turmoil in her mind and body.

Sometimes family members misunderstand the profound meaning of metaphor in therapeutic sandplay practice. I explain, before commencing sandwork, that play is another form of working things through psychologically, just as talking can be. But parents don't always hear the meaning behind that. At first, Mist seemed to feel somewhat guilty about her sandtray creations, mentioning wistfully that "Mom says I'm not here to play." Mist had just created one of the most gorgeous and elegantly simple trays I've ever witnessed: a rose on a mound, surrounded by a circle. My heart broke open after experiencing how grindingly hard both mother and daughter worked to get things utterly "right." Mist's mother's work ethic was as profoundly exhaustive for herself as for her eldest daughter. Working with her mom to round out Mist's experience and therapeutic journey, I was able to begin to dispel the idea that Mist was "just playing around" when engaged in sandplay. This, in turn, allowed Mist to more fully engage in the therapy process, wherever that led her.

Sand Journeys

Mist participated in 17 therapy sessions over the course of 8 months. She completed a total of 10 sandtrays, occasionally creating two trays (both wet and dry) at a time. Her sand journey was replete with fairy-tale images and archetypal figures: Princesses, Princes, a dark King, the Divine Child, mermaids, dragons who guard the treasure, a castle, lots of vibrant, growing plants, and a blooming flower. A Wise Woman-Witch figure appeared at celebratory festivities and provided a connection with healthy Mother energies as well. My Mother-self rejoiced in her spirit and reached out to her with my full heart. I love fairy tales and storytelling. I found that creative, vibrant Mist thrived in a heroic journey of her own in spite of great challenges.

"In sandplay a self-directed, natural process of meaning making occurs . . . The sandplay therapist does not direct or interpret the creative process, but rather supports through attuned presence, curiosity and awaiting receptivity" (Freedle, 2019, p. 97). A sandplay scene may be created with an idea in mind (top-down), or a person might just put their hands in the sand and start doing whatever they are moved to do (bottom-up). Bottom-up processing, such as sensory work with hands in the sand making patterns, candle lighting, and burning activities, occupied some of Mist's sessions. Top-down mechanisms of change, such as storytelling about relational activities with friends and "frenemies," as well as journey and celebration trays, occupied others. Single-subject neuroimaging studies (Foo et al., 2020; Akimoto et al., 2018) have begun to advance support for these mechanisms with specific regard to sandplay.

The multisensory aspects of working in sand revealed patterns which Freedle termed sandplay's sensory feedback loop (Freedle, 2007). This feedback loop encompasses the multisensory experience of a client (in the presence of a "generously attuned" therapist) seeing, touching, and moving the sand, which promotes neural integration through the experience of connection to the brain, body, and emotions. This processing experience can subsequently open up creative energies and lead to self-discovery and new possibilities for change. Badenoch posits that world-building in sand with a trusted therapist engages both hemispheres in a ". . . confluence of sensory streams . . . and the whole experience encourages vertical brain integration, linking body, limbic region, and cortex in the right hemisphere" (2008, p. 221).

Over time, in a sheltered environment where multisensory play, focused symbol representation in trays, self-disclosure, and self-reflection on the part of clients flourishes, a healing – and even transformative – sandplay process may be achieved. Freedle maintains that

With activation and repetition bodily sensations, emotions, and thoughts may be experienced and re-processed in the context of new associations. Neural pathways develop and brain regions begin to synchronize. Connections are made that promote emotional regulation, neural integration, meaning making and expanded consciousness. (Freedle, 2019, p. 91)

Mist began her therapeutic journey as a complex mix of young girl and the woman she was to become. This process of individuation was aptly understood by Erickson in his theory of the psychosocial stages of growth (1994). At the time of therapy, Mist began to move into adolescence, beginning to make decisions for herself, develop an internal value system, and prepare a more coherent and integrated sense of self. In other words, the developmental task challenging her was to establish and maintain a *personal identity* (Erikson, 1994, p. 22). Mist's journey of self-discovery would lead her through forests, battles, meetings with the wise aspect of her psyche, through to an engaged and separate sense of herself as a young woman, the eldest daughter of a woman warrior of valor (being a mom who survived against all odds and fought to return to her family).

Exploring Mist's Trays

The Sandplay Journey Map is used here to outline Mist's progression of 10 trays. This map delineates four gateways in a mandala shape, which sets the framework for the series of trays (i.e., the sandplay process) in a circular journey. The middle section of the mandala contains the numinous experience of the Self through images and symbols which illustrate the beauty and power of touching the archetypal wisdom of "the light within" ourselves symbolically. The gateways and Sandplay Journey Map can be seen in Figure 8.1.

Gateway 1 Pathways: Choosing to Journey

[The first gateway] includes trays that illustrate the initial stage of the journey. The Sandplay Journey Map presupposes that the client has decided to take the hero or heroine's journey. From that moment on, the client begins the path in the first gateway. This includes, in effect, the client's decision to address his or her presenting issue. (Heiko, 2018, p. 35)

Tray 1 (Gateway 1)

Mist began her sandplay journey in a tray where she placed two mythological figures – a white dragon and a red phoenix. They seemed, at first glance, to be fighting for supremacy. Treasures in the form of a pot filled

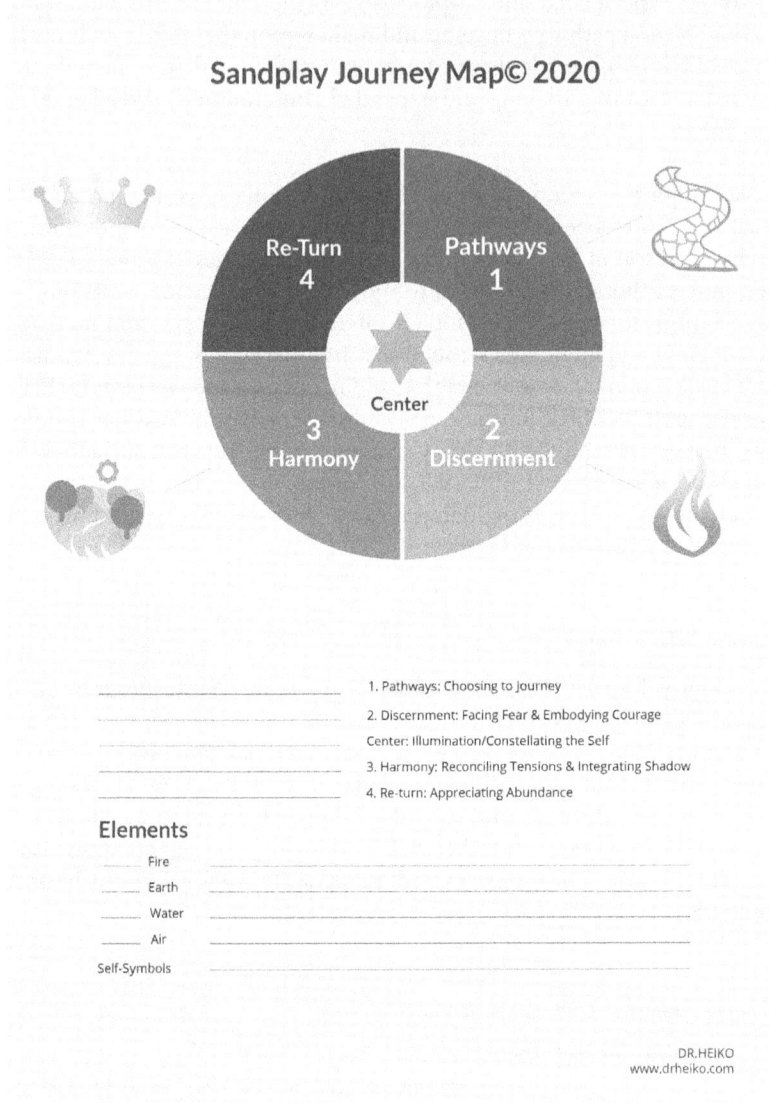

Figure 8.1 The four gateways of the Sandplay Journey Map.

with jewels, a large egg-shaped pyrite, and a volcano with lava were scattered around. Mist added water to the tray. Adding water at this juncture, possibly representing the unconscious or the emotional aspect of being, was unusual for a girl her age. It may have spoken to her sense of overwhelm and consequent drive to express sorrow.

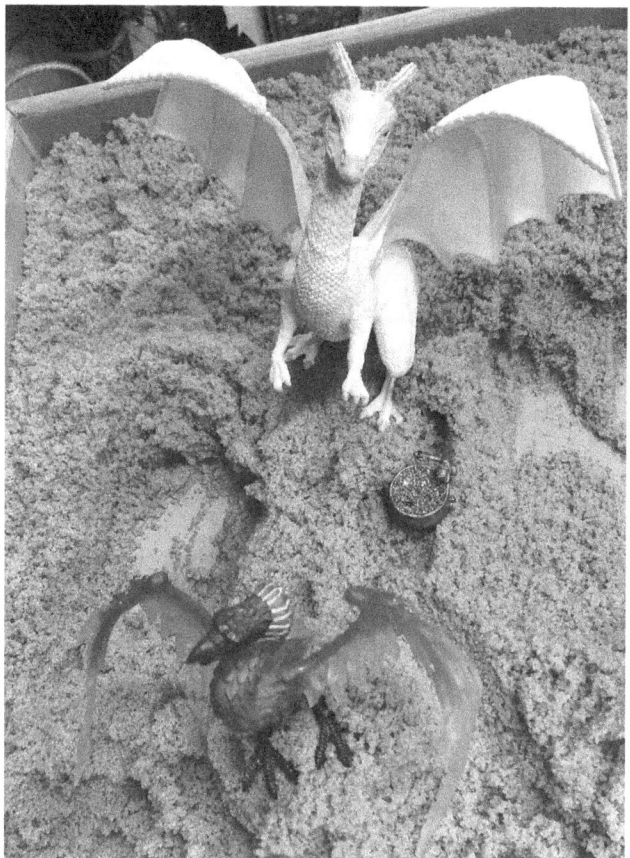

Figure 8.2 The Sandplay Journey begins in Tray 1.

The phoenix is a being that rises from the ashes of her funeral pyre. Mist's tray showed evidence of claw marks in the earth amid the creature's shooting fire and flapping wings, a great energy. Is Mist thinking of her mother here, coming back from death just as the phoenix does? What is fascinating about this creation is that the phoenix has her back to the white dragon at the end of the tray creation. The phoenix appears to lead the way on a path that points inward, towards Mist. The dragon takes an almost protective stance toward the phoenix, who is in a uniquely vulnerable position in relation to the dragon at her back. Is Mist's eyelash and hair pulling, as well as the overt tension between Mist and her mother, represented here in this way? I could only breathe into my questions silently and wait patiently for the creations to emerge.

Gateway 2 Discernment: Facing Fear and Embodying Courage

In the second gateway, the client works with differentiating the opposite emotions of whatever they must face (e.g., love/hate; dependency/independence; mastery/fear; loss/new possibilities), called "the tension of the opposites." During this process, the client confronts and integrates their shadow material (i.e., that part of ourselves we are not yet ready to acknowledge or assimilate) and the tension of opposite needs, emotions, and experiences within what Joseph Campbell refers to in story and myth as the hero's journey (Campbell, 2008). Here in sandplay, clients play out symbolic battles with enemies and create essential meetings with helper figures. In this gateway, literal and metaphorical pathways appear, fractured and wounded themes emerge, and clients work symbolically to burn away fears and also to dissolve them in order to make way for more integrated and healthy problem-solving and regulation.

Tray 2 (Gateway 2)

Mist's second tray, created in the dry sand, reflects a quieter conflict than her first. Although it was ostensibly a garden scene with a large castle in the background, I was impressed by Mist's many-layered quality of thinking and emotional responses. The figure of a psychotic boy-king figure, vicious and dismissive, stands on one side of a large stone gate. In this being's universe, he was poisoned quite suddenly. Facing him is a representation of a princess with a dragon on her shoulder, a soft, gentle figure. Next to the young woman is a peacock with its train outstretched. The peacock is associated with the Mother-Wife goddess Hera (*The Book of Symbols: Reflections on Archetypal Images*, 2010, p. 260), as well as the compassionate mother goddesses of the Hindu tradition (Lakshmi and Saraswati) and the Buddhist Kwan Yin (Cooper, 1978, p. 127). There are so many eyes on that peacock's tail. Is Mist making a connection between her eyelash pulling here and her need for connection and compassion?

Sitting down next to me, close to the sandtray, Mist spoke about her love of dance and the discipline required of her to practice for many hours a day. As she talked, she moved to find and place a pink-tutu'd ballerina next to a bride with a mirror behind her. The dancer was placed looking directly into the mirror. The bride was looking ahead, possibly to her future. What hard-won courage and effort it took for Mist to strive to attain her goal of becoming a professional dancer, to yearn for what her very beloved mother acquired: a professional degree and accomplishments along with the devotion of a husband and children. In the process of individuation, of self-exploration, is Mist beginning to look with anticipation toward her own future? Of course, the symbolic representation here of the bride doesn't necessarily mean wife and motherhood; it may specifically relate to the archetypal aspect of union with the self in the literal reflection of that dancer.

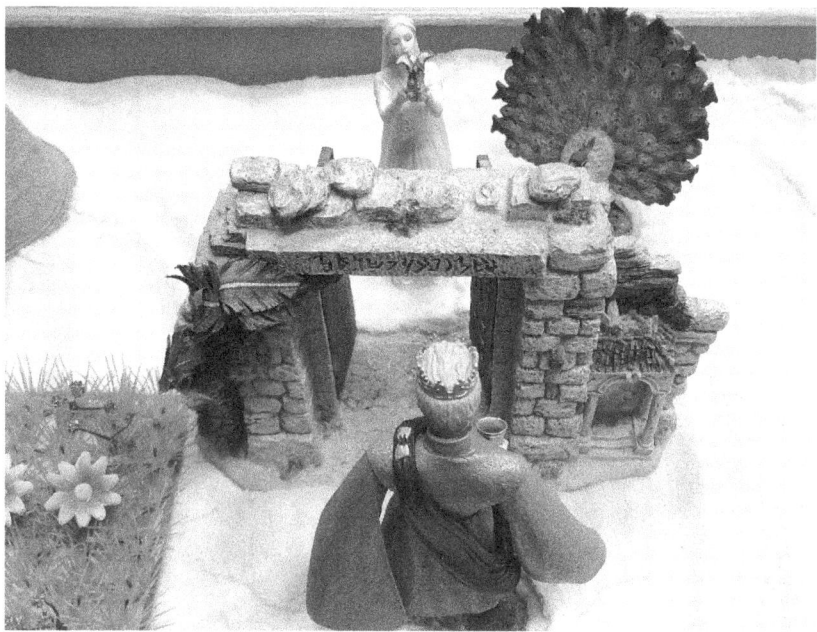

Figure 8.3 A quieter conflict is seen in Tray 2.

Center: Illumination and Constellating the Self

The center of the Sandplay Journey Map is open to all four gateways at any time. In Jungian terms, when the Self is allowed to emerge (i.e., in trays which symbolically represent the "constellation of the Self," where the numinous quality of self-expression is present), more peaceful and centered representations emerge (E. Gil, personal communication, 2014). The result of this centering can help bring clients to a state of wholeness through an integration of the tension of the opposites. Here, the client shows themselves the beauty of and connection to the sacred, the constellation of the Self that appears in images of mandalas (Gontard, 2011; Heiko, 2004, 2008, 2018; Weinrib, 1983).

Tray 3 (Center) and Tray 4 (Gateway 2), Created the Same Day

Mist came into the session looking despondent and feeling discouraged. She shared that she was still picking at her eyelashes. She created her next two trays on that day. During the first part of this session, Mist spoke of a terrifying dream: she was in a cornfield, where a man driving a tractor was coming towards her. She remembered running from him but found that she could not get far. She connected that dream with her wish to be perfect, never

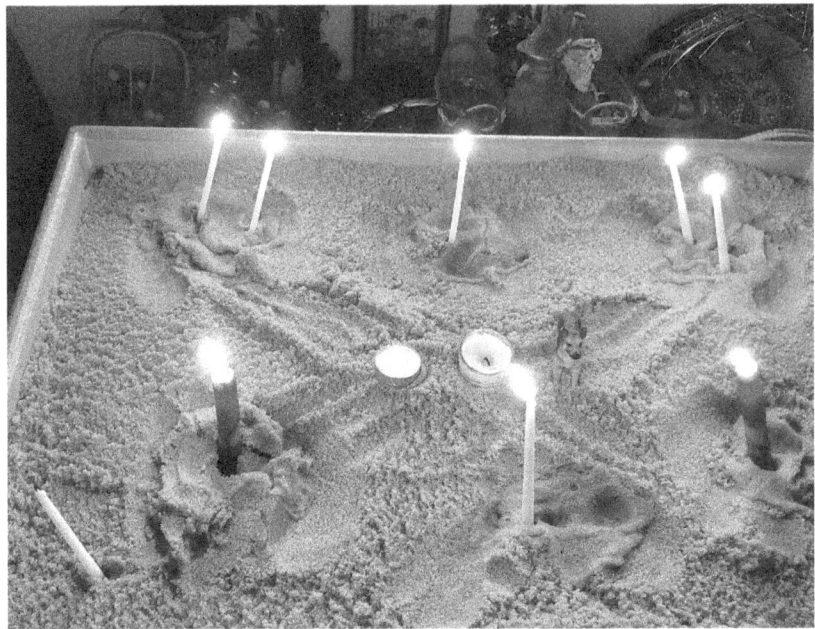

Figure 8.4 In Tray 3 Mist touches the center in a ritual of fire and water.

quite getting to that place of absolute control: whether it was occasional fights with a sibling, having trouble with other dancers in the ubercompetitive dance world she inhabited, or falling short of her self-directed goals. Mist then spoke of the death of a beloved dog and raced to the waiting room to ask her mother to find pictures of the pet on her mother's phone to show me.

Mist's first tray creation that day, Tray 3 , brought her to the center of the Journey Map. It contained 11 candles, each one set in mounds of sand, which she then watered. She lit 10 of the candles in a lovely ritual of light and water, uniting the elements in a hushed display of honoring a sacred moment. Mist placed a German Shepherd dog next to two candles in the center. Was this dog a representation of the strength and loyalty of her connection to those she loves? She left one of the candles unlit, perhaps to nudge her psyche's remembrance of the last year and its attendant tumultuous, terrifying medical drama for her mother and family. Mist spoke of *La Ofrenda* and taught me gently that day about her family's way of honoring their dead.

As if to underscore her grief over her dog's death and possibly the horror of almost losing her parent, Mist swiftly created a second tray (Tray 4) that session in the second gateway. It looks as though an agitated face opens up in the tray, eyes wide with fear, arms outstretched. Was her psyche

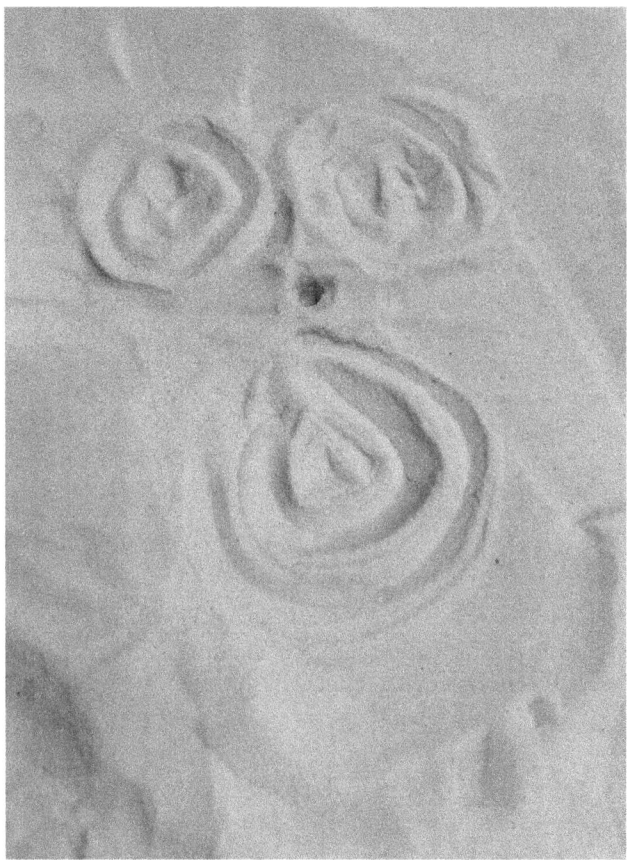

Figure 8.5 A fearful face peers out in Tray 4.

metaphorically screaming for help with managing her overwhelming anxiety, manifested by her hair plucking and pulling, her dream-filled nights and fears?

Gateway 3 Harmony: Reconciling Tensions and Integrating Shadow

The trays in the third gateway tend to work on resolving conflict and mediating an acceptance of the tension of the opposites. Clients continue to reconcile those dynamic tensions, work through psychological conflicts, and organize the psyche (Heiko, 2018, pp. 43–44). In this gateway, healing themes predominate with a sense of integral connection. Images of mending broken parts of the psyche symbolically appear. Marriage ceremonies materialize, the images of hieros gamos (i.e., the "sacred marriage"), which can symbolize the harmonious joining of masculine and feminine aspects of the self (Heiko, 2018).

Tray 5 (Gateway 3)

About a month after touching anguish in Tray 4, Mist explored the tension of the opposites in the creation of Tray 5. She constructed a tray that separated out two mounds with five lit candles on top of each mound and one candle lit between them. She surrounded the mounds, which looked like two islands, with plastic wrap and gently poured water around the base of each. This tray felt like an integration of the two separate mounds by allowing the energy of water and fire to rest in a harmonious balance in the tray. Was it a way to define and celebrate her relationship with her mother as it had been in the year before the medical emergencies and attendant trauma? Mist talked about her determination and commitment to succeed with her training in dance. Her eyes gleamed: the pride in her competence and capacity with her gift of movement was apparent.

Going In and Out of Gateways in the Journey: The Path Unfolds Back and Forth and Through the Center

Just as the path of individuation and self-identity is not a straightforward path, the Sandplay Journey Map reflects this motion of "two steps forward,

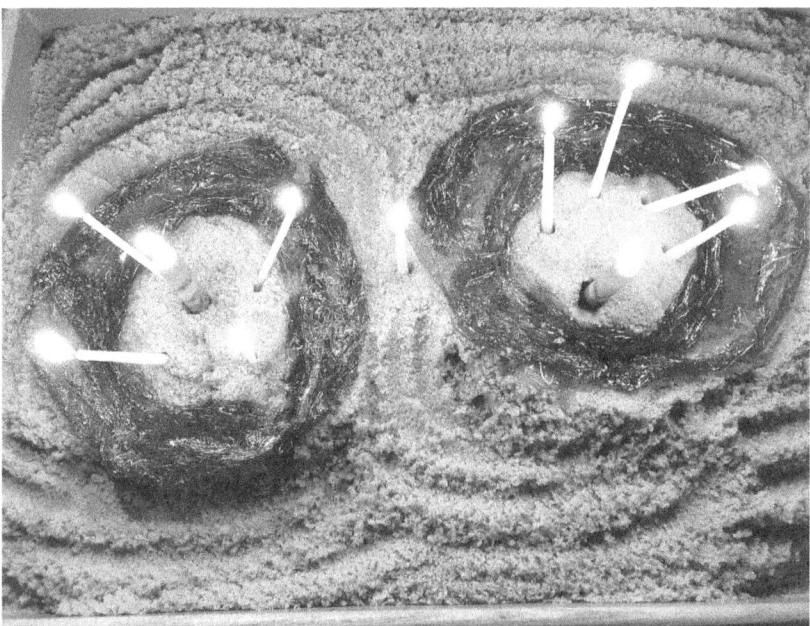

Figure 8.6 Mist creates two islands in harmony in Tray 5.

four steps backward" in the psyche's reach for growth. Trays weave back and forth in the Gateways, particularly in Gateways 2 through 4, throughout the mapping process. Mist self-identified as a teen yet still retained childish behaviors and emotional reactions with her mother at times.

Trays 6 and 7 (Back Into the Center of the Sandplay Journey Map)

The next two trays reflect the beauty and peace that can be found in connection, especially in the abstract form of Tray 7. Tray 6 was created a month after Tray 5. The mood of this tray was of a celebration, with colorful fans, umbrellas, and glass stones placed all over. Ropes of pearls, those treasures of the deep, wound around two different mermaid figures, both set under large protective umbrellas. Battery-operated candles were placed throughout the tray, lighting up the whole scene. A lovely princess figure and a handsome prince were gathered around a baby in a decorated cradle; and a youthful and smiling witch dressed in purple greeted them near a garden archway. Here, Mist seems to be connecting to the helper figure of the Wise Woman in this tray, who moves out toward the three figures in the center.

Here, we can focus on the child in the cradle in the center area of the tray. Cooper suggests that the image of the child directly engages ". . . the embodiment of potentialities; possibilities of the future. . . (and) also symbolizes a higher transformation of the individuality, the self-transmuted and reborn into perfection" (1978, p. 35). Does the baby represent the energies

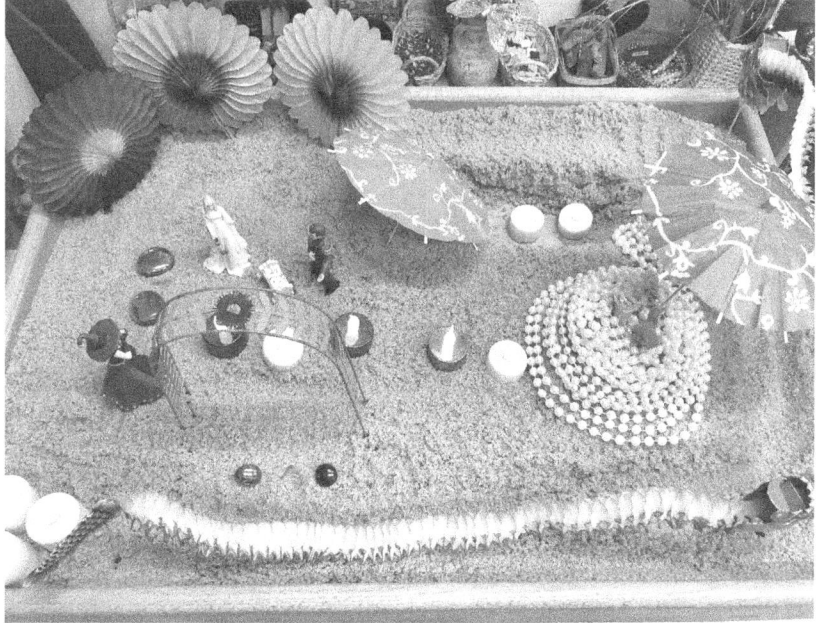

Figure 8.7 Mist constructs a constellation of the self in Tray 6.

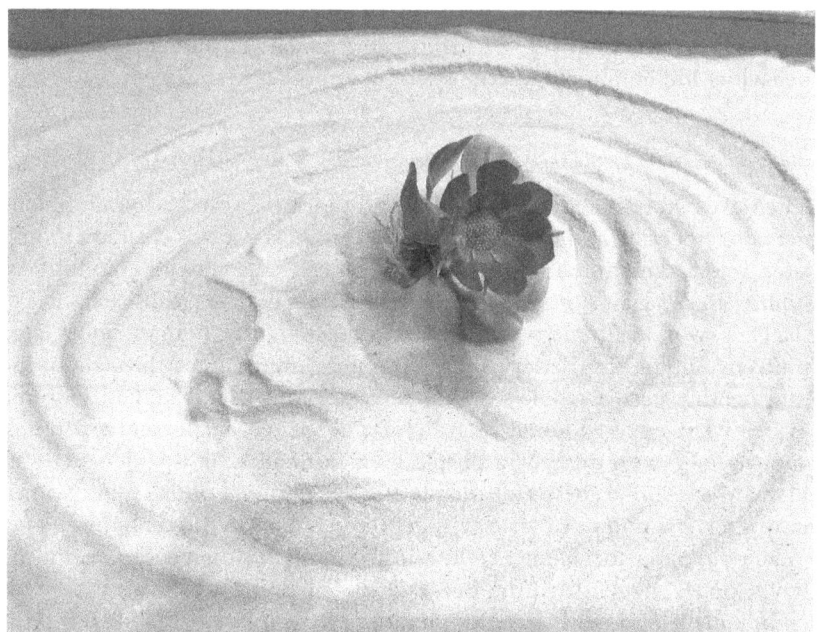

Figure 8.8 In Tray 7 a place of beauty and peace is found.

of this Divine Child archetype? The Prince and Princess appear to be paying homage to her. Mist asked me to turn the lights out in the sand room, and we sat quietly while the lights reflected on the faces of the figures, the pearls, the umbrellas, and the sand.

A week later, Mist created Tray 7. She placed a rose in the center of the tray and set it in a circular design of sand. A bit of the blue at the bottom of the tray can be seen as well. A sense of tranquility was evident in the calm of our session that day. All of us need places to rest in the psyche that nourish our sense of inner peace and equanimity. Mist appeared to reach that place.

Tray 8 (Gateway 3 Again)

In this tray, a dark-colored dragon was carefully placed on top of a castle. The dragon overlooks the scene. Was the figure guarding the "treasure" of the wisdom that the headmaster of Hogwarts was imparting to his students and assistant in a meeting taking place in the courtyard below? According to Cooper, dragons are ". . . guardians of treasures and of the portals of esoteric knowledge. The struggle with the dragon symbolizes the difficulties to be overcome in gaining the treasures of inner knowledge" (1978, pp. 55–56). Was this dragon's placement a way for Mist to symbolize coming to accept the darker, deeper aspects of her emotional reactions to loss and fear and to incorporate them into her psyche?

After creating this tray, Mist constructed a lovely treasure box for herself. As she painted it, she spoke about a recent dream where "Dad came home from the hospital with [her brother]. I looked at him in the face and thought to myself 'that's not my dad.' I asked him, 'whatcha gonna give me for a present?' It was a Superman . . . I then found my dad in a closet back in the hospital." She seemed puzzled and ambivalent about her father's role in helping her and her mother work through the struggle of her mother's medical traumas. Was she possibly wishing him to have the superpower of "fixing" her mother yet knowing that was not possible? As we mature, we come to realize our parents are not magical beings but are fallible.

Gateway 4 Re-turn: Appreciating Abundance

The fourth gateway represents an integration of the psychological material worked through in the journey and a relativistic return to everyday life. Often, there are fewer trays in this gateway (Heiko, 2018, pp. 45–46). Trays reflect a return to home and community with the treasure of wisdom, acquired through confronting the shadow and resolving some of the client's internal suffering.

Trays 9 and 10 (Gateway 4)

A week after creating her eighth tray, Mist spoke of a dream in which she had literally picked her mother up off the floor but quickly "put my mom down because we couldn't save her, I tried calling my dad, but he didn't answer. My mom's ghost said, 'push the green button.'" At times, working with Mist, I felt the full burden of her grief come through my body. Throughout this process, Mist's fear and sorrow at having her emotional life derailed did feel unbearable to me. Mist's parents experienced their own trauma as well, and the subsequent familial grief was often unshared and unspoken. I worked hard to contain my own sadness as I sat with Mist and bore witness to her pain.

Mist remembered a second dream from that same night. "The best one!" she exclaimed. "I loved a Spanish guy named Victor. My name was Myra. We got married and had a child named Connor." Does the direction of her dream indicate that victory can be grasped by dreaming of possible futures?

Mist then constructed a tray composed only of sand. The rippling, sand forms seemed to represent the divine dance of wind and water . Mist appears to be embodying the grace and harmony inherent in her passion for dance and her newfound reconnection with internal regulation and steadiness. Additionally, she placed a figure in the sand, a woman with her head resting on a platform, her hand moving up to her neck. This woman is incredibly similar to the figure of the Sleeping Princess of Malta, ". . . a priestess engaged in dream incubation, adept in giving oracles, interpreting dreams, or suggesting cures for illness" (Biaggi, 1986, p. 137). The ability to

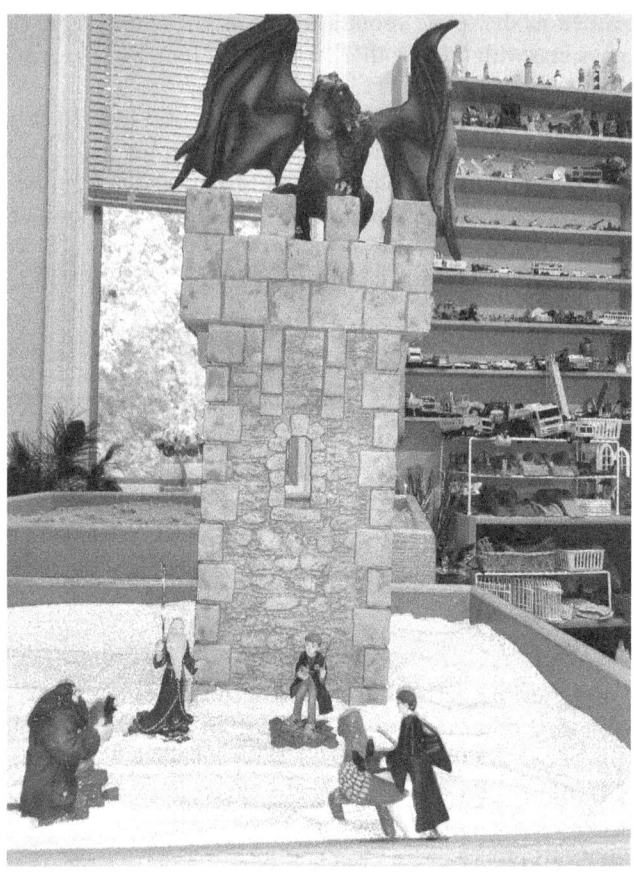

Figure 8.9 A dragon guards the treasure in Tray 8.

engage in dream incubation is vital to the development of self-identity and self-expression.

In the same session, Mist created a mermaid out of polymer clay. She had a smiling face and looked like she was about to speak. Wang refers to the mermaid figures as having

> . . . often sacrificed their own needs, desires, hopes, and longings in return for love and attention from others . . . These clients all found it difficult to say "no" to others, to listen to their inner voice and intuition, and to build . . . ego strength in order to develop a more conscious sense of self. . . (2017, p. 133)

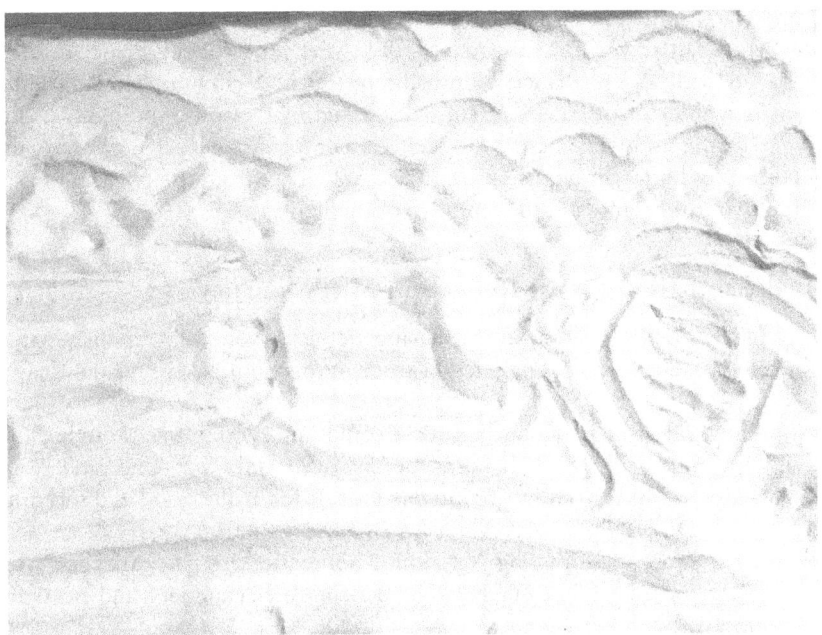

Figure 8.10 Mist shapes the divine dance of wind and water in Tray 9.

Wang also referred to the process of differentiation, when a girl develops discernment about what constitutes her inner and outer worlds, learning to reclaim her voice, ". . . Assisting and allowing each client to know herself and to help each to express herself verbally and through sandplay" (Wang, 2017, pp. 133–134).

Perhaps the mermaids in Tray 6 and in Mist's clay construction reflect images that represent the unconscious feminine familiar with the depth and breadth of navigating "emotional seas"? Was Mist connecting with her intuitive sense of knowing and possibly with a more comfortable stance of expressing her fears and anxieties? As therapy progressed, she and I verbally explored many of her inner conflicts about loss and disconnection, as well as her burgeoning feelings of self-assurance and self-confidence in navigating emotional waters.

At our last session, Mist mentioned her dreams. "I can't save Mom," she said. "One time I was sleepwalking in my dream and the ghost of Mom already told me how it ends. She blacks out. And the next morning I told my Mom that I was afraid my Dad won't be around, that's my biggest scare. I used to think my Dad forgot about what happened [at all the hospitalizations], but Mom told him to treat her like nothing happened." Mist was coming to a more mature understanding of her parents' sometimes panicked and fear-charged reactions.

Mist's last tray, (Tray 10), reflects the sweet unity of the Prince seen in Tray 8 with a new Princess, both figures set in a circle of glowing lights in the center of the tray . Again, Mist asked that I douse the lights in the sand room; and we watched the scene in companionable silence. Here, the course of the tray progression has come full circle: from the two dragons to the two lovers enjoying the embrace of the lights.

Mist and Her Mother Reflect on Mist's Journey

When I contacted Mist about sharing her experience in sandplay, (after receiving permission to include her story in this book), Mist related that

> the sand, it helped a lot because I could put my negative thoughts into art, and in the sand. It could be displayed and seen. The sand really helped. I liked to trace my fingers in it. It felt really good and relaxing.

The hair and eyelash pulling was almost nonexistent by this time, and Mist had strategies she comfortably used to manage her anxiety and need for connection with her parents.

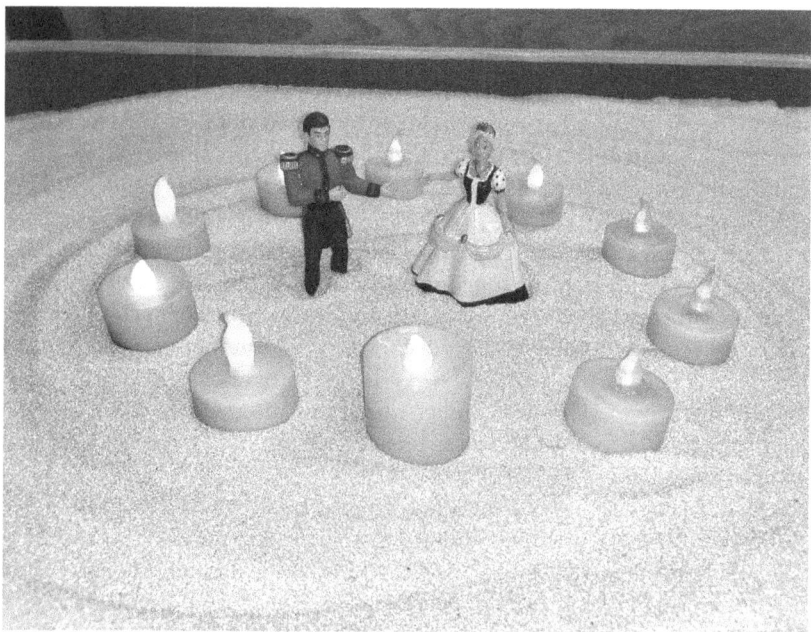

Figure 8.11 In Tray 10 we find sweet unity in the celebration of the figures of Prince and Princess.

Mist's mother spoke about family changes for healthy connection and exercise:

> I'm working on myself . . . Kicked up exercising and trying to be physically active overall. It's been keeping me more focused and motivated . . . [Mist] is doing really well. No (hair)pulling for [quite a while] now. She's calmer overall, which I attribute to her personal growth but also to seeing me kicking up my own physical health. We are even working out together and laughing more.

What I Know as a Therapist . . . and What I Have Learned From Mist

When I first began working with children and families, I believed it was my job to try to help "fix" what was diagnostically "wrong" with children's behaviors. I arrogantly thought I knew how folks should go about changing their lives for the better. I knew little at that point about the true heart of therapy. If Mist's parents had come to see me in my practice at that time, I might have primarily focused on the clinical strategies of overcoming trichotillomania through solely relying upon a clinical hypnosis protocol and behavioral goals. After 40 years of practice, I am certain that we beings carry a potential for wholeness and integration of mind, body, and spirit. Kalff expressed, "The psyche carries within itself a tendency for healing. Preparing a pathway for that healing is the task confronting the therapist" (2020, p. 30). There is no greater truth for me professionally. My "superpower" is my compassion. As Ram Dass said, "We're all just walking each other home" (Dass, 2018). I am so grateful that Mist and I walked that path together.

I was able to support Mist's parents, particularly her mother, in allowing Mist more freedoms as the oldest of four children and in her coming of age as a young woman. One big change that signaled Mist's taking more ownership of her capacities and maturity was the judicious use of fire and fire symbols. Learning to light candles played a large part in this. At first, Mist was unsure she was responsible enough to light candles herself. Such a simple task, yet so fraught with nuance and importance. Mist's mother generously allowed her daughter this privilege. I spoke with Mist and her mother about her choice to light candles, and her mother was open and generous with permissions.

I reflected on my own experience of my mother and I lighting Shabbat candles on Friday nights. I shared with Mist how I watched and learned from my mom how to confidently strike a match, both of us watching the flame grow as we said the blessings together in a time-honored ritual. For Mist to use fire in the playroom and then at home under her mother's supervision, was a bold, beautiful step in her process of trusting and strengthening herself as well as sharing her newfound status with her family.

Mist continues to lead a very full life. Her professional dance regimen has been quite complicated and sophisticated; her classes and teachers require extensive focus and dedication beyond that to which most girls her age might commit. She demands perfection of herself in very complex ways. She also is friends with other girls in training, even though the competition is fierce. The sand and symbols offer a place to embody healing and rest in very deceptively simple ways. Mist was able to relax her guard and permit herself to share emotions and thoughts after tray creations, to express emotions without overly censoring herself. She could allow herself to feel some of the "shadow" emotions and own them – envy, hurt, guilt, anger, grief.

The neural encoding process of trauma (explained in detail in Grayson's Chapter 3 of this book), explains Mist's felt sense of aloneness and disconnection, which was stored in neural circuits in her brain and body. Grayson notes that "Sandtray therapy offers a safe way to invite embodied trauma, opening the possibility of disconfirmation" (p. 33). In my role as quiet observer, I was inviting this creative play for Mist to experience being alone in the forgotten presence of the therapist. As Winnicott discussed,

> . . . this experience is that of being alone, as an infant and small child, in the presence of mother. Thus, the basis of the capacity to be alone is a paradox; it is the experience of being alone while someone else is present. (1958, p. 417)

This called forth Mist's recognition of some very painful, deep-seated fears about almost losing her mother at a time when she was entering young womanhood and allowed her to reach out to her father for the nurturance and support only he could provide. These therapeutic encounters of therapist witnessing and client engaging in symbolic play, within the temenos (container) of safety, allowed Mist to regulate her arousal and reprocess her traumatic experiences. In turn, this led to her moving through suffering to feelings of acceptance and connection. She was always a good person, and good enough. She just had to hold that inside for a time and feel it powerfully – right down into and through the light inside of her. In our work together, she did just that and did it gorgeously.

References

Akimoto, M., Furukawa, K., & Ito, J. (2018). Exploring the sandplayer's brain: A single case study. *Archives of Sandplay Therapy, 30*(3), 73–84.

Badenoch, B. (2008). *Being a brain-wise therapist: A practical guide to interpersonal neurobiology*. W. W. Norton & Company, Inc.

Biaggi, C. (2020, September 12). *The significance of the nudity obesity and sexuality of the Maltese goddess figures*. L-Università Ta' Malta. Retrived September 12, 2020, from www.um.edu.mt/library/oar/bitstream/123456789/38232/1/The_significance_of_the_nudity_obesity_and_sexuality_of_the_Maltese_goddess_figures_1986.pdf

The Book of Symbols: Reflections on Archetypal Images. (2010). Taschen.

Campbell, J. A. (2008). *The hero with a thousand faces.* New World Library.

Cooper, J. C. (1978). *An illustrated encyclopaedia of traditional symbols.* Thames and Hudson Ltd.

Dass, R., & Bush, M. (2018). *Walking each other home: Conversations on loving and dying.* Sounds True Publishing.

Erikson, E. H. (1994). *Identity and the life cycle.* W. W. Norton & Company, Inc.

Foo, M., Freedle, L. R., Sani, R., & Fonda, G. (2020). The effect of sandplay therapy on the thalamus in the treatment of generalized anxiety disorder: A case report. *International Journal of Play Therapy, 29*(4), 191–200. https://doi.org/10.1037/pla0000137

Freedle, L. R. (2007). Sandplay therapy with brain-injured adults: An exploratory qualitative study. *Journal of Sandplay Therapy, 16*(2), 115–133.

Freedle, L. R. (2019). Making connections: Sandplay therapy and the neurosequential model of therapeutics®. *Journal of Sandplay Therapy, 28*(1), 91–109.

Gontard, A. von. (2011). The numinous in sandplay therapy with children and adolescents. *Journal of Sandplay Therapy, 20*(2), 103–126.

Heiko, R. L. (2004). Children's birthday party sandplays. *Journal of Sandplay Therapy, 13*(2), 44–53.

Heiko, R. L. (2008). Finding the treasure within: The sandplay journey of stella. *Journal of Sandplay Therapy, 17*(1), 97–113.

Heiko, R. L. (2018). *A therapist's guide to mapping the girl heroine's journey in sandplay.* Rowman & Littlefield Publishers.

Kalff, D. M. (2020). *Sandplay: A psychotherapeutic approach to the psyche* (Boris L. Matthews Trans., Sandplay ed.). Analytical Psychology Press.

Simmons, R. (2009). *The curse of the good girl: Raising authentic girls with courage and confidence.* Penguin.

Wang, Y. (2017). The little mermaid: Cultural expectations of the feminine. *Journal of Sandplay Therapy, 26*(2), 133–134.

Weinrib, E. L. (1983). *Images of the self: The sandplay therapy process.* Sigo Press.

Winnicott, D. W. (1958). The capacity to be alone. *The International Journal of Psychoanalysis, 39*, 416–420.

9   Being With What Is

Touching Grief in the Sand

Barbara Jones Warrick

An Introduction to Children's Grief

It is inevitable that death touches children's lives, for they are the children, siblings, grandchildren, family, friends, and neighbors of a person who has died. Children are the ones mourning a beloved pet or classmate. Children are also touched by the death of people they don't know when those deaths are covered in the media.

> In fact, death is always present in children's and adolescents' lives . . . They observe many things they cannot name. Thus, they may sense the cycle of life and death but not yet have words for it. They can also sense that there are forbidden subjects that should not be talked about. As children get older, they begin to realize that they themselves will die. They learn that people grow old and die, but they may not learn how to acknowledge and deal with their sadness and what this loss means to them. (Silverman, 2000, p. 2)

What this means to them will differ depending on their relationship with the person who died and their experience with death, as well as their age and stage of development. It will also differ depending on the reactions of those around them. In particular, the ability of adults to engage in emotional regulation will, through the action of mirror neurons (Schermer, 2019; Siegel, 2008, Disc 6, Section 5), increase the "neuroception of safety" (Geller & Porges, 2014, p. 186).

Willis (2002) has identified four factors associated with children's cognitive understanding of death: irreversibility, finality, inevitability, and causality. The literature identifies various stages of cognition and suggests that up to the age of 7, children understand death as temporary or impermanent (Lowenstein, 2006; McKissock, 2004). As Fitzgerald (1992) suggests, preschoolers cannot comprehend abstract time concepts like forever, never, and always, so they may persist in asking when the deceased is coming back. Around age 7, children are beginning to develop a sense of death

DOI: 10.4324/9781003055808-11

as a permanent state and have a different set of questions about how this could happen and why and whether it will happen to them. Harris (2018) found that as children reach latency, their understanding of death includes biological and religious notions, such as the possibility of life after death and questions about God's role in death. By the time children reach adolescence, their ideas about death include solidified concepts of its permanence and inevitability. Although death continues to evoke experiences of loss, it now has an additional focus on making meaning out of life.

Emotionally, children and adolescents are described as grieving differently from adults (Hidalgo, 2017; Wolfelt, 2001). This is consistent with what I have observed in my work with children and families, where parents describe their children as crying or sad one moment and happily playing with their friends the next. Intense, brief periods of grief are typical in pre-schoolers. In subsequent stages of development, grief may also include: a sense of responsibility/ guilt, confusion, and distress (up to age 7 years); anger, worry for others, mourning (latency); and depression (adolescence) (Lowenstein, 2006, p. 8). In addition to dealing with the intellectual and emotional tasks of grieving, death and loss come with increased risks for mental health. Hidalgo (2017), identified increases in anxiety among children who had experienced the loss of a parent/caregiver or sibling at all stages of grief. Kaplow et al. (2012) have written about increased incidents of depression and other bereavement-related disorders as well as posttraumatic stress disorder (PTSD) in cases of complicated grief (Brown et al., 2019; Herring, 2013; Iglesias & Iglesias, 2005). From this summary, it is clear that children and adolescents need supports in order to navigate the loss and grief associated with death.

Responding to Children's Grief

Through our work in children's mental health and with Bereaved Families of Ontario, my colleague Julie Regan and I became aware of the needs of children and adolescents who have experienced grief and loss due to the death of a family member. For many of these children, parents indicated that they did not know how to respond to their children's specific needs regarding grief. Because they too had experienced the loss, they frequently acknowledged feeling overwhelmed by their own grief. Additionally, parents reported feeling confused by their children's inconsistent responses to death, fearful they would make things worse by talking about death with children who seemed to be coping, and worried that not talking would give their children the wrong message. In response to this need, we developed the Children's Grief Group. The goal of the group was to provide children who had lost a family member an opportunity to experience support from professionals and peers in processing their experience of death. Children were referred by their parents/caregivers. Additional criteria included the child's ability to acknowledge the death and be able to talk about it; to be in a stable, supportive living situation; and to commit to participate in the six weekly sessions of the group. Given my training and experience in sandtray therapy, Julie suggested that we offer a group sandtray experience as one of our weekly activities. Building on my study with Gisela De Domenico in sandtray-worldplay, the narrative therapy work of David Epston and Michael White, and McGill and Topham's (2008) relational healing continuum (a group therapy model employed in my work as a sexual assault counselor), I developed a one-session, group sandtray approach for our session on funerals. The benefits of sandtray included providing an opportunity for participants to have a shared experience of grief and to reduce the sense of isolation with their experiences of loss within a structured, predictable activity that was contained within the physical confines of the tray. The physical nature of constructing a shared world also served to engage the participants' full brains rather than limiting them to a verbal and intellectual experience. The structure of the group allowed participants to choose the activity for the final session, in which the theme was Remembering Our Loved Ones, Remembering the Person who Died. Frequently, participants asked to do another sandtray. The rest of this chapter will look at the theory, practice and outcome of these sandtray experiences.

More recently, this work is informed by an understanding of the neurobiology of trauma (including Ogden & Fischer, 2015; Ogden et al., 2006; Porges, 2017; Schore, 2003) and interpersonal neurobiology (Gantt & Badenoch, 2019; Siegel, 2008). Much of Ogden's work in the field of sensorimotor psychotherapy points to engaging the brain in ways that acknowledge and honor the physical nature of experience. The act of world building is a physical one, providing both movement in the selection, placement and moving of objects and, more subtly, in the gestures, postures, and inferred movement of the objects themselves. The role of the vagal system includes the ability of a regulated caregiver to mitigate the effects of distress, supporting a child's ability to shift from more primitive (reptilian) function to a more developed/regulated (mammalian) function through sympathetic gaze, vocalizations, and gestures (Schore, 2003, p. 167). Such responses by group facilitators and participants serve a similar function in the group sandtray process. And as we shall see, within a mindfulness framework, the frequent opportunities provided by the group sandtray structure to pause and notice the world, the changes and the experiences support the builders in stepping out of a "privatized view of a separate self. . . [to] become more open to a broader, deeper reality" (Siegel, 2008, p. 322). The presence of these many factors leads to a clearer understanding of the effectiveness of sandtray, particularly group sandtray.

Why Sandtray? A Rationale

The question often arises "Why sandtray?" In general, the benefit of sandtray therapy is its ability to bypass the reliance on verbal processing typically associated with "talk" therapies. In addition, the sandtray serves as a physical container in which one may address the seemingly boundless thoughts and feelings associated with an event. Finally, sandtray makes visible and concrete experiences beyond our grasp.

For those touched by grief, emotions can feel overwhelming, making finding words difficult. The process of selecting objects is, in itself, an exercise in meaning making, a process Frankl (1984) describes as essential to healing. In sandtray therapy, the objects stand in for words, and the images hold powerful, emotional resonance. The selection, placement, and exploration of the objects, individually and as a whole, allow access to material on both the conscious/concrete level and the unconscious/metaphoric level. This in turn, supports connection to explicit and implicit memory. Additionally, unlike art therapy, in which clients may encounter the creation of images as a barrier, the sandtray therapy collection of figures provides ready-made images.

Sandtray allows access to the tactile senses that many find soothing. These experiences of comforting touch may serve as a balm to the grieving individual. In the absence of being able to touch the loved one, touching the sand and the figures may provide a sense of reconnection to the person who died.

Sandtray is physical and, in its capacity for sensorimotor engagement, offers participants opportunities for "Working 'beneath the words', it elucidates ways the body contributes to the challenges of the individual and the group, including aspects that may not be apparent through the lens of more traditional psychotherapies" (Mark-Goldstein & Ogden, 2019, p. 123). Additionally, the ability to manipulate objects offers an opportunity for physical control in response to death and loss. Ogden and Fischer (2015) and Van der Kolk (2014) suggest that we ignore the body at our peril. The embodied experience of sandtray provides access to the tactile and sensorimotor experiences of grief encoded as implicit memory. As noted in Grayson's chapter on neurobiology in this book, sandtray therapy supports emotional regulation while allowing access to memories that are both unconscious and painful. As such, using the sandtray is well suited to grief work.

Group sandtray has the added benefit of providing the participants with a shared visual, tactile, and interactive experience. The death of a loved one can leave people feeling alone. This is both a response to physical loss and the sense that there is no one who understands the intensity of their grief. Truly, the bereft are not always able to articulate this, and so we circle back to the need for an approach that does not depend on an ability to talk about it. In building a shared world, participants in a group sandtray session are accompanied by others with a similar experience, contributing to a greater sense of connection, of being understood and accepted. When considered from a neurobiological perspective, it is important to remember that:

> One of the strengths of group therapy is the high likelihood that the
> neural networks holding early implicit experience will be triggered as

other members bring their struggles into the group. At the same time, group can become an empathy-rich environment for holding the pain and fear that emerges. (Badenoch & Cox, 2019, p. 6)

An important aspect of the process described in this chapter is the "change phase" of building. Change can be a particularly painful part of death, loss, and grief. When we include a "change phase" in this process, participants are provided an opportunity to experience change as part of the healing journey.

In preparing to offer this activity, it is important to select guiding stories and symbolic figures that will support those touched by loss and grief. For the purposes of the children's grief groups, we chose guiding stories or themes directly related to death: The Funeral and Remembering Our Loved Ones; The Person Who Died. Other topics might include present- and future-focused guiding stories such as: How I am Doing Now; My Worries/Hopes for the Future; as well as collective stories when there have been multiple or public deaths in a community such as natural disasters or the recent killings of racialized individuals by police.

The selection of figures will provide participants with items one would expect to find in a typical sandtray collection, even if they do not appear to be associated with death. This allows for the expression of the day-to-day context of people's lives, as well as for surprises along the way. Additionally, it is important to include diverse representations of death and dying in the collection of images to be used. These include (but are not limited to) hospital, medical, and other items that may have been part of the dying process, as well as grave markers, coffins, and objects associated with funerals. Figures, structures, and symbols from various religions and faith communities may also be important.

The Approach: A Description of the Group Sandtray Process

In the first group session, the focus is on establishing a foundation of safety and connection. This includes developing guidelines about confidentiality and respect and providing psychoeducation about death and loss. This process draws on and supports "both the therapist's holding capacity and the group members' mindful awareness . . . as well as their empathic awareness of one another" (Badenoch & Cox, 2019, p. 2), contributing to healthy interpersonal neurobiological interactions. In a six-week group, these factors provide a sense of containment, which is essential in order to address the topic in a meaningful way. In the third session, our focus is on funerals, and this was where sandtray was incorporated in our weekly group activity.

Building Phase

Participants were invited to choose three objects from the collection to create a sandtray about The Funeral. They then took turns placing these objects in the tray, with the clear instruction that they were not allowed to touch or move other participants' objects. They were also advised that while the "no touch" rule was in place at this stage, there would later be an opportunity to make changes to the sandtray that could include adding objects to the sandtray, moving objects within the sandtray (their own or those of others), removing objects from the sandtray (their own or those of others), or any other change they wanted to make. At any point or phase, participants have the option to pass.

Throughout this process of selecting and placing objects, participants were invited to:

> notice what it's like when: someone else has taken the object you wanted; you can't find an object you would like; you are limited to three objects; someone takes the spot in the sandtray that you wanted; someone places their object(s) near yours.

This noticing provides an opportunity to engage in mindfulness. Participants did not need to speak about what they noticed. Rather, we hoped that by integrating a mindfulness aspect into the activity, we would help participants attend to their internal process without the need for words. Additionally, the inclusion of the "practice of mindfully viewing these continual changes in our states of mind can be revolutionary for group members who have felt helplessly caught up in the flow of implicit experience" (Badenoch & Cox, 2019, p. 14). This freeing from old constraints of mindless thought benefits the participants.

It is also important to note that for each round of placing objects in the building phase, the change phase, and the narrative/story phase, a different person went first. In order to accomplish this, participants number off so that in the first round, person 1 goes first, in the second round, person 2 goes first, and so on. The intention is to assure fairness and to provide a sense of predictability and control. Death is not fair, and although certain (in that it comes to all living things), it is frequently not within our control, nor is its trajectory predictable. As such, the design of this structure provides a reparative experience – to touch an aspect of death (in this case, The Funeral) in a measured way.

Change Phase

Prior to beginning, participants are reminded that the "no touch" rule is no longer in play. Starting with person 4, each participant is invited to make a change to the sandtray; they could add a new object, move an object (their own or another's), remove an object (their own or another's), or make any other change they wanted. They continued to have the option to pass. Throughout this process of change, participants were again invited to:

> notice what it's like when: an object is added; someone places their object(s) near yours; someone moves/removes one of your objects; you are limited to one change.

This allowed for the continued integration of mindfulness into the overall process.

Death is change. It comes with loss; it sometimes comes with additions, both wanted and unwanted. The inclusion of change and its associated losses in the therapeutic process is paradoxical, drawing from both explicit and implicit reminders of death. As such, it carries both painful experiences of change and the potential for healing that pain. The ability of this sandtray process to meet both needs provides a reparative experience (or what has been referred to in Grayson's chapter as "disconfirming"). Additionally, it opens the possibility to an alternate understanding of change. This is particularly powerful within the context of a supportive, nonjudgmental group that serves to reduce the risks of shaming or of pathologizing the builders' existing relationships with change. Paired with the mindfulness approach noted earlier, participants learn *in vivo* to observe and note the experience, shifting from a reactive response to awakening implicit memory to an integration of the implicit and explicit. In being able to recognize the temporal location of stimuli in the past, there is a resulting reduction of distress in response to triggers. From a neurobiological perspective, these embodied experiences support the development of new, healing pathways in the brain.

Narrative/Story Phase

Sandtrays tell stories. By "Enlisting young people's imaginations in service of their values and preferred vision for their lives . . . Calling on community to witness young people's imaginative feats" (Marsten et al., 2016, p. xviii), they offer the possibility of new narratives and alternate accounts of their lives and experiences. In addition, "group therapy probably makes one of its greatest contributions as an ample container for collaborative storytelling" (Badenoch & Cox, 2019, p. 17). In the narrative/story phase, participants are invited to put words to their experiences in the sandtray. The role of narrative in grief work has been articulated by White (1989), who introduced the idea of "saying hullo again." White presented this as an opportunity to reauthor our experience of loss, shifting it from the dominant, cultural narrative that is typically limited to saying good-bye to one that allows us to honor our connections to those who have died and feel less alone in our grief. The sandtray process employed in the children's grief group supports this reauthoring.

On a flip chart, white board, or at a location where everyone can see, the therapist/facilitator writes down the original title (for example: The Funeral). Starting with person 5, each participant is invited to consider the sandtray experience as a whole and to give it a name, title, or descriptive phrase. As in the previous phases, participants have the option to pass. The group facilitator writes down all the words that are generated. Having worked "beneath the words," participants now have access to those words. Having engaged in the physical acts of building and change, participants now engage in "Curiosity and mindful attention to the present moment [that] are as important in sensorimotor psychotherapy as the narrative" (Mark-Goldstein & Ogden, 2019, p. 126). Thus, it is important to note that these words need only make sense to the individual who has offered them. Next comes the winnowing process.

Starting with person 6, participants are asked to consider all the words and to select one word that they feel is essential. Participants may select a word from their own title or someone else's. More than one participant may select the same word. Using a different color of ink, the facilitator circles each word selected. Starting with person 7, participants are invited to craft a new sentence using the circled words. There are no right or wrong answers, and agreement is not necessary (although in my experience, consensus is typically reached). This "wordsmithing" process includes the option of changing nouns to verbs, adjectives, or adverbs (or the other way around); changing verb tense; adding articles and pronouns; and the use of linking verbs such as is/are. For example, when using a similar process with students in a counseling program working with the theme Becoming a Play Therapist, the final words of *mystery, challenge, safety, journey, healing* became: Becoming a play therapist is the mystery and challenge of a safe, healing journey. Whether you have one title or eight, the facilitator reads back the entirety of each title, summarizing and affirming the work done and the conclusion reached. When working with younger children, whose wordsmithing skills may be limited, the facilitator may offer some examples to model the process. It is important that the tray not be dismantled at this point.

The final part of this phase is a debrief of the group sandtray. It is included in the narrative/story phase, as it is an opportunity to reflect further on the process, the narrative/story, and to put words to the experience. Within a narrative/story context, this serves a similar function to an epilogue. Starting with person 8, each participant is invited to share something about the experience. It may include a rationale for something they did during the building or change phases, an observation, a question, or some other comment. Again, participants may choose to pass. The act of mindful reflection that follows on a mostly wordless process supports the integration of an implicit experience with explicit memory. When we center this activity within a supportive group, where each participant is empowered to engage their "imaginative know-how," participants have another reparative experience in their relationship with death, loss, and grief. It has been my observation that when participants share their internal process with each other, some of the most powerful and healing changes occur. This is illustrated in the next section, which examines two sandtray journeys.

The Sandtray Journey Into Grief: Two Stories

This section will look at two sandtray journeys from the children's grief groups described earlier. In order to protect the privacy of the participants, descriptions and narrative details used represent compilations of a number of sandtrays, with identifying information removed. Similarly, images are reconstructions of the actual trays in respect for confidentiality.

The participants typically included children who had lost a sibling, parent, or grandparent within the past six months to a year. Causes of death frequently included old age, illness (often cancer), and motor vehicle and other accidents. Occasionally, participants had experienced a loss due to violence or suicide. Although we screened for compatibility, we did not screen for age because we did not want to break up sibling groups. As a result, participants ranged in age from 5 to 15, although typically the age range was within five years from youngest to oldest.

The Funeral

Participants were invited to select images based on their experience of The Funeral. They chose a church, a fence, grave markers, a coffin, a number of other figures, and various people including a baby, a crying Buddha, a fairy, and a nun (see Figure 9.1). Funeral worlds typically include some way of marking the grave, denoting a funeral service, and the inclusion of people to represent mourners. Though less prevalent, representations of religious/faith communities, belief systems, and an afterlife are also common. While participants have demonstrated creativity, imagination, and adaptability in their use of the available objects, it is important to include relevant, topic-related objects in the collection when specific themes are explored.

Participants worked through the building phase with relative ease, engaging in thoughtful selection and placement of their objects. It is common during the change phase for participants to react to the changes, expressing anxiety when their object is moved or removed by another participant and delight when they view a change as adding to either their objects or the overall scene. Reactions are expressed through gestures, sounds, and comments that give other participants a sense of what is going on within the group. Sometimes, a reaction may prompt a participant to change their mind about a change, particularly when they have chosen to remove another person's

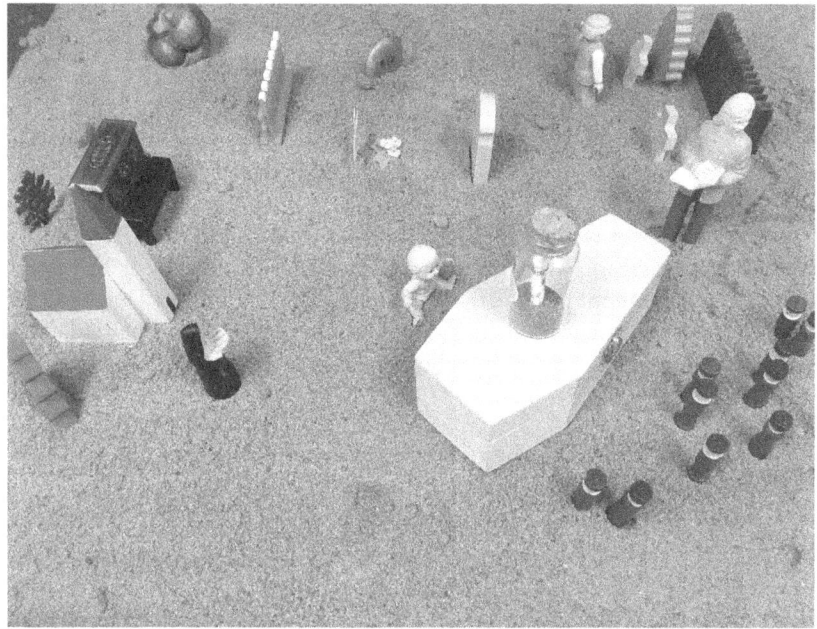

Figure 9.1 The Funeral: overview.

object. In such interactions, we see mirror neurons at work. A friendly smile, a supportive nod signals to the other participant(s) that they are seen, that they belong, that someone else understands. This in turn, supports self-reflection, self-acceptance, and self-knowing.

In this sandtray, the rearrangement of headstones prompted little reaction. The removal of the nun was initially responded to with a sigh of dismay until the participant who had originally placed it remembered they had not yet had their turn in the change phase. With this realization, the participant smiled confidently and, at their turn, returned the nun to the sandtray with an expression of triumph. This was met with smiles from the other participants. The removal of the fairy elicited a gasp from the participant who had placed it there. Looks and words of sympathy were offered. However, because they had taken their turn and there was no opportunity to replace the object, it remained out of the sandtray.

In the narrative/story phase, participants generated statements about The Funeral sandtray such as:

- Saying **good-bye** is **hard**
- I felt sad

- It was **harder** and easier than I thought
- Lots of people said nice things
- I **wish** I hadn't gone/could have gone
- Funerals can **help**

A sample of the words selected in the winnowing process are shown in bold italics. The summative statement became "The Funeral: A wish goodbye is hard and it helps."

In the debrief, participants shared their reactions, reflections, and questions. The participant who had removed the fairy asked why it had been included. It turned out that the fairy was intended to be an angel who would watch over the person who died and the people who were left behind. The participant noted they had wished the angel was suspended over the sandtray

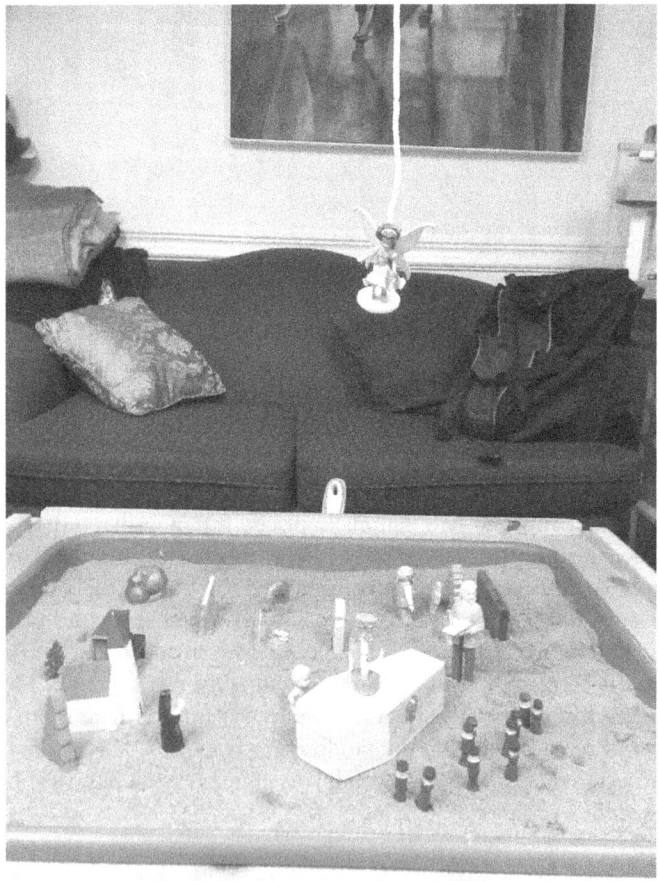

Figure 9.2 The Funeral: detail.

rather than having it stand near the edge, agreeing that it didn't really belong *in* the sandtray. At this point, the participant who had removed the "fairy" got some yarn from the craft box, tied it around the object and, climbing up on the table, figured out how to suspend the angel from the ceiling (see Figure 9.2). This met with applause and smiles of approval from all the participants. The spontaneity of this response is an example of how attending to the body's physical impulses "can foster curiosity as members reflect upon their bodily experiences . . . become aware of their sensorimotor process . . . [that] opens the door for the body itself to lead them into constructive resolution" (Mark-Goldstein & Ogden, 2019, p. 125).

Remembering Our Loved Ones/the Person Who Died

Participants were invited to select figures based on their memories of the person who died. Unlike selections for The Funeral, the selection of images tends to be client centric, reflecting the specific relationship between the participant and the deceased loved one. This has been particularly evident in the selection of images by siblings who chose to represent their own unique memories in the sandtray. The importance of having a diverse collection of figures is reinforced by participants selecting or asking for specific, sometimes surprising objects. Having plasticine or some other mouldable material proved helpful.

When used in the children's grief group, this sandtray commemorating the loved one who died is completed in the final session. By this time, participants know some of each other's stories, including details about the person who died, the circumstances of their death, and the nature of the relationship between the participant and their loved one. The figures selected tend to vary widely, reflecting the multifaceted life of the deceased. As pieces are selected and placed in the sandtray, the reactions of others included nods of recognition, puzzled curiosity, and a general sense of calm and focus. For this sandtray, there is typically little evidence of distress in the building phase.

The change phase was quite a different story. In the building phase for The Funeral sandtray, objects were moved, removed, and added in a relatively calm, methodical manner. However, the idiosyncrasies of individual participants played out in more pronounced ways in the sandtrays about Remembering Our Loved Ones during the change phase. In one of these sandtrays, a frog that was placed during the building phase was removed, returned, and removed again, remaining out of the final sandtray. It was evident from the participants' facial gestures and vocalizations that there was an "ick" factor at play. Even the sibling of the participant who had contributed the frog looked puzzled by its inclusion in a tray about their deceased family member. In this and other Remembering Our Loved Ones sandtrays, tensions often ran high as significant objects were moved, removed, and replaced. It is important in these moments for the facilitator to acknowledge the reactions and to remind participants that there will be an opportunity to talk about the experience later. In employing the "name it to tame it" strategy (Siegel, 2012, p. 27), we engage in storying the child's experience. This allows us to connect our emotionally regulated self with their capacity for emotional regulation. This is a key element in the journey of grief and healing and another example of how neurobiology is at play in this work.

In the narrative/story phase, participants generated statements about the Remembering Out Loved Ones sandtray including:

- I miss him/her/them
- ***Remembering*** them feels . . .
- They're still in my ***heart***
- Memories ***keep*** them ***alive***/with me
- We did a lot of cool/fun/crazy things together
- He/she/they were the only one who . . .
- It's ***hard*** to let go

A sample of the words selected in the winnowing process are shown in bold italics. The summative statement became "Remembering our loved ones: it's hard but it keeps them alive in our hearts."

In the debrief, for this sandtray, the older sibling asked about the frog that had been in and out of the sandtray, remaining out at its conclusion. The younger sibling described going fishing with the person who died and how they would put the live bait on the hook. With that, one of the participants who had clearly had an "ick" response marched over to the frog and returned it to the sandtray in a central position, affirming the importance of its inclusion in the world (see Figure 9.3). Needless to say, there were smiles all around. At this point, participants shared other stories about the selected objects and their connection to the loved one. Rather than the earlier tensions of the change phase, this sharing carried an energy of caring and compassion. It is also another example of impulses in action. As this was the final activity of the final session, this sandtray served to strengthen the sense of connection in a moment where we were about to say good-bye.

Client Outcomes

Children who have lost a family member to death experience what the Alberta Family Wellness Initiative (n.d.) refers to as "tolerable stress"; stress that is unpleasant, unavoidable, and generally time limited. When experienced in a supportive environment, the presence of stress hormones, such as adrenalin and cortisol, are buffered, and the impact is not lasting. However, when caregivers are unable to "buffer" their child's distress, when they are dysregulated and their own distress adds to the child's, the presence of stress hormones in the child's brain persists and remains at elevated, unhealthy levels. This leads to "toxic stress" (AFWI, n.d.). Consequently, the child's need

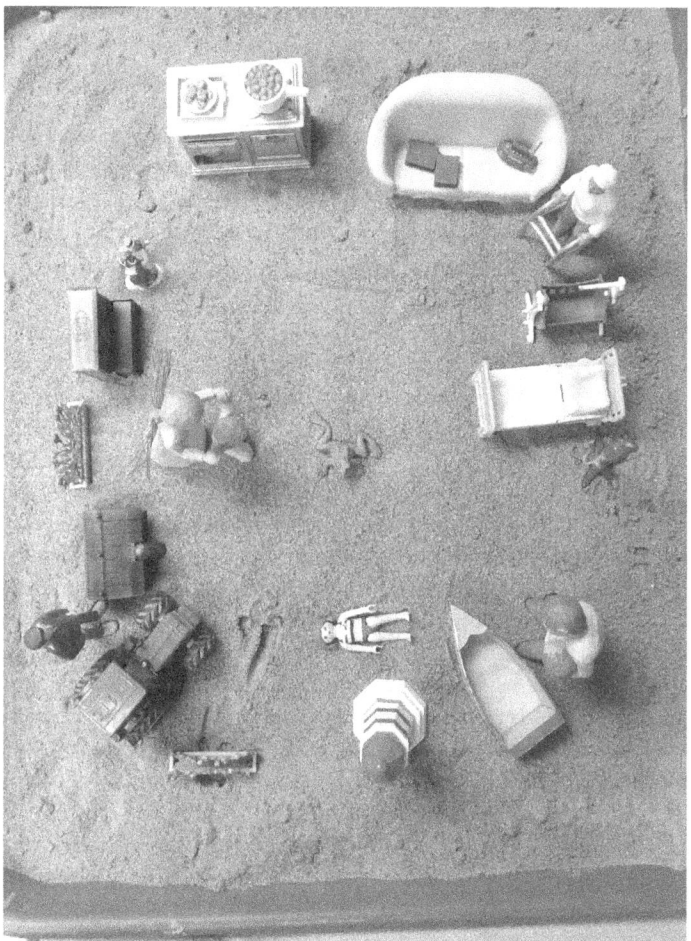

Figure 9.3 Remembering Our Loved Ones: overview.

for reassurance, to see themselves reflected and accepted by the adult, may be compromised. Although we did not evaluate levels of stress or take other measures for these groups, the research suggests that opportunities to engage in activities that support a reorientation to the stressful experience, in a supportive and emotionally regulated context, have the capacity to change (or build new) neural pathways and promote healing (Badenoch & Cox, 2019). The sandtray activities employed in the children's grief group provided these opportunities to the participants.

The group sandtray approach described here allows the child to revisit the distressing experience and promotes healing. Due to the physically contained nature of sandtray, the potential for sandtray to offer soothing (regulating) touch, and the ability of sandtray to draw on implicit memory, participants have access to a reparative experience that serves to build new pathways in the brain. These pathways are further reinforced through the use of narrative/story.

It is noteworthy that in employing this intervention, the outcomes to both The Funeral and Remembering Our Loved Ones sandtrays were healing. As has been suggested in the literature, "Often, instead of reacting with aggravation or fear when another person is activated, the other group members may be able to come from a more kind, regulated, clear-seeing perspective; a state that is good for everyone in the room" (Badenoch & Cox, 2019, p. 7). This is consistent with our observations. While it is true that throughout the process, participants experienced some big emotions, these were viewed as healthy expressions, and the response of other participants was supportive. Although the sandtrays were focused on experiences of death, grief, and loss, the final narratives were invariably about hope.

Based on the frequent requests for a second sandtray session, it is clear that participants appreciate what sandtray therapy has to offer. In The Funeral sandtray sessions, participants remain engaged in all phases of the process, express emotions, and support one another. In the narrative/story phase, they were able to give words to their experiences. With respect to their experiences of the actual funeral and their relationship with the person who died, the participants reported a number of improvements. Several children noted their ability to name and talk about their feelings. It was not uncommon to hear children who had been afraid of their feelings report, "I was afraid the sadness would last forever; now I'm not so afraid" and "I thought I was the only one who was angry [that they died] and now I know I'm not." These changes were also observed by the children's parents/caregivers and are indicators of a number of gains. These included increases in mindfulness where participant memories became integrated with explicit memory (and less triggering); improvements in emotional regulation in participants' ability to express and manage emotions; the development of new neural pathways; and cohesive narratives, as seen in the reauthoring of participants' stories of grief.

Similarly, children responded to the Remembering Our Loved Ones sandtray with positive comments. They noted that they liked being able to show rather than tell about their relationship with the person who died; that it was "like I got to introduce them to my lost one. That was cool!" This is consistent with our understanding of the capacity of mirror neurons to "support the notion of an innate pre-linguistic responsiveness to others (Schermer, 2019, pp. 30–32). Following this group sandtray, parents who had been unsure of how to talk about the deceased with their children noted how the sandtray opened a door to those conversations, saying things like, "they came home talking about this sandtray and telling me about how much they missed their loved one. And I knew we'd be okay." In the case of more recent deaths, some parents reported that it was the first time they'd seen their child laugh/cry since the death/the funeral and that they viewed their child's response as an indication of healthy grieving. On a practical level, both adults and children reported that the sandtrays gave them something concrete to talk about and that these conversations bridged chasms of silence, pain, and confusion.

Interactions such as the repositioning of the fairy-angel and the return of the frog suggest that participants are attuned to one another. The role of mirror neurons and resonance circuits is evident in these interactions, in which there was strong evidence of "empathy and identification . . . in which individuals model, reflect upon and learn from each other" (Schermer, 2019, p. 26). Through the sandtray activity, participants' ability to draw on their shared experience of grief supports them in offering and receiving meaningful, empathic responses.

A final and unexpected benefit was the ways children understood and responded to the limited number of objects they could choose for the building phase and change phase. Although this did not happen in all sandtrays, participants frequently chose a grouping of objects to represent a single choice. For example, a collection of small neutral figures was used by one participant to represent the mourners in The Funeral sandtray (see Figures 9.1 and 9.2). As facilitators, we understood this was no accident, and we did not move to stop the choice. Instead, we understood the knowingness with which they acted to be a healthy way of exercising some control, expressing a desire, and getting their needs met. This is another example of mirror neurons at work, of participants benefitting when "an individual engages in goal directed activity or observes someone else doing so" (Schermer, 2019, p. 29) because their action is met with an empathic response. A child who is able to make the rules fit their needs rather than fitting themself to rules that may feel arbitrary is a child who is in the process of reclaiming their life from grief.

Personal Reflections

When we offered the first children's grief group, Julie's invitation to include a sandtray activity was an exciting opportunity. We had trained together in play therapy and in the Erica method of sandtray assessment and were both eager to put our skills to use. However, the group models that were available to us did not include sandtray, and the sandtray training we had was largely focused on individuals. This was an experiment, an adventure in bringing together skill and creativity in service to our clients. While uncertain of the outcome, we were confident in our ability to provide a contained group activity that supported participants in exploring a potentially painful experience.

When I look back, I recall how the sandtray engaged the curiosity and imagination of the children. I remember how the participants brought thoughtfulness and playfulness to the activity. In my professional experience, these are essential components in healing. The respectful, supportive, and attuned responses of the children to each other affirmed my experience from adult group therapy that healing is indeed relational. I reflect that when we are presented with life experiences such as death, it is powerful to know that someone else not only walks with you on the journey to healing, they draw from the best in themselves and the best in you. The tray in which the frog returned to the world at the end and the tray in which the angel was suspended over the world are two examples of this. In recalling these examples for this chapter, I continue to be moved by these stories.

In approaching the sandtray activities, I noticed how the children became more like children than clients, engaging with one another in a relaxed manner. This was different from the varying degrees of guardedness observed in some of them during the pregroup interviews, when, I imagine, they had a sense they were being assessed (they were). During the sandtray activities, the children appeared curious about what was unfolding: leaning in, responding with spontaneous expressions of delight, surprise, and sometimes quizzical or concerned looks. I feel fortunate to have shared these moments of discovery with them; discovery about death, each other, and themselves.

A number of years have passed since the mid to late 1990s, when Julie and I facilitated children's grief groups. In that time, a great deal has been learned about neurobiology. What I have learned about the mind suggests that my instincts about how to structure the group sandtray were spot-on. In particular, I believe the inclusion of noticing drew on the brain's capacity for mindfulness. By slowing down the building process through taking turns, stopping to notice both the physical construction that was emerging and the internal emotions that were arising, participants were able to connect with intrinsic memories that could be integrated into a sense of wholeness. The presence of peers who reflected them and their process supported their ability to recognize they were going to be okay. I now understand that to be not just encouragement and support but a function of the interpersonal resonance within the group. I am encouraged by this look back, as it reminds me that even when we have yet to discover the science that proves something, it is important to follow one's instincts to experiment, to test out hypotheses, to learn, to grow, and to heal.

References

Alberta Family Wellness Initiative. (n.d). A brief introduction to toxic stress. *The Brain Story*, Module 5, Video 1, 2:26. https://d1vy0qa05cdjr5.cloudfront.net/a10e61ae-

422c-44cd-85d7–004150123c2/Brain%20Story%20Certification%20Course/Module%2005N/Video%2201%20Transcript%20M05–03%20A%20Brief%20Introduction%20toToxic%20Stress.pdf

Badenoch, B., & Cox, P. (2019). Integrating interpersonal neurobiology with group psychotherapy. In S. Gantt & B. Badenoch (Eds.), *The interpersonal neurobiology of group psychotherapy and group process* (pp. 1–18). Routledge.

Brown, E., Goodman, R., Shira, F., & Swiedicki, C. C. (2019). Psychometrics of the PTSD and depressions screener for bereaved youth. *Death Studies, 43*(1), 20–31.

Fitzgerald, H. (1992). *The grieving child, A parent's guide.* Fireside.

Frankl, V. (1984). *Man's dearch for meaning.* Revised and Updated. Washington Square Press.

Gantt, S., & Badenoch, B. (Eds.). (2019). *The interpersonal neurobiology of group psychotherapy and group process.* Routledge.

Geller, S., & Porges, S. (2014). Therapeutic presence: Nuerophysiological mechanism mediating feeling safe in therapeutic relationships. *Journal of Psychotherapy Integration, 24*(3), 178–192.

Harris, P. L. (2018). Children's understanding of death: From biology to religion. *Philosophical Transactions of the Royal Society of London. Series B, Biological Sciences, 373*(1754).

Herring, J. (2013). *Does PTSD interfere in reconciling grief after childhood bereavement? An evaluation of a grief-focused group intervention.* ProQuest LCC.

Hidalgo, I. (2017). *The effects of children's spiritual coping after parent, grandparent or sibling death on children's grief, personal growth, and mental health.* ProQuest LCC.

Iglesias, A., & Iglesias, A. (2005). Hypnotic treatment of PTSD in children who have complicated bereavement. *The American Journal of Clinical Hypnosis, 48*(2–3), 183–189.

Kaplow, J., Layne, C., Pynoos, R., Cohen, J., & Lieberman, A. (2012). DSM-V diagnostic criteria for bereavement-related disorders in children and adolescents: Developmental considerations. *Psychiatry, 75*(3), 243–266.

Lowenstein, L. (2006). *Creative interventions for bereaved children.* Champion Press.

Mark-Goldstein, B., & Ogden, P. (2019). Sensorimotor psychotherapy as a foundation of group therapy with younger clients. In S. Gantt & B. Badenoch (Eds.), *The interpersonal neurobiology of group psychotherapy and group process* (pp. 123–145). Routledge.

Marsten, D., Epston, D., & Markham, L. (2016). *Narrative therapy in wonderland: Connecting with children's imaginative know-how.* W. W. Norton & Company, Inc.

McGill, M., & Topham, A. (2008). *The relational healing continuum: A group counselling model for adult survivors of childhood sexual abuse and adult sexual assault.* Sexual Assault Centre London.

McKissock, D. (2004). *Kids grief, a handbook for group leaders.* Compassion Books.

Ogden, P., & Fischer, J. (2015). *Sensorimotor psychotherapy: Interventions for trauma and attachment.* W. W. Norton & Company, Inc.

Ogden, P., Minton, K., & Pain, C. (2006). *Trauma and the body: A sensorimotor approach to psychotherapy.* W. W. Norton & Company, Inc.

Porges, S. (2017). *The pocket guide to polyvagal theory: The transformative power of feeling safe.* W. W. Norton & Company, Inc.

Schermer, V. (2019). Mirror neurons: Their implications for group psychotherapy. In S. Gantt & B. Badenoch (Eds.), *The interpersonal neurobiology of group psychotherapy and group Process* (pp. 25–49). Routledge.

Schore, A. (2003). *Affect regulation and the repair of the self.* W. W. Norton & Company, Inc.

Siegel, D. (2008). *The neurobiology of "WE": How relationships, the mind, and the brain interact to shape who we are.* Sounds True.

Siegel, D. (2012). *The whole-brain child: 12 revolutionary strategies to nurture your child's developing mind.* Bantam Books.

Silverman, P. R. (2000). *Never too young to know: Death in children's lives.* Oxford University Press, Inc.

Van der Kolk, B. (2014). *The body keeps the score: Brain, mind, and body in the healing of trauma.* Viking.

White, M. (1989). Saying hullo again. In *Selected papers* (pp. 29–36). Dulwhich Centre Publications.

Willis, C. A. (2002). The grieving process in children: Strategies for understanding, educating, and reconciling children's perceptions of death. *Early Childhood Education Journal, 29,* 221–226.

Wolfelt, A. D. (2001). *Healing a teen's grieving heart: 100 practical ideas for families, friends and caregivers.* Companion Press.

10 Rediscovering Balance

Combining Sandtray Therapy and EMDR

Elaine Wittmann and Jacqueline Aldridge

This chapter was written about one child's journey as witnessed by two trained and experienced sandtray therapists who are fully trained in eye movement desensitization and reprocessing (EMDR). Elaine worked directly with the child, and Jacqueline supported Elaine in the role of a peer consultant and witness to Elaine's tray. This chapter cannot adequately instruct on how to use EMDR. For more information on EMDR and training opportunities, consult the EMDR Institute at www.emdr.com.

Elaine's Story

I first knew Asa while he was still in utero. His mother was helping me plan and decorate my new home as she and her husband were anticipating the joy of first-time parenthood. The surprise came when his arrival into the world was early, as two-pound-seven-ounce Asa left the warm, safe place of his mother's womb and was thrust into the chaos of the neonatal intensive care unit (NICU).

His little body battled as his care team administered procedures that could have been painful and confusing. He experienced alterations in temperature and noise as well as disruptions in sleep states, all in the efforts to save little Asa (Lovett, 2015, pp. 123, 135). The valiant efforts of the medical professionals were necessary though intrusive to the infant and could be "indistinguishable from the pain of child abuse" (Gardener et al., 1993, p. 604). Medically challenged low-weight babies may suffer from a variety of complications including respiratory distress, bleeding of the brain, and vision problems, and the immature nervous system is particularly vulnerable to neonatal brain injury (Nosaarti et al., 2012). Toxic stress in the developing brain of the preterm child may impact the functioning of neuroendocrine and autonomic nervous systems and neuroplasticity of the immature infant's brain (Maroney, 2003). After the NICU, children can experience the stress of coping with continuing medical issues (Lovett, 2015; Zelkowitz, 2017).

Traumatic stress for parents of preterm infants is well documented. As the newborn is physically separated from the parent in the NICU, there is a risk of maternal depression that may impact parenting behavior (Zelkowitz,

DOI: 10.4324/9781003055808-12

2017). Concerns for the normal bonding between parent and child may be interrupted, and both parents and babies may experience toxic stress (Sanders & Hall, 2018) as a result of the preterm birth and the experience of the NICU.

Asa's Therapy – Round One

When I met Asa again, he was 8 years old. I learned that his premature arrival resulted in a diagnosis of mild cerebral palsy and a nocturnal seizure disorder from an early brain bleed. Asa's parents appeared to place a great deal of responsibility on themselves for Asa's difficulties. Both cried as they anguished over decisions they made in their parenting such as giving too much attention to their son's medical needs and not paying enough attention to advice they had received along the way, as well as the emotional impact of his baby brother's birth.

Asa presented as an anxious, angry child who took his frustrations out at home, where his mother appeared to be the primary target. Asa's parents reported that his teachers did not seem to understand the frustration he was feeling in the classroom, since Asa seemed to be a committed and intelligent student. With his physical disabilities, Asa could not compete on equal ground with his peers in many ways. The competition in and out of the classroom that led to "playground politics" (Greenspan, 1993, p. 36) left Asa feeling jealous and envious of his classmates. At 8 years old, he did not have the skills to appropriately defend himself, and the consequences were a global threat to his self-esteem. In addition, Asa struggled with the attention his parents paid to his younger brother.

Asa was introduced to the play therapy room and the sandtray. There, he fought battles in the sand with army figures, tanks, cannons, bombs, and battering rams, with bunkers to hide behind and hills to climb. At first, the "other team" won battle after battle, and slowly, the "good guys" (his team) won battles and eventually won the war. Not a word was said about the play-ground battles, but school became less of an issue. As Asa worked hard in the sand, his parents learned new skills in addressing Asa's outbursts, handling their own emotional regulation, and giving Asa the attention he needed at home. Within a few months, the family successfully finished therapy.

Asa's Therapy – Round Two

Two years passed before I heard from Asa and his family again. By this time, Asa was 10 years old. On the surface, things were going well. He had just completed a successful school year, connecting with his male teacher and making all A's. Behavior problems at home had decreased. However, Asa was experiencing stomachaches that were difficult to manage, and his parents were concerned that they might be stress related. Once again, Asa was subjected to invasive medical tests, including a colonoscopy and an endoscopy. His doctors found no physical source for his pain and cleared him medically. According to Maroney (2003), it is not unusual for preterm infants to continue to have a variety of physiological difficulties, including gastrointestinal disorders and somatic complaints.

When Asa returned to therapy, I was fully trained in eye movement reprocessing and desensitization (EMDR). I considered how his current symptoms might relate to his preterm birth, given the possibility of early trauma due to his experiences in the NICU. It was helpful that I had worked with him previously, as I was aware of his early childhood history of medical issues and anxiety. His parents reported that the stomachaches had started about six months ago, seemingly "without any trigger." In fact, Asa was doing well at home and in school except for some competition with his now active 2-year-old brother. Asa's parents were pleased with how Asa loved his brother and paid positive attention to him, but they also noted that Asa seemed to need more attention lately. I speculated that the birth of his little brother may have awakened some implicit memories of Asa's own difficult birth, offering a subconscious or conscious reminder of his own limitations. Asa now witnessed and competed with the everyday "activity" of his little brother.

Maroney (2003) tells us that premature babies "can easily become 'imbalanced' due to invasive procedures and stress" (p. 679). How might that early imbalance be manifesting for Asa now? Trauma-informed therapy looks at current behaviors in the light of previous traumas (Sanders & Hall, 2018). Could Asa's stomachaches be related to events he experienced as an infant? Green et al. (2010) report that the "early memory system with which infants and preverbal children store affective and behavioral experiences, is known as the implicit emotional memory system . . ." (p. 97). Early experiences of perceived maltreatment may result in permanently disturbing the normal development of the brain, and the trauma may never be stored verbally. The object then is to have integration of "memory fragments from implicit memory to explicit memory" (Green et al., 2010, p. 99). According to Green et al., when provided a safe environment in relationship with a secure person, children can "play out" implicit memories of the original trauma and develop a narrative for their experience leading to empowerment and self-worth. Could increasing Asa's own feelings of Self – his own inner authority – help Asa in his relationship with his younger brother? How might I access the preverbal memory and the possibility of early trauma as well as the ongoing trauma of medical problems and somatic symptoms (Norton et al., 2011)? Reworking and mastery of the traumatic events with EMDR and sandtray appeared to be the answer.

I introduced EMDR to Asa's parents as a psychotherapy treatment that was designed to relieve distress and explained that the process was well researched and proven to be successful with a variety of disorders, including somatic concerns (Shapiro, 2001, 2012, 2014; Shapiro & Merlis, 2014; Shapiro, 2016). I explained that with the use of bilateral stimulation (BLS), EMDR may activate processing in both hemispheres at once. I illustrated alternating left-right eye-movements with Asa's father. Asa's parents knew their son had been receptive to sandtray therapy in the past and saw the value in combining it with something new.

EMDR is guided by adaptive information processing (AIP), a learning theory that postulates that memory networks store information through images, thoughts, feelings, and body sensations. When a stressful situation is successfully processed, "it is adaptively stored" (Shapiro, 2016, p. 6), and the individual is able to move toward a resolution. If an overwhelming or traumatic event is inadequately or maladaptively stored, healthy processing does not continue, and current situations may be linked to the responses of the earlier implicit memory. Siegel and Brcezyski (2014) describe that "trauma impairs the brain's memory systems by blocking the integrative role of the hippocampus to take implicit puzzle pieces and weave them together into explicit memory" (p. 10). A distressing current situation can be linked to a past experience, bringing up the physical sensations, felt emotions, and perceptions of the past event without conscious control. While the brain is developing, it is the most vulnerable to trauma (Siegel & Brcezyski, 2014). When working with preverbal trauma and implicit memory, the goal is not retrieval, but instead, we work with any present symptoms of distress (Went & Struik, 2010). Siegel and Brcezyski (2014) suggest that it is reintegration that repairs the brain (p. 6). The goal of EMDR is reintegration.

Standard protocol takes the EMDR process through eight phases: history taking, preparation, assessment, desensitization, installation, body scan, closure, and reevaluation. Bilateral stimulation (BLS) is a hallmark of EMDR (Shapiro, 2016). With the external implementation of lateral right-left eye movements by following the fingers of the therapist (or an object), the two sides of the brain are activated. While early research focused on the eye movements, other forms of bilateral stimulation – tactile, auditory, or a combination – were found to work equally well, especially with children (Adler-Tapia & Settle, 2008; Adler-Tapia, 2017). EMDR for children must be developmentally appropriate in language and use of creative materials (Shapiro, 2016, pp. 58–59; Beckley-Forest, 2016), and the inclusion of sandtray seemed appropriate. By identifying the current target, or experience to be addressed, the clinician elicits a negative cognition or self-belief associated with the target as well as an alternative cognition in the form of a positive self-belief. Cognitive restructuring is an essential part of the assessment phase of EMDR. By identifying irrational beliefs, restructuring and reframing the negative cognitions into more adaptive positive self-beliefs, the therapeutic process is enhanced (Shapiro, 2001; Shapiro & Merlis, 2014; Shapiro, 2012, 2016).

When the emotion connected with the target is identified, the client is asked to give the subjective units of disturbance (SUD), a scale of 0 to 10 that indicates the intensity of distress currently experienced by the individual. Another self-report, developed by Francine Shapiro, requests the client to assess the validity of cognition (VOC) on a scale that runs from 1 to 7. One represents what is totally unbelievable, and goes to 7, which is totally believable (Shapiro & Merlis, 2014). Adults will usually be able to use the numbers for each scale, but children often express their levels of distress or believability in other ways. Distances shown by a chart, drawing, or a spread of hands may also work for children (Adler-Tapia & Settle, 2008).

Gomez (2019) describes

> EMDR clinicians need to be open to other forms of communication in cases when the left verbal brain is silenced by trauma. EMDR therapy, combined with Sandtray strategies, embraces the language of the right hemisphere and its ability to utilize metaphors, archetypes, symbols, and stories. (p. 35)

The use of EMDR and sandtray seemed to be the best therapy for Asa's difficulties.

Asa's father brought him to his first session of this treatment episode. His father explained that the family was worried about Asa's stomachaches and thought that I might be able to help. Asa described his stomachaches and told me that testing had ruled out any physical causes. He made it clear that he did not want any other medical procedures! I reassured Asa that there would not be anything invasive in this therapy and reminded him about the toys and the sandtray room. I then told Asa of a new way we could work together that might help with his stomach pain, called EMDR. Based on Asa's history of nocturnal seizures, I decided not to use the traditional "eye movements" but to use another form of bilateral stimulation called "tapping."

Because early trauma is stored in the body, O'Shea and Paulson (2009) report that in reprocessing early trauma, a light touch on the knees and hands allows relaxation, and the client can feel the presence of the thera-pist. They also suggest that "a heartbeat cadence seems useful for prenatal and birth time periods" (p. 18). The Association for Play Therapy (2012) advises that while touch is a "powerful form of communication" therapists must evaluate each child's situation, the caregiver's perception of touch, and the therapeutic need for the intervention. A consent for touching may be included in the consent for treatment. (p. 1). One must be aware of the controversy of touch and take into consideration each state's licensing board's rules on physical touch. In cases where touch is not appropriate, a client may tap themself. With Asa's permission and his father watching, I illustrated alternate tapping on my knees first and then on his knees. Both Asa and his father agreed to allow me to do the tapping.

Asa's non-verbal communication demonstrated to me that Asa was not inter-ested in this new thing called EMDR. His father attempted to encourage Asa by telling him that he had to "buy into this," reminding him of the hypnosis he'd had as a child which he found helpful. I reassured Asa that, unlike hypnosis, he did not necessarily have to buy into EMDR. In fact, he was already engaging in bilateral stimulation every night as his eyes moved back and forth during REM sleep. When I tapped his shoulders in our sandtray sessions, I would just be help-ing him with the back and forth. While both EMDR and hypnosis may suc-cessfully work in healing trauma, EMDR is based on biophysical components and does not require a relaxed state of consciousness as with hypnosis (Tinker & Wilson, 1999). EMDR focuses on the client being more aware and conscious so that "memories are able to jump from one eye element of the memory to another" (Shapiro, 2001, p. 326).

First, I facilitated conscious "belly breathing" and directed Asa's awareness to his senses and inner stillness. I asked him to notice where he felt any distress in his body and to breathe the discomfort away (Higgins-Klein, 2013). Gently, I encouraged Asa to clear his mind and imagine a special safe place – a place of security – where distracting thoughts are cleared; next, I invited him to use the sandtray. Asa remembered the sandtray from his earlier treatment and was pleased to return to the sandtray room. He explored the figures, remembering some and commenting on what he thought was new. Asa then quietly and methodically chose figures and placed them in two side-by-side trays. He put the calm and safety he needed into the tray and defended it with a fence, a knight on a horse, a row of armed soldiers, and a closed gate in a tall wall.

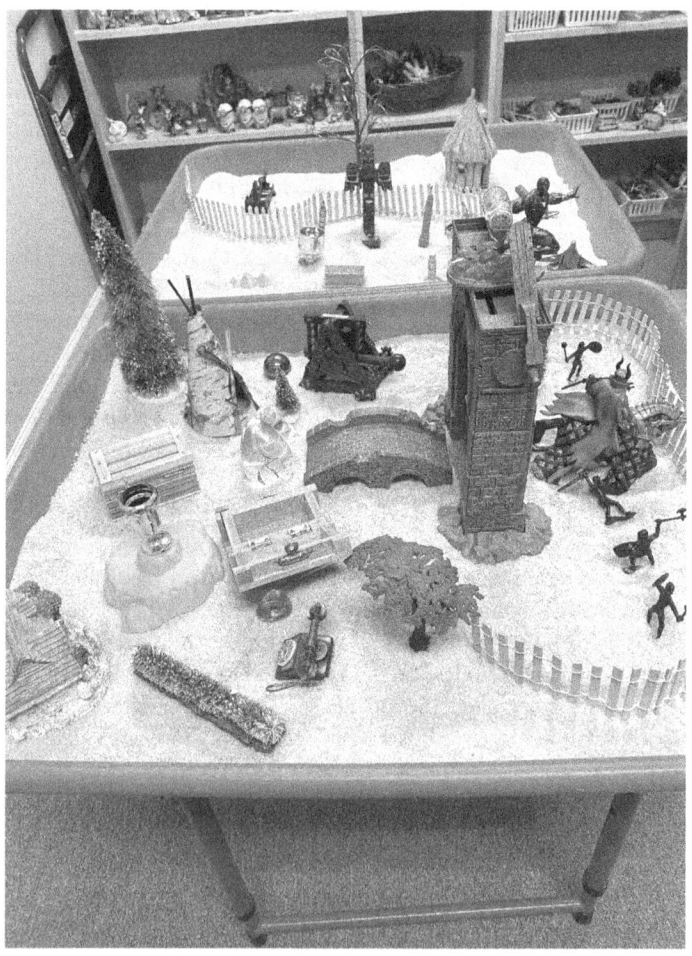

Figure 10.1 Calm and safety (tray in back) are well defended (tray in front).

As Asa processed the trays verbally, he had difficulty describing the "evil" that was outside the tray. The unconscious was felt but had no words. Because language is primarily a left hemisphere function and sandtray engages the right hemisphere, it is not uncommon for words to be elusive. The "evil" was strong but could not penetrate the walls of the fortress, and the treasures that lie within remained protected. Asa named the superhero who defended the castle Flash. He stood on the top of the wall and possessed the superpower of speed, "even faster than Superman!" Asa added "magic" (glitter in a bottle) for Flash to use as a weapon against the "evil."

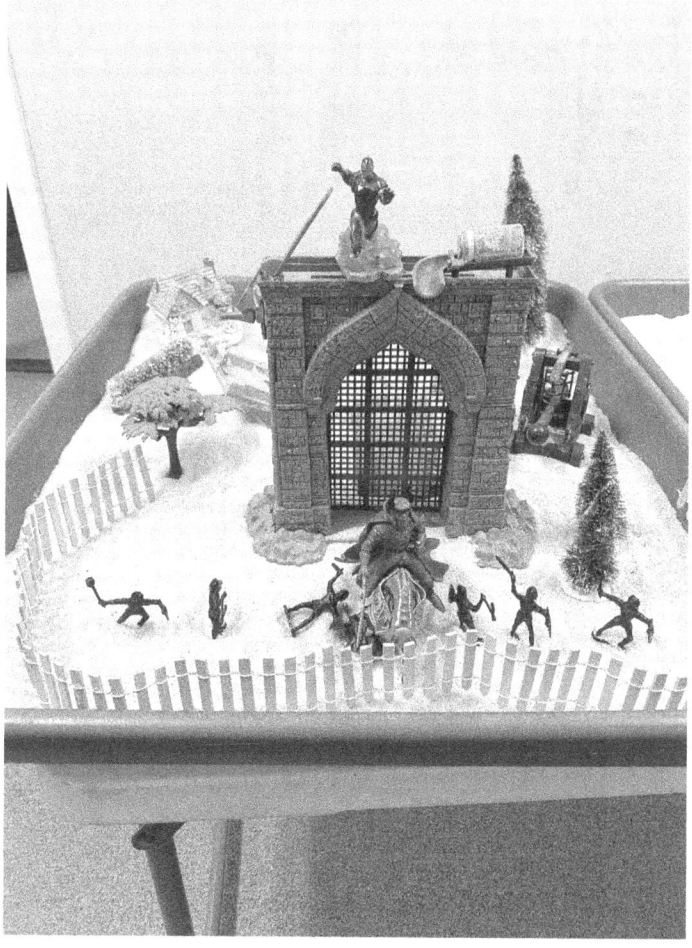

Figure 10.2 Flash, on top of the gate, adds extra protection against evil.

Asa noticed that there was a bridge from the defenses to the treasures on the other side. The treasures, or resources, could lead him to the calm/special place in the second tray. A fence assured that the calm was safely protected. The special place included a higher power, triumph, and the "future of success."

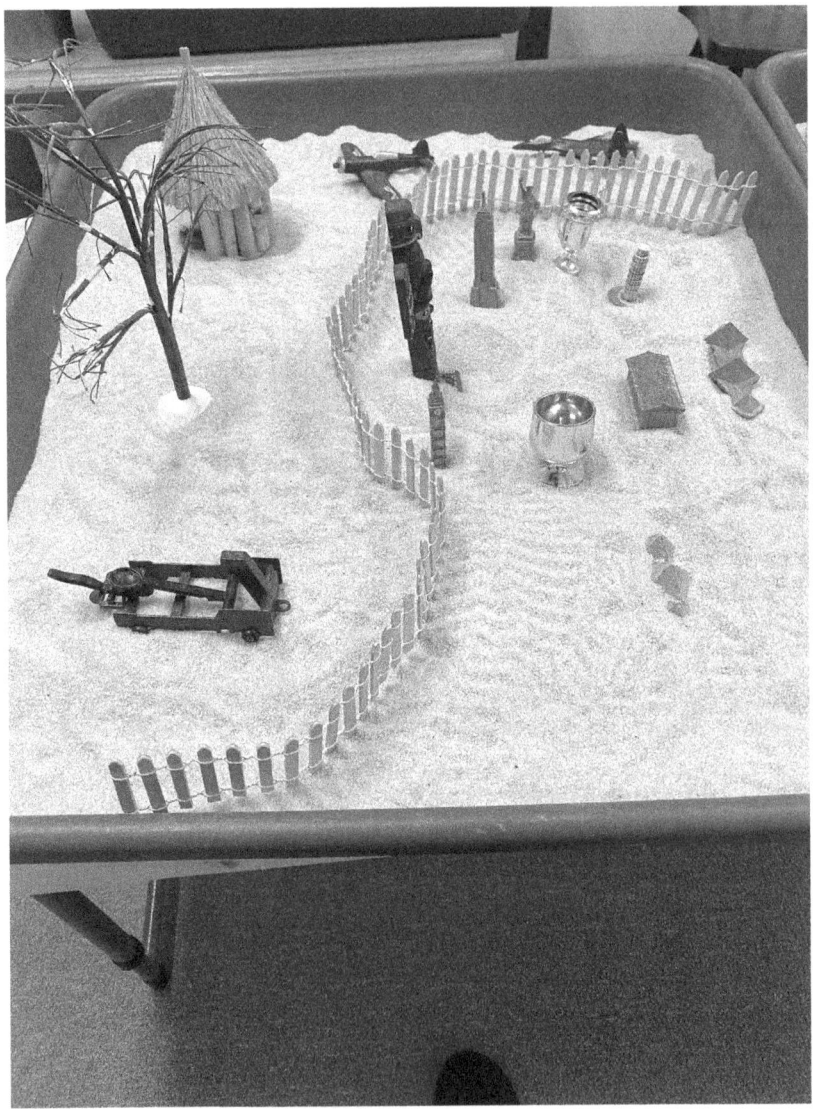

Figure 10.3 Asa's special place includes a higher power, triumph, and the "future of success."

As Asa processed, I used bilateral stimulation in the form of tapping on his shoulders and reminded him to "be with the feeling" or "just feel that feeling": the sensory connection to the speed of Flash, the powers to protect, the safety of the defenses, the resources that he could use to find his way, and the resources of a higher power and dreams for the future. Asa needed a tall wall, a gate (that could be open or closed), the power of magic, and a superhero to protect him from the forces of evil that he felt but could not see. Asa chose a superhero with the power of speed, a power that Asa did not possess given his disabilities. The word Asa chose to describe this place was "special." Using sensory experiences in the sand, creating a container in the tray, as well as a container in the supportive therapeutic relationship, fragments in the unconscious could be processed, and a new narrative could be written. I reminded Asa and his family that he could use the felt sense of this "special" place to help soothe himself and be calm in future sessions and at home as well.

The next time Asa returned to my office, we recalled his "special" place, and I reminded him he could return there whenever he needed. He was still having stomachaches, and Asa told me that his distress was at a level 10 on a scale of 0 to 10. "They hurt a lot," and he believed that they would hurt for a long time. I asked Asa what "yucky" thoughts he might have about his stomachaches. Referring to his extensive history of medical problems, most recently his belly pain, Asa sighed and said, "My body is against me." For children, negative beliefs are often concrete (Adler-Tapia & Settle, 2008). Asa's father was focused on the stomachaches, but Asa's concern was more global. If this was where Asa needed to go, this was where we would go. In response to the negative thought about his body I asked Asa to consider a positive one. At first, he gave me an incredulous look, then he said, "Of course, my body is not against me." This expectation may not have been realistic as a goal, but this was his positive thought at the moment.

I then invited Asa into the sandtray room and asked him to create a world for the negative and the positive thoughts. I expected trays full of figures, but Asa chose only two, both of which were from *Star Wars*. Kylo Ren, a male figure, stood in for "my body is against me." Rey, a female figure, took on the position "you have no power over me!" As the figures confronted one another in the sandtray, Asa's negative cognition softened, and he found his way to a more achievable positive thought. Asa could not conceive that his body was not against him, but he began to imagine that he had power over its constraints. As Kylo Ren and Rey battled in the sand, Asa became very animated and excited. Rey "pounded" Kylo Ren until he was covered with sand. At this point in the play, Asa realized that, in the heat of the battle, Rey's leg had broken. Asa looked at me with concern. I reassured him that

Rey fought the battle that needed to be fought and prevailed over Kylo Ren and that her injuries could be fixed. Again, I tapped Asa on his shoulders, reminding him to feel the experiences of the *Star Wars* figures in his own body. This symbol-driven installation could be experienced in Asa's body sensations, his thoughts, and his feelings. Asa left the session stating that his discomfort level was only half of what it was earlier and that he had a more positive attitude about the possible truth that he had power over the constraints of his body.

Asa continued his story in the following session. He asked if Rey had been fixed, and I had to admit I had not done so. Asa closely examined Rey then proceeded to put the two figures in the sand as he had done in the past. Asa and I discussed how Rey might be repaired, and Asa spotted a box of "inspirational adhesive bandages." He chose a bandage that read "You have the heart of a champion." We discussed the definition of the word "champion" and what it means to have the "heart of a champion." Asa carefully wrapped the bandage around Rey's broken leg, telling me that she had fought hard, had overpowered Kylo Ren, and that she was, in fact, a champion.

Bilaterally tapping on Asa's shoulders, I focused on the empowerment of the figures and instilled Asa's recognition of strength and power. I used the analogy for how Asa had battled his adversities and had the heart of a champion as well. Asa looked around for a box that could contain Kylo Ren and, not finding one, eventually settled on a paper bag. He placed the black, sand-covered figure of Kylo Ren in the bag and sealed it shut. He chose Hello Kitty™ duct tape, saying Kylo Ren "would not like the tape," and proceeded to tie the bag with purple and pink ribbons. There was no way Kylo Ren was going to get out!

I gave Asa the bag as well as the figure of Rey to remind him of his powers and his championship. This time, when I asked him to pick a word to describe how he felt, he chose the emotion "power." Wrapping up our session, I asked Asa to give an indicator of his level of disturbance, and he pointed to the drawing of a thermometer I use for children to show me their anxiety levels. Asa declared that "my body is against me" was at 0 and that his validity of cognition, or truth to the statement, was "only a little bit."

Installing a positive cognition via bilateral stimulation gave Asa the opportunity to reprocess stuck memories. I encouraged him to embody the word "power" that he held within himself and reminded him that he could recall the feeling of Rey's triumph over Kylo Ren whenever he had the thought that his "body was against him." As with Asa, children often reprocess quickly, given their less extensive memory networks (Adler-Tapia & Settle, 2008).

As Gomez (2019) suggests, the left hemisphere, silenced by trauma, can allow the right hemisphere to speak the language of metaphor through EMDR and intuitive expressions in the sand. Kestly (2014) reports that the "right-left-right progression as a child plays" can integrate the "divided brain" (pp. 123–124). Processing in both sides of the brain can facilitate resolution of a distressing experience through play, sandtray, and EMDR. Together, they have great potential and power.

Asa returned for several more sessions, and I inquired about the whereabouts of Kylo Ren and Rey and how he was using them. He told me that the bag with the figures was in a safe place, away from younger fingers, and that Asa and his parents talk about the figures and associated metaphors at home. Asa stated that Kylo Ren and Rey would need to stay where they were hidden but assured me he could find them if he needed them.

Much to their delight, the family reported that Asa was no longer complaining of stomachaches. Each week, Asa reported no distress about "my body is against me" and a firm belief when it came to "you have no power over me!" His stomachaches had gone away and not returned. Every time we met, I "scanned" his body for any physical connections to his target cognition and continued to use bilateral stimulation, either on his knees or shoulders, to strengthen and hold of the positive cognition ("you have no power over me").

In this phase of his therapy, Asa did not return to the sandtray. He used building materials and created elaborate structures. In his mastery over the materials, he embodied the word "power." He experienced his "power" as he beat me in basketball games and tossing a ball. I taught Asa to use "Dragon Wings," crossing his body with his arms and tapping his own shoulders as a self-calming technique. When Asa complained about his "annoying" little brother, I reminded him that he had the "heart of a champion" and could find ways to deal with a 2-year-old.

At the end of his therapy, Asa, his parents, and I had a party to celebrate his accomplhishments. We each contributed to the story of Asa and his journey in therapy. His father remarked that at first, Asa was resistant to coming to therapy; that he did not think that therapy could help a stomachache. His mother reported that she heard about the process of EMDR but had not attended any of the sessions in which it was used. Asa appeared pleased to talk to his mother about the journey of Rey and Kylo Ren and showed her how to use bilateral stimulation. I wrote Asa a letter, as I do with therapy endings, that told Asa what I had learned about him and offered wishes for the future. In the letter, I reminded Asa that he could use what he learned and could ask for help in the future. Asa reminded me that he "would probably have problems," so he would return.

Peer Consultation

I gasped when Asa stated, "My body is against me". Asa had just spoken the words describing my association with my body at the time. When I enter into a therapy session, my expectations include finding out something about the client and how they came to be where they are in the present moment, discovering something about the process of therapy, and sometimes I am handed the gift of unearthing something about me. Yes, thank you!

I have been a therapist for many years and have witnessed thousands of sandtray journeys, yet I still seek out the accompaniment of a peer who can support me in navigating the moments when professional and personal intersect. Asa's reaction to having a body that created limitations in his life touched me on a deeply personal level. It was time to explore the statement "My body is against me" in the sand. I reached out to my colleague and fellow sandtray therapist, Jacqueline, to accompany me on the journey. What follows is Jacqueline's experience of our work together.

Jacqueline Bears Witness

Elaine described how she chose the figure of the black oak tree to embody "my body is against me" and Rey (placed next to and facing the tree) to capture the words "you have no power over me." Elaine recognized that the aches and pains of getting older were behind her gasp in response to hearing "My body is against me." There were several pieces of gold placed throughout the tray, and Elaine made a connection with the gold used in past trays. There was a theme of gold, making gold, and the alchemy of making gold. With this connection, Elaine noticed that there were many pieces of gold in her world, which meant there was more to her than "my body is against me." The gasp of "my body is against me" is real, as is the unknown that

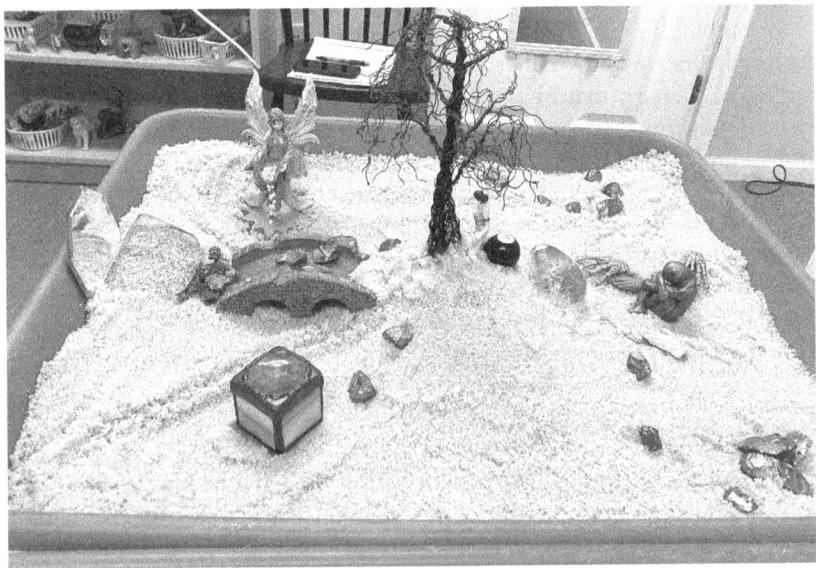

Figure 10.4 Elaine's tray processing "my body is against me."

comes with it. Elaine said, "my hope is that I have a Rey, fighting for me"; that she carries a Rey on the inside who will be with her, fighting whatever comes next.

Shifting focus to other parts of her sandtray world moved Elaine beyond the fear, where she discovered a bridge scattered with gold. Here, Elaine was able to sense that these gold pieces were resources. At first, the journey went over the bridge, but then she realized it was not a straight shot. Along the journey, there are many gifts, treasures, and boxes, but ultimately, there is death. As this reality settled in her body, Elaine focused on Rey and reflected, "My body is not going to determine where I am at this moment." Rey keeps telling the black oak tree, "You have no power over me." Rey is feeling powerful and is able to articulate that you are not defined by your body. The world within the tray can see what is happening and accept it. Death (the figure before the ultimate gold in the tray) is able to acknowledge that, yes, there is physical death, but there are many other deaths along the way, like the death of the negative belief for Asa. Her client, Asa, certainly struggled during his birth and through his developmental stages, just as Elaine struggled with the aches and pains of her developmental stage. Things have beginnings and endings, and all along the way, there is the gold.

After processing the tray with Elaine, I had a thought about the figures that Asa had chosen. Whether he was aware or not, Asa chose Rey and Kylo Ren from *Star Wars*. The story (and movies) of *Star Wars* borrows from mythology in the search for meaning, and a hero's journey in which the characters overcome adversities that challenge, sacrificing themselves for something larger. In this power of good over evil, the message is one of hope. Along the journey for these two characters, there are many deaths. Kylo Ren, at the end, used his own energy/body to save the life of Rey. This allowed Rey to heal, but it meant the end of Kylo Ren. This was witnessed in the journey for Asa. His body was against him, but along his journey, he was able to find the strength and power of Rey to heal. Through Asa's process, Elaine was given permission to consider the changes throughout a lifetime, beginnings and endings, and always gold.

Conclusion

I ran into Asa's parents in the community a couple years after he ended his therapy with me, and I learned that Asa had undergone surgery to correct his alignment and gait. He was recovering from the surgery and had had no unexplained stomachaches since our sessions. In preparation for writing this chapter, I contacted the family again. Asa was now in high school, doing well academically and interested in sports. While unable to participate in sports, he was knowledgeable about the teams, the players, and the stats on each one. He was planning to use this interest in sports as the foundation for a future career, or he just might decide to develop computer games instead! When asked what he remembered about our time together, Asa recalled,

"Playing with *Star Wars* and playing basketball on the door of your office and that I won!" Yes he did, and so did I.

Through the stages of EMDR, the battle of Rey and Kylo Ren in the sandtray, and ultimately the reprocessing of negative to positive beliefs (cognitions), Asa moved on from the pain and implicitly held trauma of his early life to create a new narrative. I could look at the aches and pains of aging and was reminded of the "gold" along the way, as well as beginnings and endings, births and deaths, and that we always have the power of connection and inner strength.

References

Adler-Tapia, R. (2017). *EMDR and the art of psychotherapy with children: Infants to adolescents treatment manual* (2nd ed.). Springer Publishing Company.

Adler-Tapia, R., & Settle, C. (2008). *EMDR and the art of psychotherapy with children* (1st ed.). Springer Publishing Company.

Association for Play Therapy. (2012). *Paper on touch: Clinical, professional & ethical issues.* www.a4pt.org/resource/resmgr/Publications/Paper_On_Touch.pdf

Beckley-Forest, A. (2016). Play therapy and EMDR. *Play Therapy, 10*(3), 11–14.

Gardener, S. L., Barland, K. R., Merenstein, S. L., & Lubchenco, L. O. (1993). The neonate and the environment: Impact on development. In G. B. Merenstein & S. L. Gardener (Eds.), *Handbook of neonatal intensive care* (3rd ed., pp. 564–608). Mosby Year Book.

Gomez, A. M. (2019). The world of stories and symbols: The EMDR sandtray protocol. *EMDR Magazine, 24*(1), 35–38.

Green, E. J., Crenshaw, D. A., & Kolos, A. C. (2010). Counseling children with preverbal trauma. *International Journal of Play Therapy, 19*(2), 95–105.

Greenspan, S. (1993). *Playground politics: Understanding the emotional life of school-age children.* Perseus Books Group.

Higgins-Klein, D. (2013). *Mindfulness-based play-family therapy: Theory and practice* (Illustrated ed.). W. W. Norton & Company, Inc.

Kestly, T. A. (2014). *The interpersonal neurobiology of play: Brain-building interventions for emotional well-being (Norton series on interpersonal neurobiology (Hardcover))* (1st ed.). W. W. Norton & Company, Inc.

Lovett, J. (2015). *Trauma-attachment tangle: Modifying EMDR to help children resolve trauma and develop loving relationships.* Routledge.

Maroney, D. (2003). Recognizing the potential effects of stress and trauma on premature infants in the NICU: How are outcomes affected. *Journal of Perinatol, 23*, 679–683. www.nature.com/articles/7211010

Norton, B., Ferriegel, M., & Norton, C. (2011). Somatic expressions of traumas in experiential play therapy. *International Journal of Play Therapy, 20*(3), 138–152.

Nosaarti, D., Reichenberg, A., Murray, R. M., Cnattingious, S., Lambe, M. P., Yin, L., MacCabe, J., Rifin, L., & Hultman, C. M. (2012). Preterm birth and psychiatric disorders in young adult life. *Archives of General Psychiatry, 69*(6), 610–617.

O'Shea, K., & Paulson, S. (2009). *When there are no words: Reprocessing early trauma & neglect held in implicit memory.* Sfrankelgroup.com. http://www.sfrankelgroup.com/courses/emdria/wtanw/WHEN%20NO%20WORDS%20handout%20text.pdf

Sanders, M. R., & Hall, S. L. (2018). Trauma-informed care in the newborn intensive unit: Promoting safety, security and connectedness. *Journal of Perinatology, 38*(1), 3–10. https://pubmed.ncbi.nlm.nih.gov/28817114/

Shapiro, F. (2001). *Eye movement desensitation and reprocessing: Basic principles, protocols, and procedures.* The Guilford Press.

Shapiro, F. (2012). *Getting past your past: Take control of your life with help techniques from EMDR therapy.* Rodale, Inc.

Shapiro, F. (2014). The role of eye movement desensitization and reprocessing (EMDR) therapy in medicine: Addressing the psychological and physical symptoms stemming from adverse life experiences. *Perm Winter, 18*(1), 71–77. www.ncbi.nlm.nih.gov/pmc/articles/PMC3951033/

Shapiro, F. (2016). *EMDR institute basic training course: Weekend 1 of the two party EMDR therapy basic training.* EMDR Institute.

Shapiro, F., & Merlis, D. L. (2014). *EMDR institute basic training course: Weekend 2 of the two party EMDR therapy basic training.* EMDR Institute.

Siegel, D., & Brcezyski, R. (2014). *(Permanenton-line series) rethinking trauma with Daniel Siegel, MD and Ruth Buczynski, PhD national institute for the clinical application of behavioral medicine how to use brain science to help patients accelerate healing after trauma.* https://s3.amazonaws.com/nicabm-stealthseminar/Rethinking-trauma-new/Dan/NICABM-DanSiegel_Part5-Transcript2.pdf

Tinker, B. A., & Wilson, S. A. (1999). *Through the eyes of a child (Norton professional books)* (Illustrated ed.). W. W. Norton & Company, Inc.

Went, M., & Struik, A. L. (2010). *The use of EMDR with infants.* Presentation at the 11th EMDR Europe Association Conference, Hamburg, Germany and retrieved from EMDR International Association, Francine Sharpiro Library: Creating Global Healing, Health and Hope.

Zelkowitz, P. (2017, April). *Prematurity | Prematurity and its impact on psychosocial and emotional development in children.* Encyclopedia on Early Childhood Development. www.child-encyclopedia.com/prematurity/according-experts/prematurity-and-its-impact-psychosocial-and-emotional-development#:%7E:text=These%20infants%20can%20also%20be,this%20may%20affect%20parenting%20behaviour

11 Working Across Cultures

Finding Common Ground in the Sand

Joanne Marie Wicks

Before we start, I would like to acknowledge the Aboriginal and Torres Strait Islander peoples as the traditional custodians of Australia's land and waters. I pay my respects to their Elders past and present and to the children who are their leaders of tomorrow. I acknowledge their history and the many thousands of years in which they have raised their children to be safe and strong (Australian Childhood Foundation, 2020). This Acknowledgment of Country is a crucial part of Australian culture when conducting a meeting or work on Australian land. I also feel it to be appropriate to disclose that I am a white Australian who does not claim to have expertise in Aboriginal culture. I wrote this chapter from the honorable experiences I have been granted throughout my career by being invited into many Aboriginal communities, homes, and families by Elders and Aboriginal community members.

I want to recognize and honor that no single Aboriginal culture represents any others. Although I will use the word *Aboriginal* to refer to Aboriginal peoples in this chapter generally, I respect that Aboriginal and Torres Strait Islander peoples comprise many languages, kinships, tribes, and ways of living (Atkinson, 2002). The term *communities* acknowledges Aboriginal peoples' diversity in Australia, each corresponding to unique histories, languages, political dynamics, cultural characteristics, economic resources, social situations, and Aboriginal Lore (Atkinson, 2002). For Aboriginal people, 'Country' does not just mean Australia as a whole. But instead, Country refers to many different and distinct groups, making up Australia. In Aboriginal ways, Country refers to the rivers, rock, hills, waterholes, as well as all living things; 'it is both a place of belonging and a way of believing' (Kwaymullina, 2005).

Australia is a vibrant, multicultural country. In 2016, two-thirds, roughly 65%, of the Australian population were born in Australia (Australian Bureau of Statistics, 2016). Nearly half, 49%, of Australians, had either been born overseas or had a parent born overseas (Australian Bureau of Statistics, 2016). With Australia's rich culture comes many multiple languages. There are more than 300 separately identified languages spoken in Australia, with about 20% of Australians speaking a language other than English at

DOI: 10.4324/9781003055808-13

home. After English, the next most common languages spoken at home are Mandarin, Arabic, Cantonese, and Vietnamese. Although Tasmania had the highest rate of people speaking only English at home with 88%, the Northern Territory (NT), where I live, had the lowest rate of about 60% of English-speaking households (Australian Bureau of Statistics, 2016). This means that I would commonly work with multi-lingual people. Therefore, using an interpreter, whether it is for an Aboriginal family or migrated family, is something that I am very familiar with in my therapeutic practice. This also means that relying on mediums of therapy that prize non-verbal communication, such as sandtray therapy or play therapy, allows me to access the world of many people, which other services might have to refer out, due to language barriers.

Sandtray therapy is a powerful healing tool that offers the client an opportunity to communicate their experiences without requiring them to speak verbally. Throughout this chapter, you will be introduced to two clients of mine. Their names, ages, identities, gender, and details have been changed substantially to protect their confidentiality; despite the permission, they have granted me to use their stories for teaching purposes. The pictures of their sandtrays have also been re-created by me as an attempt to protect their privacy further. Aliyah's story involves a small young girl who sought asylum in Australia with her family. She experienced terror beyond her capabilities, where her mind and body struggled with managing the experiences. Sandtray therapy provided an opportunity for her to share her world when her voice failed her. Samantha's story explores the world of a young girl who is wise beyond her years, mainly because her Aboriginal ancestors are always with her, guiding her.

Australia

In Australia, Aboriginal people represent 3.3% of the Australian population and 30% of the Northern Territory people – the highest proportion of any state or territory in Australia (Australian Bureau of Statistics, 2016). Aboriginal people's and families' contemporary life should be considered in the context of colonization, displacement from Country, assimilation policies, intergenerational trauma, deprivation, transgenerational forced child removals, and current discrimination. Aboriginal peoples are arguably the most disadvantaged group in Australia and have suffered extensive adversity (Atkinson, 2002; Hunter, 2007; Silburn et al., 2006). Additionally, Aboriginal children are over-represented in child protection and out-of-home care services compared to non-Indigenous (Australian Bureau of Statistics, 2016). For example, one in six Aboriginal and Torres Strait Islander children received child protection services, which is 6.5 times more than non-Indigenous children. However, Aboriginal peoples and their communities' have a long history of resilience and growth in the face of adversity and trauma (Dudgeon & Kelly, 2014). These powerful characteristics are also passed down transgenerationally.

Aboriginal families and communities are built around the Aboriginal identity, which includes belonging to an Aboriginal community, deep connection to Country, cooperation governed by sophisticated kinship systems, and participation in custodial ceremonies (Dudgeon & Kelly, 2014). The Aboriginal identity is often a source of strength, growth, and empowerment for Aboriginal people, serving as a protective factor from adverse experiences. Rich in their culture is the power of storytelling; this includes sand stories. Dating back to 1915, the first description of Australian Aboriginal sand stories emerged when missionary Carl Strehlow described a sand story game involving leaves, which Western Arrernte women played at Hermannsburg (Green, 2015). The traditional narratives that were told in the sand were a combination of gesture, speech, hand signs, and song to communicate meaningfully to each other. Deep in the language of Arrernte, Warlpiri, and Western Desert peoples in Central Australia, sand stories and sand iconographic symbols are still used as a form of language in this part of Country (Green, 2015). These stories are richly articulated in Jennifer Green's (2015) book *Drawn from the Ground* and demonstrate the potential for Sandtray to be a culturally relevant form of therapy for Aboriginal peoples.

Samantha's Story

Samantha was a girl about 7 years old. Her hair was black and curly, often half tied back from her face with a braid, and she was always wearing a smile. Samantha would walk in well before her Aunty Jean arrived at the office door. She must have bolted from the car the moment she was told it was safe to run to my door. Samantha had a bounce about her, something that made you always smile back. It was hard to believe that Samantha's first few years of life were not anything to smile about. Samantha was born and raised in Country. Her mum, a proud Aboriginal lady, was well known and respected around Community. Samantha was the third child to her mum and the first child to her dad. Samantha's dad was not well known to the community.

A few months into Samantha's life, her mum was heavily consuming drugs and alcohol. The child protection worker explained that Samantha's father had introduced her mother to drugs to keep her under his control, which child protection stated, was something he had done to previous women in previous relationships. Additionally, he was very intimidating and violent. One night, when Samantha was 6 months old, he had hurt her mum so severely that she was almost unrecognisable. This was the first time Samantha had gone into care with child protection. After a few weeks of being in care, Samantha was returned to her mum, along with her two other siblings. Several months later, the family violence happened again, and Samantha was removed, only to be returned shortly after and so on. The child protection worker said that when Samantha was 2 years old, they did not know where her mum and dad were and that Samantha was living with a relative. The story was that her parents had gone into town for a few days and had not returned. However, because Samantha was safe, alongside her siblings, and in the care of kinship, presenting as happy, that is where she would stay until her parents returned. A couple of months later, the kinship family member fell ill, and Samantha and her two siblings were placed in the foster care system, kilometres away from her Aboriginal community. After moving homes several times, with several different carers, she was placed with Aunty Jean.

Aunty Jean was patient. She was not Aboriginal but Fijian and had a lot of family around her. She had a biological son of her own, who was in his teens, and a husband who the children called Uncle and who worked away a lot. Aunty Jean had been caring for Samantha and her siblings for about 4 years by the time I met her. Aunty Jean's skin color was a lot lighter than Samantha's, but Samantha said her skin was the same color as Uncle's. Samantha said she would attend church on Sundays and went to a school that had 'church talk' in it.

Samantha's child protection worker told me that her mother was sober now and was interested in having Samantha back in her care. Over the years, the children and the mum had contact with each other, which often went well. Child protection was considering if it was time to reunify Samantha to her mum's care once they ensured it would be safe. Samantha was brought to me to support the process of reunification by providing Samantha with a space to process her experiences. I was allocated 10 therapy sessions for Samantha and several extra sessions to work with Aunty Jean and Uncle, as well as a couple of sessions allocated to work with Mum should the child protection department decide that reunification was going ahead. Samantha's siblings had therapy with other clinicians at another service. This amount of therapy sessions and multiple allocations to different therapy practice is not unusual in the Northern part of Australia.

I remember meeting Samantha; she stood close to her Aunty Jean, holding her hand tightly. She was polite and smiled for the whole time. However, her body did not show me she felt safe. Her body stood rigid as if at any moment, she was ready to run for the door. She observed me closely and at times glanced to her Aunty Jean for reassurance. I had already completed a carer's intake-consultation with Aunty Jean without Samantha present prior to this session. I ensured that Aunty had an idea of what the first session would look like for Samantha. Samantha, on the other hand, was not sure about me at all but continued to act polite and pleasing.

I started the initial session off with our greetings by explaining who I am and that many children call me 'the Feelings Doctor'. I explained my job was to play with children by helping them, if they wanted to, make stories about their feelings using sand and toys. I told Samantha that I have two other parts to my job. I explained that

> one part of my job is that I am a privacy keeper, that the things you share with me stay private, but you can share what we do and say in here, but I won't share it with other people unless you ask me too. The

other part of my job is being a safety keeper. That means I am one of the people who help to keep you and others safe. If someone is hurting you or hurting someone else, then I must tell other adults what I am worried about it, and that means I might tell other adults what you say or do in here, only if I am worried.

Samantha smiled and said 'Okay, can I see the toys and sand now?' I explained Aunty would be in the waiting room while we go into the Sandtray room and that she can go check in with Aunty if she needs to. Samantha nodded her head to indicate she understood.

In the sandtray room, Samantha was delighted. She looked at every shelf and every item. She touched what I assume where her favorite ones as she said, 'I love you and you and you and you'. My sandtray is on wheels, so she pushed it over to the shelves and kept exploring all the miniatures. Eventually, she collected a few and dropped them in the tray. She picked them up, one by one, and placed them around the tray where she thought they should go. I sat quietly, close in proximity, feeling privileged to watch her create a world. Samantha worked her way around the sandtray as if she had done this many times before. I remembered asking her Aunty and the protection worker if she had ever had therapy, and both had said she had not. Yet, she seemed comfortable and content. This isn't always a feeling experienced in the very first therapy session.

Samantha's first sandtray world was intriguing. I have re-created her tray for the purpose of this chapter. Samantha had placed a snake in the middle of the tray; the snake was red and thin and faced away from her. Around the snake were gems and diamonds and jewels. On one side of the tray, she had placed scary creatures with three heads, dragons and vicious-looking lions, tigers and monsters. Halfway down the tray, there were other mystical figures such as mermaids, ponies, rainbows and presents. She slowly placed all the items how she wanted them without speaking a word. She was careful and deliberate. At the end of the session, I asked her if she wanted to give the tray a name, and she said, 'The Snake Is Like Christmas, Only Santa Doesn't Come'. Well, I did not expect that! I had experienced her placing some evil-villain-like items in the tray, but nothing that felt as devastating as Santa not arriving on Christmas day. At the time, I thought I had done an excellent job of not showing Samantha the shock I experienced when she named the tray. I walked her back to her Aunty, said goodbye, and went back into the sandtray room to view her tray again. I was very curious but not knowing, as this was her first tray and our first connection together. Because of that, I did not want to jump to any conclusions. I wrote my notes, and next week came around very quickly.

Samantha was in her school uniform, hair neatly done, and she had her big smile worn proudly on her face. She was at the door well before Aunty. She seemed excited and ready to start. Aunty took a seat away

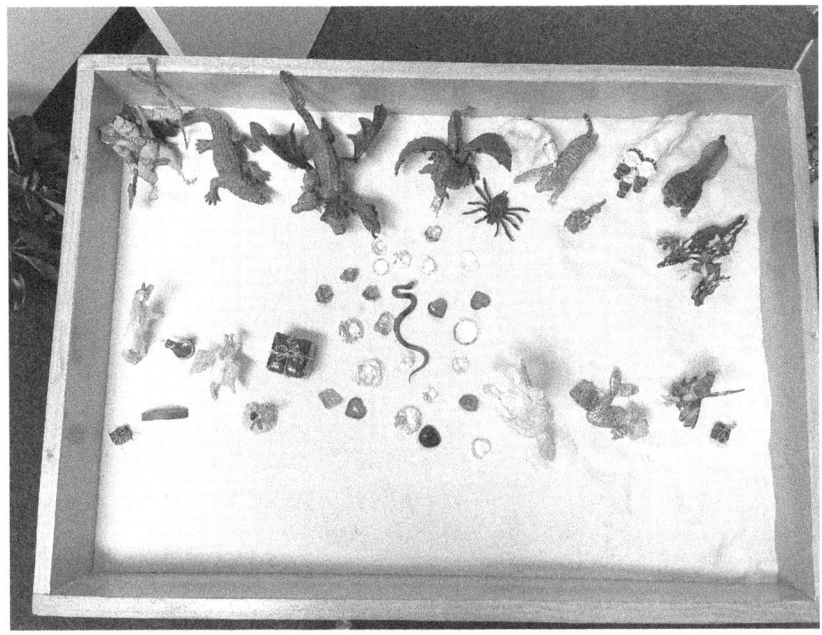

Figure 11.1 Samantha's first sandtray, titled 'The Snake Is Like Christmas, Only Santa Doesn't Come'.

from the sandtray room, and Samantha and I went into the room. Samantha collected the same mermaids, fairies, princess and queens. She placed them all around, making the tray as beautiful as she could. She didn't talk in this session, but it was apparent she was delighted by her creation. I could tell by her body language and face. The session ended, and she named it 'The Princess Valley'; there were no villains, evil or baddies, just beauties. She left the sandtray room happily. The tone of this session was significantly different from the last. Her third sessions came around as another week went by.

Her third session was similar to her second, filled with prettiness and beauty. I think she called the third session's sandtray 'The Magic Fairyland'. After this session, I was confused; something didn't feel like it did the first time I had met her. Even Aunty seemed different, but I couldn't place it. That week, I tried to reach Aunty by phone, but we kept missing each other, and before I knew, it her fourth week came around.

Samantha's fourth session started like her last three. With smiles and excitement, Samantha beat Aunty to the door and entered the sandtray

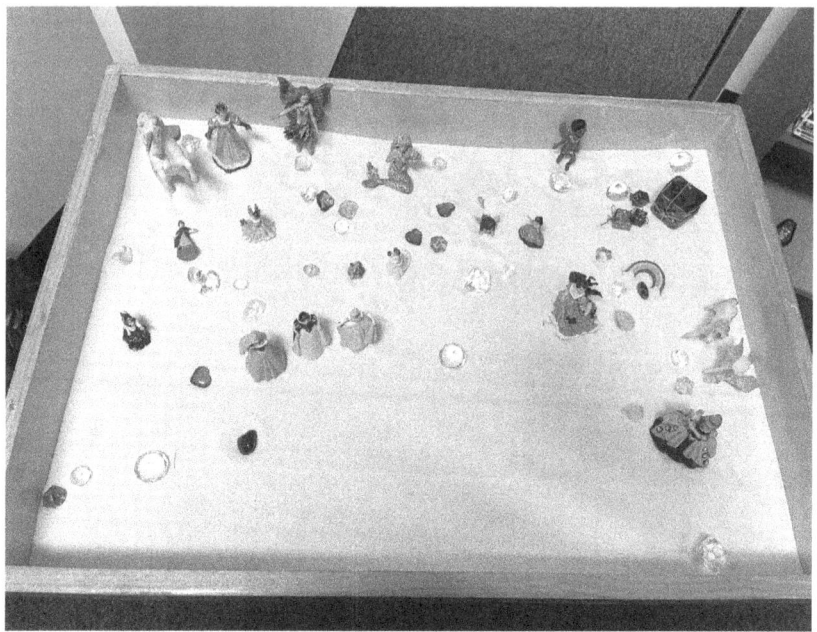

Figure 11.2 Samantha's second sandtray, titled 'The Princess Valley'.

room with enthusiasm. She picked the red snake up again for the first time since her first session. She got the gems, jewels and diamonds and sprawled them all around the snake. She picked villains and scary creatures and placed them at the bottom of the tray, and then she placed some creepy-looking items at the top of the tray. Like all her sessions, she spoke zero words. This was expected, as the miniatures were her words and creating her world was her way of telling a story. Her smile had faded as this session had progressed. It felt serious. I sat close by and watched as she built something important. She had the mermaids and princesses in the tray, but they were not near the snake. They were placed in the corner of the tray and seemed to be well out of the way. At the end of the session, I asked her to give the tray a title, and she said, 'The Best Day of Your Death'. I was very curious about this tray title, but it seemed fitting with what she had created.

Later in the week, I was able to get in touch with Aunty via phone. She explained that Samantha had been required to create a PowerPoint presentation at school about the 'best day of her life'. She filled the PowerPoint with all her favorite shows, favorite foods and favorite things. Nothing atypical that a 7-year-old would not want on their best day. Additionally, Aunty informed me that mum was going to start having more access next week.

She would have the children after school a few days a week and would be required to return them just after dinner.

During Samantha's fifth and sixth sessions, the snake was in the middle of the tray again, surrounded by baddies and mean like-creatures on the top and bottom. The beauties and princesses were placed far away to the side. She named these trays with a similar tone to her first and fourth sessions. At her seventh session, she said goodbye to Aunty in the waiting room and walked confidently into the sandtray room. She drew shapes in the sand, circles and dots. She placed the red snake in the middle and collected the evil creatures as she had in her previous sessions.

Once she put the items where they belonged, she moved the red snake closer to the evil creatures. The evil creatures picked the snake up and tossed it to the other side of the tray where other bad creatures resided. This session was alive, and the red snake moved around the tray, being tossed back and forth between the darkened miniatures. Samantha did not say much, but she did say, 'The snake is trying to join them, and they hate the snake and say no'. I reflected and said, 'Ooh, so the snake wants to be with these baddies, but they don't want it to join them'. Samantha responded, 'Yeah, they said no, and now they are hurting it, to teach it a lesson'.

This process of back and forth went on for the rest of the session. No matter how the snake tried to join the baddies, it did not succeed. The snake did not go near the beauty-like items. With no conclusion, her session ended, and she walked out to Aunty. I wondered was the snake a baddie too? And if so, why did the other baddies reject it?

Samantha's child protection worker called me a few days before her eighth session and said there had been an incident with Samantha and her mother. She informed me that while caring for the children, Samantha's mother was under the influence of drugs and had tried to get hit by cars as an attempt of suicide. Since the incident, Mum was in the care of the hospital. No one was hurt physically, but the ordeal emotionally impacted the children.

Samantha arrived for her eighth session as she had all her other sessions, excited to see me and be in the sandtray room. She created a similar scene as in her previous session, only this time, the red snake had a brown snake with it. Both were thrown back and forth, at times violently, for the remainder of the session between groupings of bad and evil miniatures. Samantha stated that 'The snakes don't know how to say "no" to the baddies first. The villains always say no to the snakes and they have to just keep trying, even though they are saying no to them'. I reflected, 'Hmm, so even though these are the baddies, the snakes want to be included with them, even though they don't do kind things'. She said, 'Yep, confusing, huh?' I nodded and agreed. I was definitely confused. I asked about the mermaids and why they were there. Samantha said, 'It's not their time yet, they have to wait until the snakes are done'. That's all that was said verbally in session eight. The session ended, and she left.

Between sessions eight and nine, I had had many conversations with Aunty Jean and the child protection worker. I had provided skills and scripts for them to hold safety conversations with Samantha about her mum's behavior on the road and why she was in hospital. I had also spoken to her school to provide support and strategies. I was aware that my allocated therapy sessions were coming to an end, and I wanted to ensure that the adults in her life felt capable and had the skills to continue to support Samantha once my therapeutic relationship finished. Because of this, I met with her school and Aunty Jean a few times over my course of treatment.

Samantha arrived for her tenth session. She knew this was her last before school holidays started and her family, with Aunty and Uncle, would go away on holidays. I was hoping I would see Samantha in the new year with an approved amount of new sessions; however, that would be two months away.

She was excited to see me, as she was for all her sessions. She created her world, using the miniatures she had always used. Only she did not pick up the snake right away; typically, that was the item she collected first. She had the baddies at the top and some at the bottom of the world, with the beauties to the side. The snake had not been placed in the tray yet . . . She seemed to have finished the building of her tray and said, 'Dr. Jo, do you notice where the snakes are?' I said in response, 'Hmm, the snakes are not where I can see them'. And she said, 'Yes they are! You have to look harder'. I got closer and looked around the tray. I knew she hadn't used the snakes because they were still on the shelf behind her, so I said, 'Samantha, I am looking very hard, but I am not able to see where the snakes are'. She then said, 'They are in the spine of the mermaid, and the legs of the princesses, and the hair of the queens, and the wings of the fairies'.

Samantha continued to say, 'The snakes are inside them all; they always have been, and no one ever knows'. She said, 'My mum is trying to tame some of her snakes right now. Snakes don't often do as they are told, even though they know right from wrong. I have some of my mum's snakes in me, and she has her mum's snakes in her, and her mum probably has her mum's snakes too'. Samantha then said she wanted to call this tray 'The Snake That Doesn't Win But Is Always There'.

Samantha continued to say,

> Dr. Jo, the gems are in the beauties too, they are from the mums and their mums. Those gems are for the mermaids, fairies and queens to give to their baby mermaids and baby fairies and baby queens. They don't own them, just keep them safe until it's not their turn to have them anymore.

I reflected, 'The beauties have an important job, to tame their snakes and to keep the gems safe until they give them to their children'. Samantha said, 'Yep, this is titled "The Gift"'. And she took the red snake off the shelf as she walked out the door, placed it in the middle of the tray and said, 'Isn't it better if we could see people's red snakes? Not keep them hidden and secret?'

The session came to an end, and we said our goodbyes and that we would hope to see each other again in the new year if she needed.

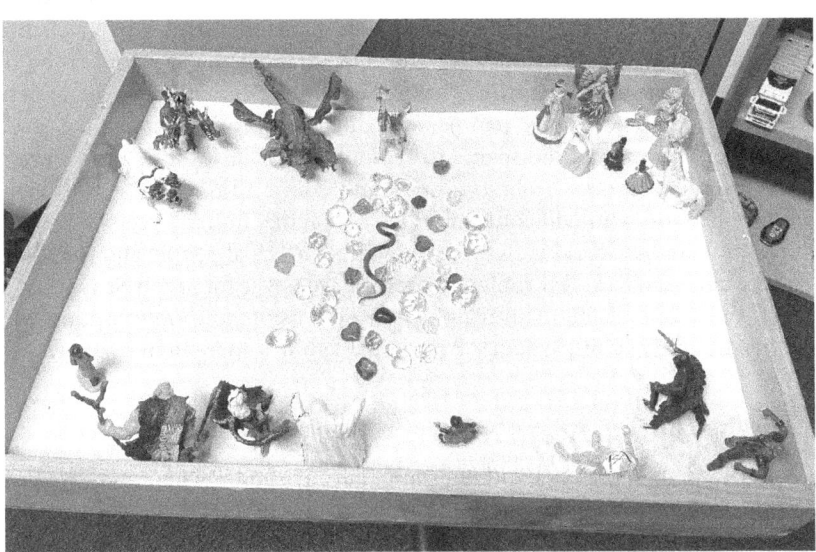

Figure 11.3 Samantha's final sandtray session, titled 'The Gift'.

My Reflection on Samantha

Samantha's sandtray sessions were primarily non-verbal. She spoke when she felt like it was needed or when I prompted her out of my deep curiosity that couldn't be ignored. I recognize that asking questions for clarification met more of my needs than the need of Samantha, but it did not seem to disrupt or distract her from her process. However, Samantha showed me that ultimately, creating and building a sandtray was enough for her and that verbally processing her world was not as important. Samantha was guided to go where she needed to go by her inner drive for healing, and I was fully present with her, so she wasn't on her own.

I didn't know precisely what the snake meant at the start of her sessions. And I must admit, I also didn't feel that the sessions that were filled with beauty, such as session two's 'The Princess Valley', were very meaningful at the time. However, as the sandtray journey progressed, I soon became aware of how important those sessions were to her. She taught me that even though I didn't have a comprehensive understanding of each world she made, they were every bit as important to her and her therapy journey.

As she described her last session for me, in spoken words, I soon understood that she, transgenerationally, brought the good and the bad with each living generation. Still, I didn't know specifically what the snakes meant before the tenth session. And the truth is, I didn't need to know for it to matter to her. Before she told me, I wanted to know, I wanted to ask 100 million questions, but how distracting and disrupting would that have been to her process? Also, would it have led me to know more than what

I know now? Samantha taught me that I did not need to know via her verbal words for her process to be useful for her. Samantha expressed grief, loss, rejection and disconnection throughout her trays as each session passed by. She did so without saying many words at all. She brought out the experience of intergenerational trauma, without probably knowing there was a word for it, and used the snakes to symbolize it. But what she also showed was transgenerational healing, growth and connection to those who came before her and who will come after her. Samantha, in her 7 years of life, was able to share her world views, the view of Aboriginal people and the values of the ancestry with few spoken words. I have never forgotten Samantha; in fact, she is one of the main reasons I am so passionate about working with different cultures, in particular Aboriginal families and children, today.

Aliyah's Story

Aliyah was an 8-year-old with a 5-year-old sister and residing in a detention centre in Australia because her mum and dad had fled their war-torn country for safety. The family had been detained in Australia for several months before I met them. Immigration detention centres were set up all around Australia to detain people seeking asylum despite asylum seeking being legal in Australia. The detention centres were controversial, and so was the work associated with them. Families often travelled by dangerously made boats to Australia from other countries. Many never completed the journey. My default stance was well articulated by Warsan Shire (*"Home" by Warsan Shire, 2009*), who said, 'you have to understand that no one puts their children in a boat unless the water is safer than the land'. Let me tell you; the water was never safe.

Aliyah showed us with every behavioral movement she made that she was not feeling safe. The medical doctors described Aliyah as 'a young girl who was riddled with anxiety and fear'. They reported that she never played in the compound playground or smiled at others who passed her by. She wet the bed every night and barely ate any food. She did not speak to anyone, including her family members, unless it was in a whisper, and still then it was minimal. She screamed and cried if her parents left her for even a moment. Her primary language is Farsi, and though her parents said she knows English well, since being detained in Australia, they were starting to doubt whether she knows any language at all due to her lack of speech.

I spent some time talking with her parents while Aliyah lay under their chairs, making very small, restricted movements. I spoke very briefly, without detail, about trauma, its impact on children and the symptoms she demonstrated. I described sandtray therapy as a non-verbal form of therapy but explained that I did not have the sand with me due to it being restricted in the compound. However, I did have the miniature toys, which can be effective without sand. I explained that they could wait outside the room for the session and that we would leave the door open so Aliyah could come in once she felt safe to do so. I explained an interpreter would be in the room with me and that I had trained the interpreter with therapeutic language to assist with her session. Her parents agreed and wanted to try it, saying they would speak with Aliyah and get back to me. Later that day, they told me she was reluctant but curious and that she had agreed to come, so we booked a session for the next day.

Because I didn't have a lot of time in this detention centre, I planned to provide Aliyah with an intensive variant of sandtray therapy, meaning we would have up to three sessions in a week. When Aliyah arrived for her first session, she came into the room holding her mum tight. I verbally greeted her with the interpreter alongside me and sat close by on the ground while the interpreter sat on a chair. I deliberately placed the interpreter on a chair because I was aware of the number of adults in one room for a single small child. I wanted to create a bit of difference between the adults. However, I feel my efforts might have been in vain because Aliyah was so focused on what she needed to do that I don't think it would have mattered where people were located in the room. Her mum gently sat her on the ground near the pile of sandtray toys. Her mum took a seat close behind her. Aliyah crept closer to the miniatures and started to move the toys around with her hand. The interpreter informed me before Aliyah arrived that she would never have seen toys like this before. Aliyah seemed curious. She very seriously and quickly placed the toys around the space. She did not look at them for long but appeared to order them how she needed them to be. After 15 to 20 minutes, she stood up and dragged her mum to the door and left. Not a single word was spoken. All the items she had placed seemed to be under threat. The small might be afraid of the large. The group might be afraid of the gang. There was no safety, only threat and danger for every item she touched.

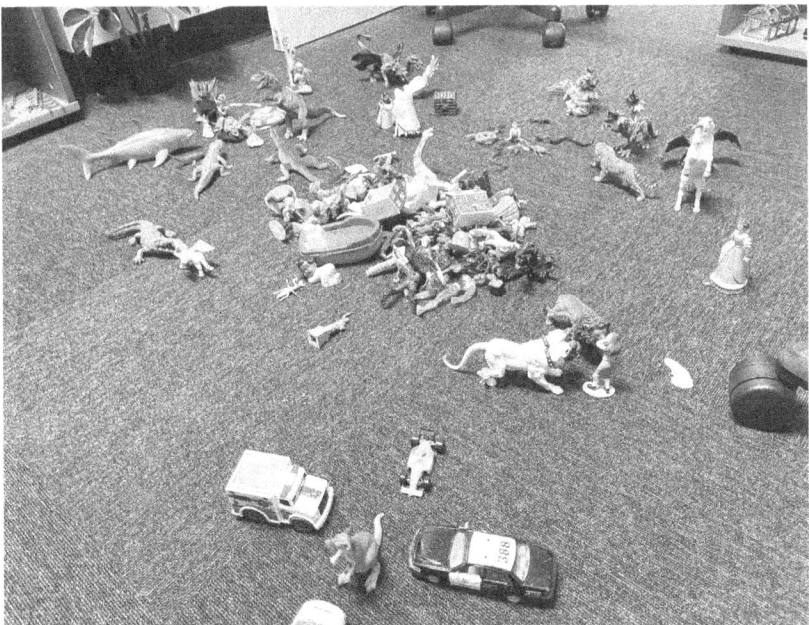

Figure 11.4 Aliyah's first encounter with sandtray figures.

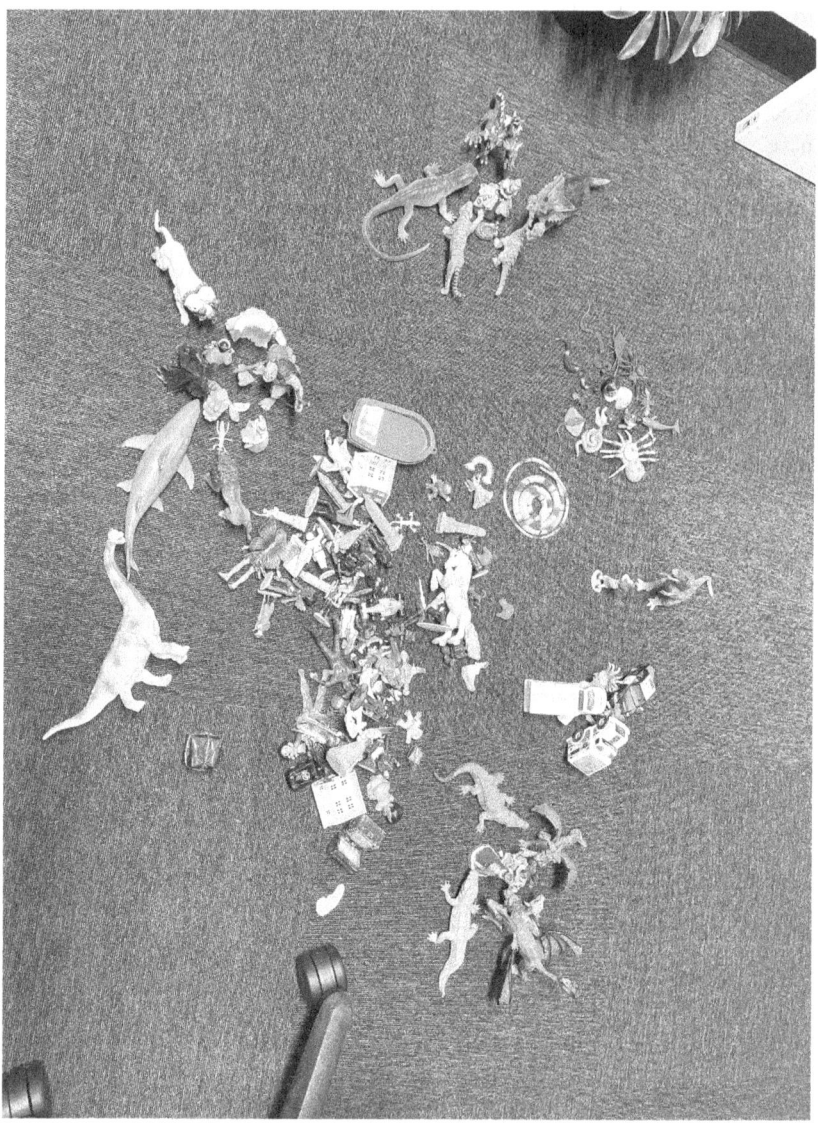

Figure 11.5 Aliyah's first arrangement seems to touch experiences of threat.

Her second session began like her first. Aliyah walked into the room clutching her mum tightly, yet she remained very curious. Like before, the miniatures were placed in the middle of the room jumbled up. She sat by them and began building. She moved the toys, placing them in a similar fashion to her first session, only this time the threat and danger were closer and more fearful.

Aliyah's third session was similar to her first two. It went for 15 to 20 minutes and used the same items, and she left the room without speaking.

I wasn't able to capture images of this session due to restrictions with phones in the compound at the time. In sessions four and five, she created the familiar scenes; however, with each session the threats came closer, bigger and more violating. The miniatures were placed with more danger, threat and harm than her previous sessions. Everything seemed to have something to be afraid of. Aliyah never spoke a word in any of her sessions. Her body was restricted, and her facial features were still and focused.

Session six was different. Not only was this our last time together, which I didn't know at the time, but my experience of her was also different. She seemed lighter, still restricted with minimal affect but more relaxed in her body. I hadn't been able to catch up with her parents or any medical personnel prior to this session but had planned to later that day. Aliyah placed the miniatures in their positions, only they had more space between them.

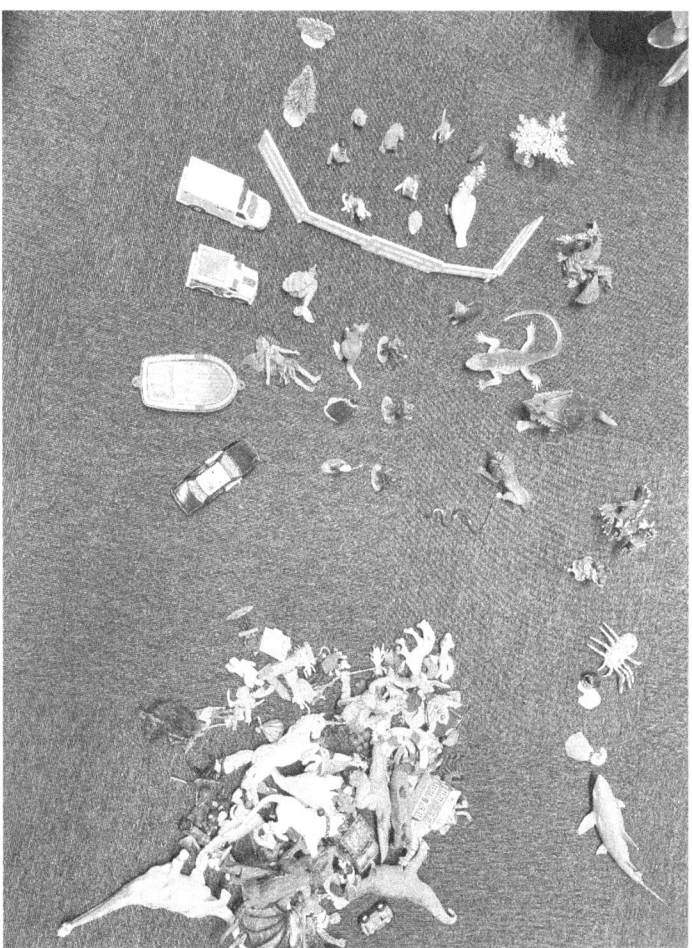

Figure 11.6 Aliyah's last session.

There were opportunities for movement, and maybe a possible escape, should they have chosen to come alive and move. She had babies grouped together now, which previously were always isolated and threatened individually by something bigger and scary. She placed smaller threats with smaller items, where previously they were surrounded by large scary figures as if, now, they were more evenly matched in their challenge.

Beside her, she placed a fence with trees and what felt like 'hope'. This was the first time she had placed any nature-life miniatures in any of her worlds. She had animals and small creatures grouped together as if they were going to be okay. She didn't verbalize this, but it was a felt sense. She also had uniformed people on the outside near the more significant threats. I wasn't sure if the uniformed people were safe or harmful, but at the time, I remember feeling as if they were placed for safety. As was her way, when Aliyah finished, she hopped up, took her mum's hand and left the room without any words. I didn't know I wasn't going to see her again, as she abruptly left the detention centre that day to reside in an Australian town. But I think of her often.

I spoke with the medical professionals who had spent time with her parents earlier that day. They reported that Aliyah had shown a significant reduction in her symptomatic behavior. They had observed her playing in the compound playground with her sister two days prior. She had kept her bed dry three nights that week and volunteered to go to the food mess with her dad to get food for the whole family. Although Aliyah wasn't entirely safe in the detention centre, it appeared that her perception of safety was increasing, and her sense of threat was decreasing. In a matter of two weeks and no more than six sessions of 20 minutes with no sand or words, Aliyah was able to show a glimpse of her world and begin to experience the possibility of moving into a potentially safe future. After all, this was what her parents hoped for when they choose to put their two small children and themselves into the water to travel to Australia.

My Reflection on Aliyah

Aliyah solidified my appreciation for an intensive model of therapy. She showed that with only a few sessions, in a short amount of time, a non-verbal medium of therapy can be helpful. Her use of words, through the miniatures, ones she would have likely not been exposed to before, still spoke to her and therefore spoke to me. This therapeutic exchange is what sets sandtray therapy apart from any verbal-based therapy.

Working with interpreters has its benefits and its challenges, especially when you are attempting to deliver a medium of therapy that prizes non-verbal communication. Sometimes, I had a lot of time to prepare interpreters, explaining the therapeutic process, expectations and possible scenarios children might demonstrate in their sessions. Other times, I had no preparation time, and we would start facilitating therapeutic work together like an awkward dance. One layer that I had to consider when working with interpreters was that their personal history often had similar themes to those of the clients we worked with together. I ensured that I had space for my interpreters like I did for my clients. It was important that I held space for them to process the content of what was experienced as they helped me in my job.

It was also important for me to intentionally consider my choice of miniatures provided for my clients of diverse backgrounds, as these are their words in therapy. What this specifically looks like will be different for everyone. For example, the interpreter mentioned that Aliyah would not have seen toys like the ones I offered. While that might have been true, and Aliyah was demonstrating severe restrictive behaviors, this did not hold her back from expressing her world vividly as the sessions went on for her. This is an important component of sandtray therapy; children are capable of finding what they need to say with what is provided, whether it is familiar or completely novel, but if we can make it easier for them to communicate their world, then the felt sense of safety might arrive sooner. Finding miniatures that resemble the faith, values, animals, food, music, clothing, culture and history of the people you work with is vital and honoring to those we serve. The collection does not necessarily have to be extensive, but it does need to be intentional.

Conclusion

Primarily non-verbal therapeutic models allow you to cross communication barriers while being able to establish rapport and connection required for psychological change. The two examples provided here demonstrate the simplistic non-verbal power of sandtray therapy without undermining the complex psychological intervention that it is. Sandtray therapy can access the world of people of all ages, from all backgrounds, from all language groups, because it symbolically speaks to each individual person. They, as the client, create their stories, they create their worlds, and they share their experiences, wishes and wants, all on their terms. As it has been described throughout this book, sandtray is a dynamic therapy that is imbedded in neurobiological science, demonstrated through a therapeutic relationship, allowing people to share experiences that are often left unheard and unseen. Sandtray therapy makes the invisible visible.

References

Atkinson, J. (2002). *Trauma trails, recreating song lines: The transgenerational effects of trauma in indigenous Australia.* Spinifex Press.

Australian Bureau of Statistics. (2016). *Estimates of aboriginal and torres strait islander Australians.* Australian Bureau of Statistics.

Australian Childhood Foundation. (2020). *Personal communication.* Australian Childhood Foundation.

Dudgeon, P., & Kelly, K. (2014). Contextual factors for research on psychological therapies for aboriginal Australians. *Australian Psychologist*, *49*(1), 8–13. https://doi.org/10.1111/ap.12030

Green, J. (2015). *Drawn from the ground: Sound, sign and inscription in Central Australian sand stories: Language culture and cognition*. Series Number 13. Cambridge University Press. https://doi.org/10.1017/CBO9781139237109

"Home" by Warsan Shire. (2009). Facing History and Ourselves. www.facinghistory.org/standing-up-hatred-intolerance/warsan-shire-home

Hunter, E. (2007). Disadvantage and discontent: A review of issues relevant to the mental health of rural and remote aboriginal Australians. *The Australian Journal of Rural Health*, *15*(2), 88–93. doi:10.1111/j.1440-1584.2007.00869.x

Kwaymullina, A. (2005, May/June). Seeing the light: Aboriginal law, learning and sustainable living in country. *Indigenous Law Bulletin*, *6*(11).

Silburn, S. R., Zubrick, S. R., Lawrence, D. M., Mitrou, F. G., De Maio, J. A., Blair, E., & Hayward, C. (2006). The intergenerational effects of forced separation on the social and emotional wellbeing of aboriginal children and young people. *Family Matters*, *75*, 10–17.

12 Finding Safety

Healing Attachment Wounds in the Sandtray Therapy Process

MereAnn Reid

In this chapter, we are going to explore how the sandtray can help facilitate the healing of an attachment disruption related to adoption. An important aspect of this process is the power of visual storytelling, or work with images, as a conduit for self-reflection. Early attachment experiences have a lasting impact on how we connect and relate to one another and ourselves. Our families of origin function like relationship laboratories. Somatic, social, and emotional experiences shape our personalities and our nervous systems, establishing patterns, narratives, and coping skills we carry with us into future relationships and the wider world. Our earliest attachments carve a template for our abstract models and expectations about relationships, shaping unconscious beliefs about how the world works (Badenoch, 2008; Kestly, 2014). In this context, children born into one family who grow up in another, through adoption or foster care, are tasked early in life with retooling their initial dance of attachment, adapting to a changed environment and new relational landscape.

This pivotal life transition, even when it occurs early on, requires organizing survival needs and coping skills at a foundational level. As play therapist Dottie Higgins-Klein (2013) describes, "the process of parent–child bonding takes time and patience . . . when there has been abuse, neglect, or . . . trauma in the child's past, this bonding may be especially difficult as well as especially necessary" (p. 59). Play therapy is an ideal modality for supporting the growth of children whose beginnings have been difficult or disorganized; making sense of changing caregivers and layered losses (identity, culture, physical resemblance, geography, family history, and gestational bond, to name a few) is a process of recreating safety and repatterning regulation, empowering meaningful connection with the self and others. This is attachment work.

Amazingly, children's bodies and brains already hold an instinctive internal map, present at birth, to help them find their way. Sandtray therapy offers a sensory-rich, open-ended, expressive medium with the capacity to ground the body and support the *neuroception* of safety, a neurobiological process by which "the nervous system evaluates risk without requiring awareness" (Porges, 2017, p. 19) and invites engagement without emotional

DOI: 10.4324/9781003055808-14

flooding, helping both client and therapist to remain aware and connected (Dion, 2018). Kestly (2014) further illustrates the role of play as a conduit for the nurturing and care of our deepest emotional needs, as "the actual circuits of these systems lie deep in the brain below the neocortex, and they do not need cognitive resources to become alive" (p. 72).

Sandtray work invites our creative image-mind (right brain) to communicate emotional experiences for which we don't have adequate language (left brain) and don't require explicit memory. This brings to mind the power of unconscious dream states to draw our psyche into a realm somewhere between mindful awareness and our jumbled facts/fears/fantasy fragments of knowing. The addition of a three-dimensional sandtray canvas to bring them together in the presence of a trustworthy, regulated therapist offers engagement with a contained, symbolic, miniature-scale version of our inner world. This sense of being accompanied allows us to bring new awareness to our experience and our reactions. Badenoch's (2008) succinct description of "the integrating power of sandplay" highlights the nonverbal, neurobiological processes that occur as clients engage with the sand:

> The insula gathers all of this sensory data into an emotionally meaningful context, helping all this information converge in the middle frontal cortex, and a rich *relationship* with the sand often unfolds. People get absorbed in arranging the sand just right. This whole experience encourages vertical integration, linking body, limbic regions, and cortex in the right hemisphere (p. 221).

Having a sandtray available in the therapy room offers an opportunity to play with regulation, experimenting with new narratives and symbolic representations of interpersonal dynamics. We have an important role as therapists to hold the attunement necessary as our clients hone their internal model for positive relationships, simultaneously grounding the intensity of their somatic and experiential processing (Dion, 2018; Kestly, 2014). Helping clients integrate the complexities of adoption across the life span becomes a process of guiding them through core relational and emotional tasks, including loss, loyalty, trust, fear of abandonment, and grief (Roszia & Maxon, 2019). All of these can be depicted and observed in the image-rich language of the sand.

Pictures of Attachment

Marti, an 8-year-old African American girl, was adopted as a toddler. Her grandmother, Sharon, often cared for her as a baby, while Marti's mother struggled with depression. Marti's birth father was deceased. Sharon's emphysema made caring for a busy baby difficult, and ultimately, the family pursued an open adoption. Marti's White adoptive parents, Silvia and Van, welcomed Sharon often for visits until she died suddenly when Marti was 7.

Always a busy child, Marti struggled with sleep and body aches after her grandmother died. Within weeks, she developed a fear of the dark, worried about being alone, even at home, and bounced off the walls before bedtime. Academically capable but socially slow to engage, Marti struggled to focus and participate in class, becoming adamantly opposed to attending after-school care. Van picked her up promptly at 3 p.m., and they spent afternoons together at home, but these were not peaceful days. Marti angered easily, was frequently "bored," refused homework, and insisted on sharing her parents' bed at night but was a restless sleeper, so no one slept well. When frustrated and especially when hungry, her dysregulation escalated quickly, exploding in yelling about how she "should just die" and was "the worst one," crying uncontrollably. Marti would not allow her parents to provide physical comfort or even come near when she was this upset, often running to her room and slamming the door. This was, notably, the only time she tolerated being alone.

Marti's off-track behavior had an anxious, hypervigilant tone. I saw her dysregulation as a fear of abandonment and difficulty balancing her power with vulnerability. Therapeutic goals included more ease falling and staying asleep, less chaotic mood swings, and finding reliable outlets for relieving anxiety. She needed help to regulate.

In the intake, we explored the pattern of people missing from Marti's life. The ambiguous losses of parental depression, adoption, unknown birth father, and transracial identity development were compounded by the death of her grandmother. The relational trauma of neglect by her birth mother carried the message "you don't exist," while the complicated grief of adoption offered a confusing status of attachment figures being there but not there. The trauma of layered and repeated losses was amplified for Marti with her grandmother's death. Though the adoption had been finalized for years, Sharon's passing underscored the ambivalence and separation that came before.

In her first two years of life, when babies are establishing a secure base for attachment, Marti had alternately been neglected by her birth mother and cared for by a loving but very tired and stressed grandmother. She'd bonded with each of them in turn, and both caregiving relationships ended. By the time her grandmother died when Marti was in second grade, Marti had adjusted to the both-and relationship of open adoption – having two parents and a doting birth grandmother – but the abrupt severing of that social bond likely touched on preverbal experiences of missing care, and her separation distress surged to the front of her conscious awareness.

Dragon Battles and Truth Camp

Marti gravitated to the sandtray from our first session, her worlds showing themes of nurturing care resulting in harm or negative outcomes, including animal babies being shushed until they were buried completely and figures "getting hided [sic] to protect them" then being forgotten. What follows is a description of an early session.

After a few minutes in the sand, filling and emptying a set of stacking cups, Marti brushed off her hands and turned to the shelves. She selected whole groups of figures: farm animals lined up on one short end of the tray, a row of cats prowled the perimeter – then SWOOSH! – a fire-breathing dragon dive-bombed them, knocking the mama tiger down and flying to the corner of the tray. Marti used a shovel to pat the surface of the sand, smoothing (and soothing?) the scene of the attack. She added more dragons and *Star Wars* figures, dragons facing in, fighters facing out. In the center, she placed a heart-shaped box and a single flower, reminding me of a gravesite. Nearby, a suitcase sat next to a cave filled with food.

With 5 minutes left, she moved the only person in the scene, a White kid in a monster costume, to the steps of a nearby dollhouse. She carefully propped an hourglass and a trumpet along the back wall, then grabbed a Black mother figure from a basket, tossing her flat on her back, alone in the dollhouse upstairs. The monster-child had escaped the battle of the dragons, but she and the mother appeared oblivious to one another; they co-existed but didn't seem connected. Marti announced she was done and walked out of the office.

Marti's tray highlighted themes of escape and rescue, with a few characters showing resourcefulness and self-sufficiency but little capacity to

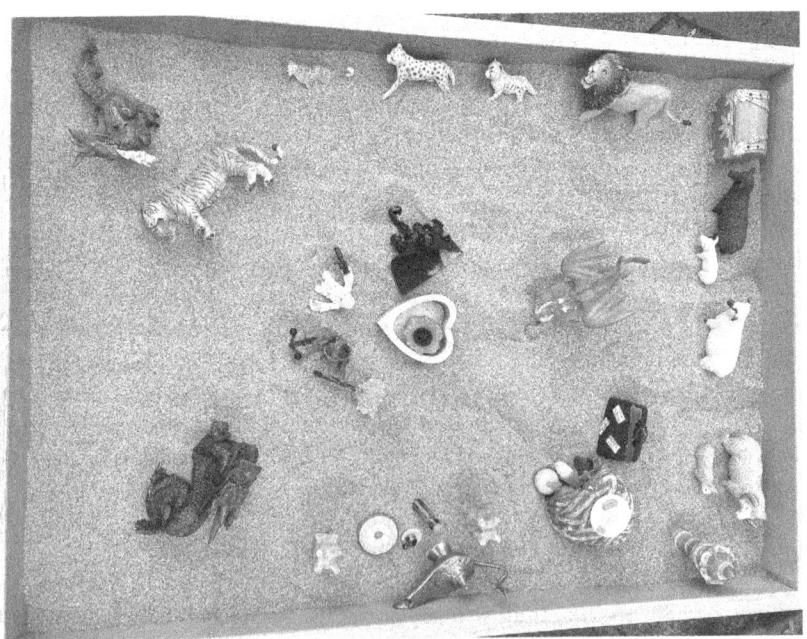

Figure 12.1 Dragon Battle by Marti.

collaborate; each band of figures held separate ground. Both the mother figures – the tiger mama with her cub and the dollhouse mom – got tossed aside as their portion of the narrative ended abruptly. I wondered if this was a picture of insecure avoidant attachment.

In brief, this style of relational regulation follows a cycle: connection with a primary caregiver is disrupted, the infant is distressed but not reliably soothed; based on this recurring pattern, trust in the availability of caregivers is diminished, the child's capacity for stress or perceived challenge is limited, and the flexibility to tolerate a range of emotions is reduced because the child does not possess a felt sense of being accompanied. Marti could stay within her *window of tolerance*, or capacity to tolerate thoughts, feelings, and sensations, without becoming overwhelmed (Dion, 2018) during much of the school day, but by the afternoon, her coping skills were exhausted, and bursts of rage came in the wake of microfrustrations built up with peers, multiple daily transitions, an afternoon dip in blood sugar, and all-day separation from caregivers, on top of poor sleep. Marti was frequently taxed by her daily rhythm and showing me her working model for relationships.

Our early experiences and memories tend to organize in patterns reflective of our first attachments. Daniel Siegel and Tina Payne Bryson (2012) offer a beautiful metaphor for understanding relationships and the brain, describing mental health as "our ability to remain in a *river of well-being*" (p. 11). On either side of a peaceful middle channel, Siegel and Bryson envision one bank representing chaos, the other rigidity, illustrated by raging rapids and stagnation, respectively. Both require adaptation, though neither extreme invites flexibility or flow.

Based on our relative window of tolerance, our metaphorical river may be wide or narrow. Memory and adaptations inform attachment and response patterns, projecting our experience-shaped responses toward chaos or rigidity onto our future relationships. A chaotic environment brings feelings of being out of control, and unpredictable or multiple changes in caregivers can shape our expectations along disorganized schemas prone to fragility and even collapse under stress. The autonomic nervous system's response is triggered in the same way it would be in a situation of imminent physical danger because the bodily system is behaving *as if* its survival is threatened in the current moment, not taking in the contextual data that's different from a truly dangerous situation.

Adaptively, traumatic experience disrupts typical memory processing, which braids together data streams of sensory input, stress hormones, memory encoding, and narrative recall. Instead, implicit and explicit data fragments are stored separately so as not to overwhelm the brain's cognitive capacity for organizing distress and incongruence; survival, not analysis, is favored in the midst of trauma. This serves the body's essential protective instincts by short-circuiting the logic and control centers of the upper cortical brain in favor of prioritizing the lower brain's limbic and brainstem-based regulating impulses. Even afterward, physiologically metabolizing and psychologically making meaning of the event – integrating the trauma – may be further derailed by the flurry of stress hormones surging through the body, depressing the function of the hippocampus (our explicit memory hub) to protect us from being fully conscious of our distress (Porges, 2017).

In short, implicit memories are held in the somatosensory network, with sensations occurring throughout the body, not just localized at a specific sense organ, prompting the body to respond to a felt sense or familiar sensory cues, even if the time, place, and people are all different. This is true of traumatic memories but also of non-verbal, implicit memories from before the age of 3. Prior to 18 months of age, toddlers construct sensory-based experiential memories encoded without conscious awareness.

Before the hippocampus comes online around age 2, normal memory processing already includes a rich tapestry of perception, emotion, bodily sensation, behavior, mental models, and *priming*, preparing the brain to respond to predictable patterns. For instance, a particular smell can bring on a visceral or emotional response associated with previous encounters with that scent, even without an explicit awareness of the context. Our brains are primed to process the sensory input based on a felt sense memory encoded implicitly and shaped by experience, rather than consciously recalled.

Between the ages of 3 and 5, as the hippocampus matures, we can begin to know about the world and actively shape our responses, creating increasingly factual and episodic memories we can recall and build on across the life span. This important development allows us to determine how to feel and act in the present as well as predict future events (Siegel, 2010; Badenoch, 2008; Kestly, 2014).

We humans navigate experiences through both conscious awareness and sensory data; together, these inform a congruent sense, or "dual awareness," of felt safety, allowing us to remain both present and regulated (Dion, 2018). How, then, does the sand provide an opportunity to increase felt safety in the autonomic nervous system? Let's explore that question as we compare Marti's earlier tray showing aggression, thwarted nurture, and hypervigilance with one of her later trays, which she dubbed "Truth Camp."

Returning from a summer break, Marti arrived with some excitement about her time at camp. After sharing briefly during our check-in with her mom, Marti got up from the couch and walked toward the sandtray shelves. As often happened while choosing her figures, Marti's forefingers and thumbs came together, the fingertips on each hand rubbing in tiny repeating circles; though silent, the persistent motion reflected a mobilization of her nervous system, a visible signal that her mind and body were syncing up to begin the building process.

Steering her focus to a basket of habitats, she selected a beaver den, igloo, treehouse, and small glass house. Placing one in each corner of the tray, she referenced a formula from her past few sessions, anchoring the corners like compass directions. As each figure entered the scene, Marti repeated a series of movements: left-hand fingers circling, pick up a figure with the right hand, smooth sand with the left hand, patting the surface, place figure with the right hand, twist the figure into position, brush stray sand from the base, clasp hands together. This ritual was repeated with each tiny dwelling: circle, lift, smooth, pat, place, twist, brush, clasp. She was like a dancer, following music only she could hear.

Still, I felt my own fingertips swirling together in my lap: I was following her lead, picking up her rhythm. I reflected this movement silently then offered an observation aloud: "Your hands are busy today; your whole body is helping you choose." She gave a single, short nod. Fingertips still circling, Marti's busy right hand selected one figure after another, collecting them in a red wicker basket. A low, quiet hum merged with a gentle sigh as she turned away from the shelves, toward the tray. Her shoulders eased, and her chin tipped up slightly to take in the geography. With this gesture of arrival, she breathed in deeply and set to work.

"They're at a camp where they have to show their true self," she started, populating each corner with pairs and trios, people and animals alike, some in their abodes, others corralled by fences. A pattern of figures emerged: matching tall and small creatures, mothers and babies, light bodies and dark bodies, giving a feeling of yin and yang balance. Marti offered that the girls in the beaver den – Dorothy of Oz and a dark-skinned angel – had the power to "know who's telling the truth" and "get their food they need." Just as I began to marvel, internally, that Marti was embracing her identity and sense of connectedness, she turned her attention to the Black Disney princess in the igloo corner. She described Tiana as "possessed by evil and not able to find her true self" and "lying." Involuntarily, my hands squeezed into tight fists beneath the table as Marti revealed, "they make her look nice when she really isn't a good princess."

My amygdala – my brain's data processor – was on high alert; I was getting threat signals from the play environment: The princess is not who she says. Marti's hands rested steadily on the edge of the tray. I inhaled a deep nostril breath and met Marti's eyes over the tray. No one blinked. I managed a small smile, and we breathed out together. In this instance, her capacity to tolerate incongruence was greater than mine; I had to slow down my implicit response in order to tune in to hers. My fists unclenched, flat palms smoothing up and down my thighs. Another breath in. And out. We blinked together. "I really hear how hard it feels to say the truth," I managed. Tuning into Marti's posture and presence told me she was regulated; this was an important tray, but it didn't feel threatening to her.

Our nervous systems were dancing together again. Attunement is an important aspect of cultivating and rehearsing the continuum of the autonomic nervous system in close relationships. Dion (2018) reminds us, "we need to stop trying to figure everything out in the playroom and begin to feel what's happening" (p. 62.). I had been present enough to track Marti's narrative and gauge her activation, simultaneously monitoring my own

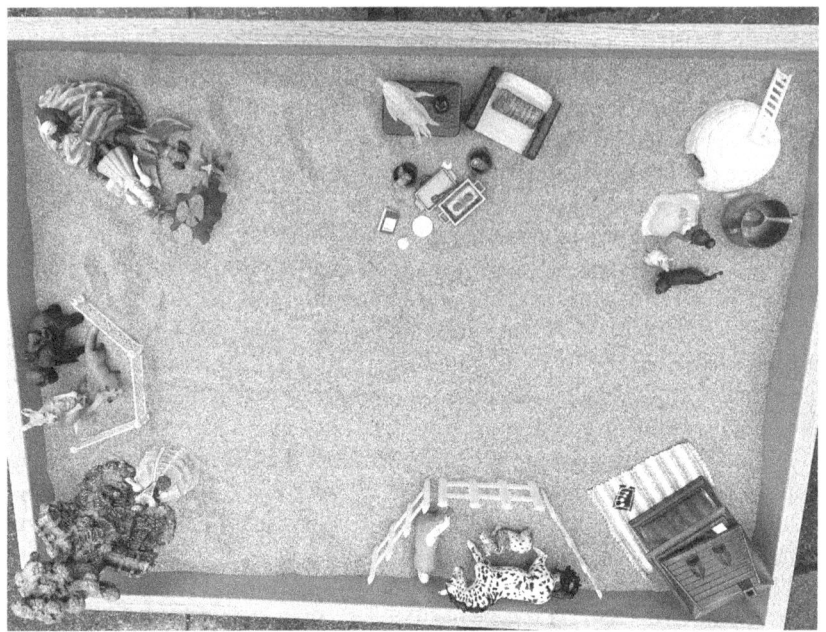

Figure 12.2 Truth Camp by Marti.

nervous system response and modulating my reaction. I had briefly borrowed her steadiness. We had come back into regulation together.

As we simultaneously track the play themes and the builder's non-verbal communication, to an important extent, we feel what the client feels. Their emotional and physiological shifts are read and reflected by mirror neurons (Porges, 2017; Dion, 2018), which observant clinicians learn to interpret through our own attachment experiences – transference and countertransference are one way to think about this felt experience, which we recognize and hone through clinical practice. I was feeling Marti's self-judgment and quest for belonging in my own body!

Back in the session, Marti walked shortly away to find a favorite sensory toy, a foam ball launcher. There was a familiar and satisfying POP! POP! as she sent a series of balls flying across the room. I watched her body unwind as she let out a sigh and flopped onto the couch.

"Tell the story!" urged Marti, a familiar closing ritual for our sessions. I recapped the sand story, using her words as much as possible. Marti declared I'd gotten the story "just right," calmly walking ahead of me down the stairs to rejoin her mom.

Back in the playroom, I took a photo of the tray and grabbed a basket to start clearing and putting figures away. Dismantling each corner in turn,

I lifted the igloo beside the Black princess and found a treasure chest brimming with jewels! When had she put that there? Had I been so distracted by the evil princess that I had missed her hidden treasure? To me, Marti's tray had been a map of all the parts of herself, all of them true and showing a range of traits. Even though I had gotten absorbed in a part of her narrative that felt incongruent – that was why it got my attention – Marti and I were able to lean into the therapeutic relationship to sustain us through my lapse in mindful presence. In fact, Kestly (2014) reminds us that "the hallmark of secure attachment is rupture and repair rather than a steady state of connection – something that can relieve our fears about not being a good enough therapist when we falter" (p. 69).

Our Bodies Know What Safety Feels Like

For many children with low affect tolerance, it can be a struggle to identify and describe emotional and somatic experiences. Healing preverbal loss has two primary building blocks: experiencing a reparative relationship (trauma and attachment therapies or therapeutic parenting) and learning ways to effectively down-regulate at the brainstem level to calm the nervous system (mindful movement, meditation, compassion practices, occupational therapy) when a surge of dysregulation arrives. Engaging the body while reflecting and modeling regulation strategies builds tolerance for a broader range of feelings, a phenomenon we see even in infant studies (Kestly, 2014; Badenoch, 2008). Dion (2018) concurs and reminds us of our role: "In order to help repattern children's nervous systems, the children first need an external regulator, someone to help them integrate the dysregulated state in their nervous system. Integrating intensity must first start with the therapist" (p. 54).

Arranging the physical environment of the playroom is one intentional way we signal safety, with attention to sensory elements and making nonverbal invitations to play readily available. We can include many contextual cues and play props in the therapy space that signal "this is a good place to play" (Kestly, 2014, p. 101) and support clients in settling into a calmer, more receptive state, helping them access "a greater regulatory capacity" (Porges, 2017, p. 83). Affective neuroscientist Jaak Panksepp (2012) tells us that mammalian brains are wired to drive toward both SEEKING and PLAY in a nested hierarchy that builds on the regulating capacity of the brainstem, rooting both child development and the therapeutic benefits of play in rhythmic, repetitive, patterned activities. Kestly (2014) describes how children's natural orientation toward curiosity and the exploratory drive of their experience-shaped brains can be invited into social engagement with the aid of percussion instruments, bouncing balls, and other toys referencing the give-and-take, call-and-response of breathing, a drum-like pulse, walking feet – all rhythms familiar from the womb.

Building on these elemental signals that the therapist is available for connection, Porges (2017) describes how "activating the social engagement system with its ventral vagal pathways enable the autonomic nervous system to support health, growth, and restoration" (p. 24). Further, he says, "Play literally becomes a functional therapeutic model that exercises the neural regulation of autonomic state through reciprocal social interactions" (p. 83). In other words, by communicating our own sense of ease in the environment and surrounding ourselves with a pleasurable range of sensory reminders of our own safety, our clients are able to detect and borrow our regulation capacity as they work to expand their own.

We teach our clients this emotional flexibility and access to regulation through joining our window of tolerance with theirs, effectively expanding what and how much they can handle before emotional flooding overtakes their capacity to cope, as described in Grayson's Chapter 3 of this book. Our neurobiological states are persistently transferrable. We constantly dip into and reflect one another's nervous systems, an adaptation that allows us to respond and connect in relationships, as humans must for survival.

According to Porges (2017), our capacity to "get" what someone else is feeling is based on our neurophysiology. Since we humans are hardwired to *neuroceive* – our neural circuits can distinguish whether people or situations are safe or not-safe – and because we therapists are trained to observe our clients closely, "we can detect and interpret how another person feels, because the nerves that control the striated muscles of the face and head are linked in the brainstem," conveying a series of facial expressions and social cues that we decode by tracking our felt sense of the interaction in concert with conscious awareness of the immediate social context and a client's history (p. 133). This is the practice of honing our dual awareness. Lisa Dion (2018) further explains how "tracking . . . these experiences is how we maintain a neuroception of safety, which allows us to stay regulated and present. The use of mindfulness, breath, moving, and naming your experience all support your ability to keep one foot in and one foot out," connecting with but not getting lost in the child's play and emotional experience; "we have to be in it and not in it, simultaneously" (p. 101).

Felt Safety Registers Internally

Joining in the play experience with a child while maintaining our own regulation and flexible capacity for potential activation allows us to accompany them through the ups and downs of the play without becoming overwhelmed ourselves. This conveys to children in a wordless exchange that we are able to join and track their play, even when it gets intense or messy. While staying attuned to their nervous system arousal and support needs, we can anchor them by managing our own activation. This communicates safety and permission for them to lean fully into the play as a neural exercise and supports them in tuning in to associated sensory cues (Porges,

2017; Kestly, 2014). As play therapists, we have many modalities for inviting children toward emotional communication and expanded coping skills. Play therapist Dottie Higgins-Klein (2013) asserts that "sandtray therapy is not a separate theoretical modality, but a combined intuitive and somatic approach to exploration and expression of the inner self" (p. 102). This process of building resilience includes, at the root, regulation of the autonomic nervous system – which we initially map on the emotional and physiological regulation system of our caregivers – cultivating a balance of trust, self-protection, and adaptability (Dion, 2018).

In turn, the aftereffects of a traumatic event or separation – both in Marti's case – shape an embodied anticipation, as described in Grayson's chapter, that comes to bear in future moments and influences behavior. Instead of the honed neural circuitry of secure attachment that leads to increasingly flexible regulation capacity, posttraumatic stress triggers a surge of scarcity thinking or deficit beliefs reinforced by breaks in attachment. This can trip a fight-flight-freeze response that becomes a road map for relationships and reactions to stress.

Whether we're moved to get out of the way of other people's anger or stop that same feeling from roiling inside us, Panksepp (2012) identified RAGE as one of seven core emotional-motivational circuits sparked by hormonal shifts and stress response. In short, this applies to attachment patterns in that "subtle situations such as the loss of love are not easy to study neuroscientifically, but RAGEfulness readily arises when our social desires are thwarted" and "can also be exacerbated by certain bodily changes such as hunger" (p. 150). Tied closely with FEAR and PANIC at being left alone, RAGE – the all-caps designation distinguishes these essential and bio-complex evolutionary and affective systems from the more subjective feeling of rage, fear, etc. – shows up as separation anxiety and "distinct social feelings that arise from social exclusion and loss" (Panksepp & Bivens, p. 323).

While babies and toddlers are far more likely to be moved to tears when these emotional-motivational systems flare, we are all at risk of default to our most primal regulation tools when emotionally flooded. The abject grief of losing a loved one, especially suddenly, can make us acutely aware of feeling out of connection and powerless to reach the person who has died or otherwise disappeared. In short, the brain networks for GRIEF can depress our circuitry for SEEKING and PLAY, effectively minimizing stimulation in areas of the brain where connection, enthusiasm, and positive vitality are promoted (Panksepp & Bivens, 2012). PLAY brings us back into connection.

As she worked on grief and complex attachment puzzles, Marti featured mother–baby pairs across her stories, and copious quantities of food showed up, illustrating themes of positive nurture, connection, loyalty, and abundance. Often, bridges appeared to connect good and bad, sea and sky, wild and home. This was reflected in her physical stance as well, shifting her weight from one foot to the other as she narrated the action – she sometimes appeared to be rocking herself, as a toddler would, to an internal tune of her own composition.

About a year into therapy, she spent eight sessions on the floor, building her story beneath the sandtable. Through this period, she expressed mild frustration that many of the figures would not stand up outside the sand, persistently propping them up, assigning them supportive companions, or patiently working to balance them – seemingly exploring how they could function independently and get help at the same time. Just as she worked through this phase, shelters and a theme of protection became important. This solidified her signature style of building in the corners. I wondered if this was a new metaphor for safety and belonging.

Bridging Marti's Sandtray Work and Daily Life

I saw Marti for play therapy and sandtray sessions over a span of 2 years. Increasingly, she was able to express mixed feelings, tuning in to her needs and sensory resources for comfort, taking space to reflect on what helped her feel at ease, and articulating her wishes and feelings. We moved from fragile grief work at intake through a phase of settling in her physical body and more restful sleep routine at home, building her stamina for collaborating on a life story book, an illustrated narrative of her adoption story.

Marti's work on expanding her window of tolerance and gaining awareness of her habits made a huge difference to her capacity for healthy risk-taking. Her teachers were supportive of daily snacks and walking breaks, often entrusting her with an errand or delivery to another classroom, further empowering and reflecting their faith in her. Marti's family built a daily sensory routine with the help of her occupational therapist, including a smart snack basket in the fridge with crunchy, chewy, protein-rich options to help steady her blood sugar.

About a year and a half into therapy, Marti had a chance to join a hip-hop dance class. Family dance parties and daily music listening after school led to Marti incorporating this form of movement as an outlet for pent-up energy and worries before bed. She eagerly participated in the class, taking the risk to try new skills and getting a chance to socialize outside school with other kids of color. She gained confidence and spent more nights sleeping on her own, even getting Van's help with a makeshift loft, creating a cozy reading corner in her room just big enough for one. She completed two seasons of soccer, where she found an important balance of strength, pride, and trust in the power of her body and the support of a team.

Siegel's Pathways of Integration detail how "connecting intimately in relationship while retaining our own sense of identity and freedom" (Kestly, 2014, p. 64) can be a bridge back to relational trust. This is important because sensory and relational input, together, invite down-regulation from mobilization (fight/flight) toward social engagement. Play is essential to human growth and social development, and storytelling is an ideal vehicle for this process. There is no better format for the crosstalk of ideas from one side of the brain to the other. The catch is: the body and the mind need to work together in order to fully inhabit and integrate the narrative. This is the digestion process of making meaning and building attachment.

As a narrative develops, new meaning can be made of events, patterns, and connections. As the client articulates their felt sense and perspective, new capacities emerge. This occurred for Marti in several ways. Patterns that showed up in the sandtray were reflected in her daily life. As I watched a process of anchoring through marking the four corners of her tray and recurring figures building alliances, Marti made a new friend at church. As she developed a habit of circumambulating her finished sandtrays, she initiated a get-well card to her birth mother. A few weeks after Marti shared her "Truth Camp" tray, she made a list of things that helped her feel calm at home. As she was finding peace in her mind and body, she was making peace with her wants and needs; as she was integrating, she found resolution. We know from the Adult Attachment Inventory that securely attached adults are able to digest their experiences enough to develop a coherent narrative of both their positive and difficult aspects (Dion, 2018; Kestly, 2014; Siegel, 2010). These are tasks of regulation.

We embarked explicitly on reducing Marti's trauma sensitivity first, inviting her body and mind to collaborate in managing the experiences and threat signals that had been overwhelming; we did this using the contained environment of the playroom, building a trusting relationship, referral to occupational therapy, and establishing an intentional sensory routine and manageable predictable daily rhythms at home and school. All these elements helped signal safety at the brainstem level, the area growing fastest and most dynamically in utero and in concert with the limbic system through the first three years of life. This provided updated brain connectivity and relational patterns so she could engage in co-authoring a chronological, accurate record of her adoption story and life up to the present day, banking on her expanded repertoire of regulation skills to help her digest both the positive and challenging aspects of her story.

My Experience Working With Marti

Just before Marti's family reached out for support, I was navigating the imminent death of my own father. In any other season, I would have excitedly agreed to take them on; Marti was an ideal client for me, and I liked her parents right away. But this was not good timing. I named all the logistical challenges our work posed – distance, cost, timing – and Silvia politely replied "we'll wait" before calling me back 6 weeks later. By that time, my dad had recovered from his most recent health crisis, and I had space to return to work.

It was not lost on me that saying "yes" to Marti meant saying "yes" to grief and attachment work in the midst of my own. We scheduled the intake, and

I took my hesitations to my supervisor, my therapist, and my consult group. And then I took my hands to the sandtray. What emerged was a wishing well surrounded by angels and the four elements. I saw right away that I had incorporated members of my inner community, whom I recognized from my intensive study with a sandtray mentor steeped in internal family systems and attachment theories. I recognized the archetypes of an angel/devil pair, a virgin/crone dyad, and figures representing the dual energies of comedy and tragedy. I hadn't wholly intended to build a tray; it was more like I found myself propelled toward my office, kneeling on the floor before the menagerie, knowing that was where I needed to be.

It didn't register until well after I'd built that impulsive tray and was deep in work with Marti that my impromptu grief tray reflected many of the aspects I'd later observe in hers: four anchored corners, paired figures representing opposite traits or forces, the presence of fire, and a ritual of building barefoot. We were linked; whether by energy, relational wounds, or universal symbology didn't matter to me. Our parallel process was an echo of one another's presence.

Over the past decade, an immense body of work in the relational neurosciences has shed organizing light on how profoundly our felt experiences and non-verbal exchanges matter. Revisiting Marti's work for this chapter finds me nearly 6 years out from our time together. As I watched her, week after week, place pairs of figures in the tray, deeply experiencing the sensory landscape, I could see her body responding in real time. This palpable engagement reminds me of a metaphor play therapist Lisa Dion (2018) often uses to describe co-regulation in the playroom: "We're rockin' babies," she says, describing how the rhythmic and repetitive motion of rocking a baby to sleep regulates both the mother and baby's nervous systems, joining them by a shared metronomic pulse. When a therapist and client co-regulate via the sandtray, this occurs through witnessing the built world together, taking in a shared landscape of texture and images, including how they relate to the sensory data of sand, water, fire, space, color, movement, and proximity to other figures. The therapist has an opportunity to feel what the client is feeling, taking it in and reflecting it back, so the client feels felt. With the passage of time and distance, I can still recall many sensory details of the exchanges Marti and I shared, because they had energy and dimension. There exists within me a felt sense of her. I can reflect on the true wisdom of the intuitive process we shared – not mine, but *our* wisdom, mine and Marti's together. I imagine she can still feel it, too.

References

Badenoch, B. (2008). *Being a brain-wise therapist: A practical guide to interpersonal neurobiology*. W. W. Norton & Company, Inc.

Dion, L. (2018). *Aggression in play therapy: A neurobiological approach for integrating intensity*. W. W. Norton & Company, Inc.

Higgins-Klein, D. (2013). *Mindfulness-based play-family therapy: Theory and practice.* W. W. Norton & Company, Inc.

Kestly, T. (2014). *The intepersonal neurobiology of play: Brain-building interventions for emotional well-being.* W. W. Norton & Company, Inc.

Panksepp, J., & Bivens, L. (2012). *The archaeology of mind: Neuroevolutionary origins of human emotions.* W. W. Norton & Company, Inc.

Porges, S. (2017). *The pocket guide to the polyvagal theory: The transformative power of feeling safe.* W. W. Norton & Company, Inc.

Roszia, S. K., & Maxon, A. D. (2019). *Seven core issues in adoption and permanency: A comprehensive guide to promoting understanding and healing in adoption, foster care, kinship families and third-party reproduction.* Jessica Kingsley Publishers.

Siegel, D. (2010). *Mindsight: The new science of personal transformation.* Bantam Books.

Siegel, D., & Bryson, T. P. (2012). *The whole-brain child: Twelve revolutionary strategies to nurture your child's developing mind.* Bantam Books.

13 Sandtray With a Mind of Its Own

Developing Trust in the Wisdom of the Process

Bonnie Badenoch

Sylvie strode into my office and, without saying hello, moved quickly to the long wall of sandtray figures. With what felt like near-panic, she searched the shelves. "Ah!" she exhaled, grabbing a small, brightly colored creature with removable parts that stick out everywhere. She clutched it awkwardly to her chest. "I was so afraid I only dreamt this . . . this . . . I don't know what to call it. I wasn't sure I had seen it here. I'm so relieved because it's been speaking to me." We began our hour together engaging with this whatever-it-was – a being who had apparently been accosting her from the shelves, just below the level of conscious awareness, for some time. Determined to be heard, she (as Sylvie began to call it) inserted herself into her dreams as a figure that was terrible and laughable at the same time. As she brought the little figure away from her chest, two of her removable pieces fell to the ground. "That's it! She keeps falling apart, and I can't make her stay together. I have to and I can't. I can't." Her voice trailed off.

She picked up the pieces, thrusting them as deeply into the holes in the little one's side as she could, only to have two pieces from the other side detach themselves. In terror, she dropped the rest of the figure on the ground. The remaining pieces scattered on the carpet. Now there was nothing but a semiround multicolored ball with two big eyes staring up at her. She cringed toward me. I had said very little so far, mostly just making listening sounds, keenly attentive to the relationship unfolding before me. "I'm here," I said. We looked at each other for a long, warm moment, something that often settled us into relationship.

Taking a shallow shaky breath, she slowly and cautiously reached down to pick up the naked ball. She was careful to keep the eyes turned toward her as she reached toward me to place this little being in my opening hands. After releasing it, she put her hands around mine so that my fingers gently closed over the upward-gazing ball. Then she was able to take a full breath followed by a long exhalation. Something had completed itself. Neither of us had any cognitive idea about what had just happened, but it felt intensely meaningful and important. For the rest of our time together, she talked about her teenage son, and she never dreamt about this little creature again.

DOI: 10.4324/9781003055808-15

During 25 years of experience with sand and miniatures, through both my own and my clients' relationships with the figures, I have learned to trust, without question, the wisdom of whatever process unfolds. Protocol has gradually given way to the fluidity that is the hallmark of right-hemisphere revelation (Badenoch, 2018). There is so much vitality and truth in this process that whether the tray is 12 × 12 inches, round, octagonal, or regulation size, the dynamic relationship between our inner world, yearning to be seen, and these sacred objects will find a way.

I once did a sandtray in-service for a facility seeking to help teens who were too troubled to be in school. Leading me to their playroom, they showed me two plastic containers filled with beach sand and a large tub that contained nothing but farm animals – multiple iterations of pigs, cows, horses, and chickens. At first, I was appalled by the lack of diversity, only to be told that these were donated supplies – all that they could afford – and that the kids' imaginations turned these humble animals into glorious kings, frightened children, fearsome lions, elegant dragons, and the occasional wall or tree. Such is the need of our inner world to find expression, to speak to us about things that words can't contain.

When we invite these figures into our offices, we are opening a space in which the wisdom of our right-hemisphere relational world can express itself with all the ingenuity and creativity and novelty that it possesses. Just having these populated shelves in our counseling rooms can mitigate our tendency to move toward left-hemisphere solutions and interventions by enlivening our right hemispheres so that we remain more whole-brained through the day. If our shelves are arranged not by category – all dogs together and so forth, as the left hemisphere suggests – but by an inner sense of who belongs with whom, the portal to the right opens wider. If we consciously engage with our figures as we arrive in our space, we can assist in that right-enlivening process. What attracts us this particular day? If we can open to simply listening as we move into relationship with what has called us, we may be quite surprised by what this being – who chose us – wants to convey. Surprise is one of the ways our right hemisphere gets our attention as it stays attentive to what is uniquely emerging in this particular moment. "Surprise" is also one of the words I hear most often when one of my people does his or her first sandtray. "I had no idea what I was doing! And look what happened!"

Letting the experience flow freely, following our people wherever they may be taking us needs to rest on a secure foundation of trust that their inner world knows the path toward healing, and knows it better than we ever can. This kind of trust rests on at least two pillars. One is doing an abundance of our own trays at the beginning of our experience with this way of working. Ideally, we will continue to do that work regularly and always accompanied. My partner and I have an ongoing practice of witnessing each other's sandtrays as a way to stay in deep connection with each other and with what is unfolding internally. Accompaniment always deepens the process because in the warm embrace of another's ventral presence, our inner world can find the safety to venture with confidence into unknown territory. Having such a sand buddy supports our ongoing investment in and amazement at what sandtray can bring us. Keeping it alive in us changes the way we offer it to our people. Then it is never just a technique we are suggesting but an embodied experience whose possibilities our people will sense because it is alive in us.

The second pillar of trust is deepening our understanding of the embodied relational brain. This gives our left hemisphere what it needs to feel secure in surrendering to the right brain's unfolding and unpredictable wisdom. Rita's chapter in this book on the neurobiology of sandtray is a wonderful beginning for that. Immersing myself in interpersonal neurobiology for the last 17 years has planted my feet more and more firmly on the solid ground of these convictions:

> each of us possesses untold resources for healing, an inherent treatment plan, if you will;
>
> what we need is the accompaniment of someone with sufficient holding capacity and wisdom for that inborn process to emerge;
>
> this accompanying person is willing and able to follow us, developing a responsive dance that honors our inner wisdom and is grounded in his or her own healing journey in the sand.

In other words, as Iain McGilchrist (2009) might say, we can best support others by fostering our right-hemisphere capacity for being present through developing an able left-hemisphere emissary who understands how and why this process can be trusted to take us where we need to go. On this solid foundation, we can more easily relax into the emerging unknown that is sandtray. When we do that, our people will sense that we have no particular expectations about what may occur when they begin to engage with the figures and the sand. With all this in mind, I now have the pleasure of sharing with you moments when some powerful and unexpected encounters arrived.

Accosted

Richard was leery of my sand and miniatures since he first came in. "Do you have cats?" he asked, looking at the two plastic, sand-filled trays on the floor. "No," I grinned. "Those are for sandtray work. It's one of the ways some people who come here choose to approach healing."

He wasn't curious about that. "Those things on the wall remind me of grandmother's smelly, cluttered house," he said with mild disgust. I silently thanked the figures for already putting him in touch with part of his history.

"Whether we engage with them or not is entirely up to you," I said.

He turned away from the shelves, only to find himself looking at them again as he chose a seat on the couch facing the wall of miniatures. My office has always been arranged so that people can be with or completely avoid having visual contact with the figures. I don't have a preferred spot, so I always offer people whatever seat feels right to them. I trust their inner world will find the most helpful place.

He began. "I'm coming to you because a friend told me you know something about neuroscience, and I hoped you might explain to me why every relationship I'm in always turns out so disappointing. I know I'm smarter than most people, but that isn't it. So it must be something with my brain, right?"

"Well, everything we experience has to have something to do with our brains, since that's the lens through which we perceive the world. Because of the kind of neuroscience I study, I'm most versed in how our earlier relationships shape that lens and influence how we experience the people in our lives." I was aligning with him, left brain to left brain, but it wasn't lost on me that his eyes were more on the shelves than on me. Since he could also have been looking out the window at the lovely park if he wanted to avoid eye contact with me, I felt pretty sure he was already in conversation with the shelves, though he may not have had any conscious awareness of it.

We talked a bit about his history and finished our first time together, making another appointment. Glancing again at the shelves, he paused as he got near the door. "I could swear that little plastic man was looking at me the whole time," he said, pointing at a red-haired, overall-clad man with furrowed eyebrows and clenched fists. "That might be important," I said. "I doubt it," he replied with a glare.

The next time he came in, he spontaneously started talking about the stepfather who had entered his life when he was 3 years old. He was from the "lower classes," according to Richard, angry and critical every day, and never showed up as a father. After we spent an hour with him and the little boy who yearned for a warm, attentive parent, I wondered if this disappointing man might well have been awakened within Richard by the figure on the shelf.

It was important for me to hold this hypothesis lightly and tenderly, not using it to steer the therapy by asking who he might be looking at on the shelves. For one thing, I wasn't sure what had happened. For another, even if it did, it might never happen again in the natural course of the healing process. I believed what would be most helpful was for me to follow him as he came in the next time.

For the next two sessions, he talked with me about his work. I remembered him telling me how smart he was the first day, and these two sessions seemed to be about cementing that firmly in my experience of him. For many of us, one of our most powerful protectors from embedded trauma is the part we show the world most consistently. As long as he was king of the intellectual hill, he didn't have to feel much. My listening to him attentively and appreciatively let that protector part know that he was respected for his important place in Richard's inner world. As far as making our way toward traumas that need healing, safety is everything, and it arises most potently from feeling that every part of us is accepted and valued.

Then came our fifth session. He seemed to have run out of easy talk. Perhaps his protectors had stepped aside a little. His eyes were again scanning the shelves, although I wasn't sure he was aware of it. His eyes landed, and after a moment of quiet, his low, sad voice said, "My mother never had any idea who I was." In tone and volume, it was so far from the matter-of-fact way he had talked about what he called his mother's "benign neglect" that it startled me a bit. Then we dropped together into the ache in his belly that had arisen as he allowed himself to feel some portion of the magnitude of his loss.

I saw Richard for about 4 years. Never once did he do a sandtray. I offered a couple of times, to be met by a disdainful, "Are you kidding?" Only once did he acknowledge the power of the figures, and that was to say jokingly that it was unfair that I kept these things to torture people. Yet he continued to sit across from them and often be captured by them, one at a time. With their help, we visited the multiple crushing disappointments he had experienced with the people closest to him. As implicit memories welled up and were met by the disconfirming care, acceptance, and attention he experienced in our relationship, he began to find more nourishing relationships coming unexpectedly into his life. We might not have been able to do it without a little help from our friends. They opened the embodied inner world of this highly intellectual, well-protected, left-hemisphere-dominant man in a way that no amount of talk could have.

A Long Story

At the other end of the spectrum of engagement with these living beings that line my shelves, Maria and I had an arc of experience from avoidance to immersion that unfolded throughout her therapy. She came to me almost entirely incapacitated by the flood of memories of a tortured childhood. For our first couple of years, her window of tolerance was so small that the profusion of characters on the shelves were profoundly disturbing, so she needed to not see the shelves. She explained to me that she always wore a hoodie to avoid upsetting sights. Even sounds were slightly muffled, she said.

She carefully arranged the chairs so that she was looking out the window at the soothing park, positioning me far enough to the right of her that I was probably just barely in her peripheral vision. After a few months, she would occasionally risk a glance at me. Hearing her history, I realized that she had had almost no experience of emotional safety, so her ventral vagal circuitry had very little practice and was extremely fragile. Her movements toward restricting incoming experience were powerful wisdom.

Maria and I practiced safety together time after time. I prepared for her arrival by inviting the internalized presence of those who have been most safe for me into my body so they could help me remain steady in the presence of the terror within her. By about 2 years in, we were making more regular eye contact, a clear sign that she could accommodate more activation without rocketing into sympathetic or collapsing into dorsal. There was much to celebrate – and we did.

One particular day, she came in, settled herself in her usual place, and said, "I feel like I want to take a peek at those folks on the shelves." I smiled in surprise. She went on, "I feel like they've been watching over me this whole time, waiting for me, wanting to help me." Little tears sprang up at the corners of my eyes. I knew these figures had a palpable presence in the room because so many people had shared that with me, but I wasn't aware that they had been touching Maria this whole time. I felt silent waves of gratitude flowing from me to them.

After that, we did sandtray work regularly for the next several years, always following her lead about the timing of the next tray. They provided blessed containment for her horrific experiences. Eventually, we both sensed it was time for her to move outward in her life, leaning into my internalized presence for accompaniment, but without regular visits. She asked if we could have a longer session – maybe 2 hours but open-ended in case "it" took longer. She didn't tell me what "it" was. Trusting the wisdom she had exhibited from our first meeting, I said a joyous yes.

When she arrived, she asked for help moving the furniture out of the way so there was a clear diagonal space across my 10×15-foot office. She was sparkling with anticipation about this secret project. Beginning at one corner of the carpet and employing the help of her friends on the shelves, she told the story of her life along that diagonal. I was riveted. As her story reached the time I entered her life, about two-thirds of the way across the office, she asked me to choose a figure for myself. From then on to the opposite corner, we built together, taking turns. With laughter, tears, long pauses in silence, moments of heart-healing eye contact, we honored how we had become a team on behalf of all parts of her. No words were spoken once she began. About a third of the figures on my long shelves had their place in this comprehensive narrative.

We sat back on the couch, side by side and hand in hand, to allow this panorama to continue to speak to us. Then we found ourselves reminiscing a bit. I told her how inspiring our time together had been for me as she diligently and courageously worked her way free of unspeakable tragedy. She said, "The most important part for me was that you seemed to trust me and my ability to heal. You didn't push me, but you didn't leave me either. It's hard to find words for it." I told her my friend, Jim Finley, says it this way: "Neither invading nor abandoning" (Finley, 2020). We paused to feel that together once again. As we parted, we both acknowledged that we had become part of each other forever.

Family

This is a short story about repetition, bonding, and endings that come too soon. A little boy named James came to our playroom having just been adopted by older parents. He had been in an orphanage and four foster homes prior to arriving with this new mother and father. None of the lost placements had been about his behavior but only about circumstances that made continuing impossible. He was actually a quiet little fellow, shy-seeming at first, with big cautious eyes. He had every reason to wonder about any new encounter. Who would leave him next?

The play therapist at our agency was quite magical with young kiddos. As she welcomed him in, she was watching to see what drew him most. The sandtray shelves were close to the door of her office, and he never got past those. Without a word, he began to assemble families in first one tray and then another – gorillas, birds, giraffes, and sometimes humans. He looked up at her, sensing whether he had permission to continue. She smiled, nodded, acknowledged him. He cleared the two trays, putting the figures back on the shelves, and did it all over again with different families. This time, she started to gently describe what she was seeing but saw him shrink away a bit, so stopped. He kept on building in the silence. This continued for 45 minutes. And then for 20 sessions, except that he did begin to greet her, and then to hug her at the beginning and end of their time together. Apart from that, the pattern never varied, and one couldn't blame her for wondering if she needed to do something to try to shift this. However, she felt – in her belly and her chest – that he was doing just what he needed to do, this little guy who desperately yearned for family and lived in fear that he would never really belong anywhere.

At the end of the 20th session, his father came in to say that they wouldn't be coming back. He gave no reason and wasn't open to a final session. With some anger and a troubled heart, she had the presence of mind to pull from the shelf a little hedgehog that James had used in every tray and thrust it into his hands. They had one final deep look at each other before he turned to walk away with his father, head down and shoulders sagging. The next day, she called James's mother to try again for a final session. The woman simply said, "He told me he liked you. I didn't think that was supposed to happen," and hung up. Something about the bond that grew between James and his counselor caused intolerable pain for this mother.

I would like to say that James's therapist later heard that everything turned out all right, but she never did. She also never forgot him. I suspect that the hedgehog and the many families and the kind woman who had the space inside herself to let him do what was needed stayed with him forever, too.

Thresholds

By now, these stories may be fostering the sense that sand and miniatures open a liminal space, a doorsill between two worlds. I wouldn't say exactly between conscious and unconscious because much that is conscious often arrives in the tray. Instead, it seems to invite a shift in perception, an orientation away from the light of certainty and toward the mysterious dark. As facilitators, if we let go of expectation about what will happen next (which is hard to do unless we have developed deep trust in the inherent healing capacity that inhabits our people and us), something else seems to step in to guide the process. When we let go of expecting a product – a completed sandtray – and follow what is arriving in the liminal space our people are entering, sand and figures sometimes reveal themselves as sacred catalysts for the next implicit opening.

Andi was about 30 when she first came to see me. She said she was continually aware of "a well of anxiety that sometimes seethes quietly and sometimes boils over. It's hard for me to make decisions." Immediately intrigued by the creatures on the shelves, she often walked over to touch one or more after we greeted each other, commenting on how she felt about them. Sometime in our early meetings, she asked about how sandtray works and felt interested in trying it soon. "Just let me know when you sense you're ready," I offered. She paused for a moment and said, "How about now?" With a smile, I suggested she put her hands in both kinds of sand (clumpy and flowy) to see which one her body might need right now. After being quite thoughtful about her experience, she indicated the clumpy sand. She moved into relationship with beeswax-coated grains and arranged them for about a minute. As she turned away, I offered a basket for the figures.

I make a practice of accompanying people to the shelves, especially their first time. As Andi got close, I felt her breathing become ragged, torn between rapid gasps and holding her breath. Tears gathered in her eyes. She looked at me in terror, whispering over and over, "I'll do it wrong. I'll do it wrong. I'll do it wrong." If she had expressed this fear from a more adult part of her before we had begun, I might have said, "It's impossible to do it wrong. Whatever happens will be what is needed in this moment to illuminate where you are, and that's just right." Now, though, with the imminence of needing to choose, she had been drawn across the liminal threshold to embody the world of a very young child whose choices always seemed to result in someone else being hurt. All that mattered in this moment was providing sanctuary for that child's terror. We made our way back to the couch and attended to the strong visceral experience that had arisen in her, awakened by the presence of the figures.

Getting into relationship with the process rather than doing a tray has been a fairly regular occurrence. A young, extremely soft-spoken man, an artist, arrived in my office precisely because he had heard that we offer sandtray at our clinic. Because there would be some kind of imagery and art, he thought it could help. Puzzled by his persistent shyness, which made him almost mute many times, he wondered if maybe being a first-born who had to manage both his parents was at the root of it. He acknowledged at the time that this didn't make much cognitive sense, but it felt possibly right.

As he engaged with the sand and figures, his early trays had no beings who he felt were him. Only his mother and father occupied the trays, in big ways. About that time, he also drew a picture of himself sitting on a chair, so transparent that we could see the slats through his body. We were feeling our way into his invisibility, bit by bit. At some point, we also began talking about inner community, how we internalize those closest to us, and this led him to wonder more directly about his parents' presence inside him. The next time we were face to face with the sand, he had difficulty finding any sense of his body needing clumpy or flowy grains. He finally shook his head and walked away, mystified. We then spent 30 minutes drifting from shelf to shelf with him being unable to choose a single object. He would occasionally, in the faintest of voices, call up a few words to describe the profound emptiness he was feeling. I stayed close, wandering with him. He eventually sat down, exhausted, and simply said, "That was my mother. That is how she is every day."

The process of sandtray had again provided a liminal space through which his mother was able to step into his body to give him her lived experience. These kinds of arrivals by others who live within us are particularly powerful when they are spontaneous, as this was. They often generate a quality of compassion that liberates us into the resolution with that person that we have longed for, particularly with people where in-person reconciliation isn't possible. What emerged for this young man was a growing sense of his distinctness from his mother. He said, "I believe most days I lived partly as her in my shyness and timidity. Now, I feel myself standing close to her, caring about the tragic lostness inside her, but it no longer grips my throat and my belly."

Sometimes the sand itself is the doorway. Dierdre was in her 60s when her growing sense of meaninglessness and despair pushed her into my office. Recently retired, she was realizing that without her work, she had nothing to cover up these feelings. She remembered them from her teens, from a postpartum depression, from a period of staying home with her daughter when she was recuperating from a badly broken leg, in the empty house after her divorce, and every time she had tried to meditate. "A trap door opens into grayness that I know will swallow me. I will die of it – or by my own hand. It's intolerable." She was just about to start her own business to fight it off again when it came to her that she really wanted it gone from inside her. Instead of feeling suicidal, she was filled with the kind of determination that set the air vibrating throughout the room.

We had been together for about half an hour, some of it spent with her inquiring about all the stuff in my room. She eyed the large tray of clumpy sand, walked over to it without saying anything to me, and began pushing the sand toward the sides of the tray, creating a huge lake in the middle. Only, as you all know, the sand wouldn't stay put. Everything from a few grains to good-sized balls kept rolling back into the lake. She became fiercer, trying to pack the sand tighter, more and more of it spilling over the edge of the tray. I was standing near her, wondering if she was even aware of me, when she burst out, "You see! You see! Everything is impossible! That's what I've been trying to tell you!" And she half-collapsed against me, overcome by the very despair she had been telling me about. She had just embodied the spiral of her life from supreme effort to collapse. Sisyphus and his impossible rock.

We made our way back to the couch so her dorsal collapse of despair could be met by my ventral holding. This was a first disconfirming step toward implicit change in that earliest wound of impossibility, which, we learned, had formed when she was unable to get her mentally ill mother's attention, probably even in the womb. Almost before Dierdre and I were acquainted, the sand offered the liminal threshold into the experience itself. She accepted the invitation. We met for several years. During that time, Dierdre often returned to the sand and was never drawn to the figures. At times, she simply plunged her hands deeply into the flowy grains as a way to regulate the alternating waves of terror and rage. At times, she spent most of the hour building elaborate structures, always with the clumpy sand. Almost without exception, the doorway to deeper embodied experience opened during these encounters.

Kleenex

The last story I have the privilege of sharing offers a unique meeting between the creative genius within us and the keen aliveness of those who live on our shelves. Daniel, an exquisitely thoughtful and quiet young man in his 20s, was an architect for a living and a graphic artist for fun. He was also terrified — not too strong a word — of becoming vulnerable with anyone, leaving him painfully lonely. He had just left a relationship that was threatening to become closer than he could tolerate, so he was perplexed about why he was even willing to come to my office. A friend of his had seen me for a number of years and suggested it, mentioning that I had some different ways of working, including sandtray. Almost against his will, he said, he found himself sitting across from me and my miniatures. This double pull of extreme caution and the urge to move forward was familiar to him. I sensed his warm-heartedness hiding behind the soft but profoundly intellectual way he presented himself.

As he shared his history with me, it was pretty unremarkable. Born in the Midwest, he had a mother who sounded somewhat narcissistic and self-absorbed and a strict but mostly kind father whom he appreciated for inculcating a solid sense of human values. He and his younger brother had romped through childhood in the woods and rivers with their friends. To this day, he loves going back to Madison to feel the unique qualities of the air and land and water. "None of this explains to me why I can hardly tolerate being really seen, much less being close to someone," he said. It was mysterious to me, too.

I offered that sandtray work often lets us see into the corners of our inner world that intellect can't penetrate. He turned pale and stopped breathing for a moment. "No rush," I said, making a note that something big no doubt lived within that dark, unseen space – threatening enough to pull him toward a dorsal state merely from the suggestion of touching it.

The hallmark of our work together was "slowly, slowly." Long conversations about what mattered to him, philosophical discussions of what is true in the world and what is merely perception, deep dives into the neuroscience of trauma and healing, accompanied by brief mentions of his profound loneliness. Then, one day, he was suddenly ready to work in the sand. I was curious about what had changed but kept that to myself. He chose quite a number of figures and placed them meticulously, changing their places in micromovements until they were exactly where he needed them to be.

That day, a strange thing happened. I had been doing this work for at least a decade by then, and without exception, I had always felt a connection with what was arriving in the tray. Some combination of what I knew about the person's history, the relationships between the figures, and ways that my own inner world was being touched made for a lively conversation in my body and emotions. I was always cautious because I knew what I was experiencing was invariably colored by my own perceptual lens, so it was vital that I remain open and curious as they shared more with me. However, in this moment, I felt nothing at all except a mild confusion about why I felt nothing. Daniel said little about the tray, and we continued on with our conversation.

Over the next few months, he chose sand perhaps another six or seven times. Without exception, the trays felt absolutely meaningless to me, although he seemed to find them personally meaningful in ways he really couldn't capture in words. What he said was so vague, I found myself unable to capture anything about it in my notes afterward. By now, we had been together for a little over a year, and one day, the conversation turned to how we were doing. He said, "I feel like I'm beginning to imagine trusting you a little bit. Just imagining it, not the thing itself." I was delighted.

About two meetings after that, he said, "I need to make a confession." Long pause and then he continued. "When I do a sandtray, I pick the object next to the one I really want, but I can still see the one I chose. So when I put them into the tray, I'm seeing something completely different from what you see." I had a powerful impulse to laugh hysterically but held it back. "It's ok if you laugh," he said. "I wondered what this was like for you. But, you see, I couldn't afford for you to really see me, so it was the only way I could still do it." Laughter faded inside me as I felt some echo of his terror of being seen. Then I just felt grateful for his remarkable visual abilities, honed by years in architecture and graphic arts, now allowing him to explore his inner world without revealing himself to me.

I asked him what it was like to be telling me this. "It's part of imagining trusting you. Like you can see a little bit of me without seeing very much of me." He decided to hold off on doing sandtrays for a while. Shortly after that, he made a trip home. An elderly aunt happened to say to him, "I'm glad you're doing okay, Sonny. It was terrible how miserable your mother was when you were a babe. Hardly looked at you. I was afraid you wouldn't make it. You were so skinny." With that, she wandered off. A little more inquiry revealed that his mother became severely depressed as soon as she knew she was pregnant with Daniel. As best we can tell, carrying this child awakened the memory of her mother dying in childbirth when her sister was born. His mother had been less than 2 at the time. Given Midwestern stoicism and what Daniel knew of his grandfather, this was a loss she never had the support to grieve. His father told him that his mother had been depressed, with thoughts of suicide, until he was about 18 months old. Then she popped out of it to become her vivacious if egotistical self. Daniel was

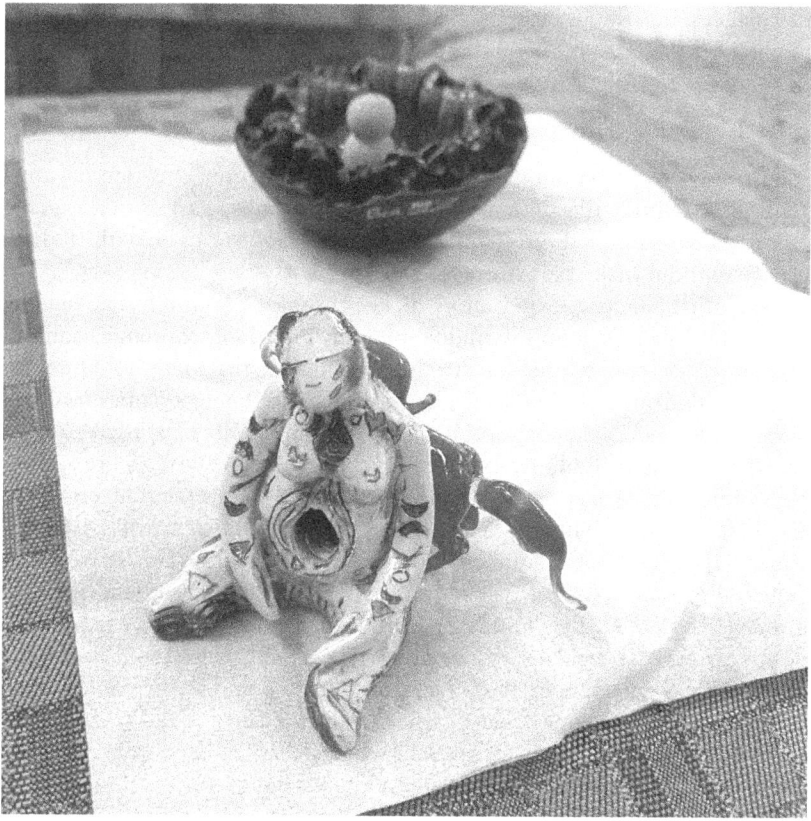

Figure 13.1 Doing Kleenex. Empty grieving mother, with a fiery horse behind her. (Do you see its blazing red and orange?) Faceless wooden child in a black lava bowl, as distant from her as he can be. He is slightly out of focus, fading away in the distance, as he surely must have seemed to her.

too young to make explicit memories of any of this, but carried the entire story in his body and relationships.

When he returned, we sat quietly with all this new information. Things made sense, we agreed. For him to come in close contact with his inner world by being vulnerable to someone else felt like it would be death-dealing. He said, "I feel like I live at the event horizon of a black hole or on a narrow ledge 3,000 feet above ground." "So is it okay if that's where we stay together for as long as it takes?" I asked. He nodded with a wry smile. "Together but without you seeing me. Weird paradox."

About 2 weeks later, he came in with a proposal. "Would it be ok with you if I did Kleenex instead of sandtray?" I wasn't sure what he meant. "Instead of the vast wide-open space of the sand, could we put a Kleenex on the ottoman? I think I can tolerate showing you that much of me." "Brilliant!" I said. And so we did. Usually about three or four figures made their appearance. Daniel spoke of them almost not at all, so he could be seen in small glances, but always protected by the veil of mystery that kept him from tumbling off the edge of the cliff. Such wisdom touches me deeply.

Some Final Thoughts

It's morning now. Spending a little time with my figures, this one has my attention. My body fills with a sense of anticipation as I gaze at her, eagerness mixed with a little dread. I am awed by her beauty. I can be with all that for now without making anything else of it.

Some other sandtray experiences flicker through my mind. The single tiny kitten placed alone in the middle of a tray after long contemplation of the shelves. She opened the door to the unshed tears that were holding this elderly man's depression in place. The solitary figure built of flames next to which was placed a small fire extinguisher. The angry, fire-starting teenager cursed sandtray and all of therapy as he did this. He never started a fire again.

The traumas we carry have a wordless dimension even if we fully remember what happened. The ongoing aliveness of this implicit world becomes clear when the memories awaken and fill our bodies with their sensations, emotions, movements, and perceptions. The presence of sand and miniatures can safely open that liminal space between knowing and experiencing, the gateway to healing. As we are privileged to witness and hold the inner worlds of our people, the process of reflection and repair comes alive between us as we provide what was needed at the time of the trauma but not available. It is truly a sacred space in which what has been split away for their safety is restored and they become more whole.

Our part in this is primarily preparation through doing our own work in the sand and becoming wise in the ways of wounding and healing. Then, as we open to our people in receptivity and trust, we become a sanctuary for every part of these courageous ones who come to us (Badenoch, 2018).

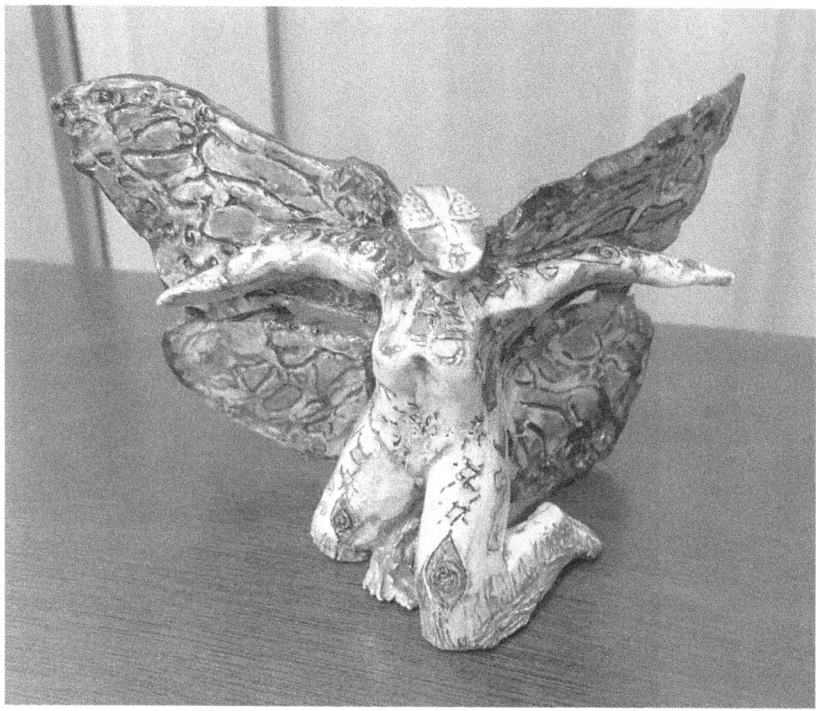

Figure 13.2 A mysterious beauty enters my inner life and stirs me in many different ways, beyond words. Opening your imagination, you might see her vibrant monarch wings.

References

Badenoch, B. (2018). *The heart of trauma: Healing the embodied brain in the context of relationships*. W. W. Norton & Company, Inc.

Finley, J. (2020, September 16). *A mutual vulnerability*. Center for Action and Contemplation. https://cac.org/author/james-finley/

McGilchrist, I. (2009). *The master and his emissary: The divided brain and the making of the western world* (2nd ed., New Expanded ed.). Yale University Press.

Part 3
Tying It All Together

14 The Heart of the Matter

Common Experiences of the Sandtray Therapist

Rita Grayson

We have arrived at the end of our sandtray story chapters. The authors have described their various experiences using the sandtray: working individually with children, adolescents, and adults; using the sandtray as part of a process group; combining it with other therapy protocols; using the sandtray as a bridge across language and culture; even reaching beyond the protocols of sandtray therapy itself to offer unique healing encounters. In each of these chapters, the authors have shared their individual responses to the work described. The overarching theme is that of deep passion and respect for all that sandtray therapy has to offer, both to the therapist and to the client. What follows is a summary of some of the more common experiences described in the preceding chapters.

Releasing

Becoming a sandtray therapist calls on us to do a lot of releasing. Initially, it may take the form of asking our left hemisphere to suspend analysis of what is happening in the tray. Prioritizing knowledge over presence pulls us away from the embodied relationship that is essential to healing. When working in the sand, we are asked to enter the process as it unfolds moment to moment. We must always be prepared to toss our well-intentioned plans for a session out the window. This asks a lot of us, as it has repercussions for our ability to account for time spent and progress made. In response to demands in the environment, and sometimes from our clients themselves, we are challenged to stand firm in favor of deep healing over quick symptom relief. Let's take a look at some of the ways our chapter authors were challenged to release.

Releasing Our Need for Certainty

For many of us, the first thing we need to release is our urge to know the meaning of the sandtray figures and their placement in the tray. When I walked into my first sandtray training, I was hoping to learn how to analyze and assign meaning to what was appearing in the tray. I mistakenly

DOI: 10.4324/9781003055808-17

believed that was what sandtray therapy was all about. It was both frustrating and liberating to learn that a particular sandtray image takes on whatever meaning the client's implicit world assigns in the moment. I was frustrated because I longed for the certainty that would come with looking up symbols in a dictionary. And I was relieved that I didn't have to rely on left-hemisphere knowledge over right-hemisphere experiencing. As we listen to Joanne's story of her work with Samantha in Chapter 11 of this book, it is possible to feel the tug of her left hemisphere. She really wants to know what the snake is all about! Eventually, Samantha let her in on the secret, but Joanne had to be very patient.

Many times, we never explicitly know what the figures or the movement in the tray means. And we don't have to. But we do have to hold steady within the mystery and not lose faith that healing experiences are manifesting.

Bonnie's story of Daniel (Chapter 13) is a great reminder of the power our clients experience, regardless of whether or not it makes sense to us. When, in an attempt to increase his felt sense of safety, Daniel chose the figure on the shelf adjacent to the one he was drawn to, Bonnie was unable to sense any connection between the sandtray world in front of her and the man on the other side of the tray. And yet, thanks to her unshakable trust in Daniel's inner world to guide the process, she was able to release any concern and know that things were unfolding in their proper time, pace, and direction.

Releasing Agendas

Every time we learn a particular therapy process, including sandtray, we learn a series of steps, be they assessment tasks or treatment interventions. There can be a great sense of settling when we can follow prescribed protocols, as they give us something concrete by which we can gauge our work. Being able to fill out a form or complete a therapeutic task provides a sense of order in what may otherwise feel messy and uncertain. Grounding therapy in the right hemisphere, as we do in sandtray, requires us to release any attachment we may hold to how things should go. We give ourselves to what is arriving in the present moment, both within the tray and between us and the people we work with.

This is not always easy, as we saw with Caron (Chapter 7). Thanks to her training and experience working with clients like Jackie, Caron knew it would be best to complete a prescribed assessment process before diving into treatment. As often happens, Jackie and her family came to therapy overwhelmed by their struggles, and their need for relief overtook the carefully crafted assessment process. Caron had no choice but to loosen her hold on assessment protocols in favor of the pressing needs the family brought with them to each session. While pivots such as these can seem frustrating and lead us to believe we are not getting anywhere, the opposite is actually true. Our ability to sense the moment-to-moment needs of our clients and respond accordingly creates connection and safety in the therapeutic relationship, which is fundamental to the healing process.

This is not to say we never follow a protocol or offer a directive. Leaning on the work of Iain McGilchrist as discussed in Chapter 3 of this book, it is a matter of immersing ourselves in the moment, tapping into the felt sense arriving in our bodies, which then arrives in the right hemisphere, and offering that experience to the left hemisphere, which may then dip into its catalog of assessment and treatment protocols and offer a "next step" that is responsive to the moment.

We see this illustrated in both Sean and Aimee's stories (Chapter 6). Aimee describes sessions with Cheryl which began with working in the sandtray, followed by Aimee offering a more directive play therapy intervention based on what had just transpired in the tray. Aimee co-experienced Cheryl's play, sensing it in her own body, which informed her right hemisphere. When she and Cheryl moved away from the sandtray, her left hemisphere was able to offer some possible directive activities that were responsive to what had just been experienced in the sandtray. Similarly, in discussing his work with Jackson, Sean recounts a successful suggestion he made about joining the theatre program at school. The idea did not come out of the blue. Instead, it was sourced from Sean's deep understanding of Jackson and his dilemma, based on the time they had spent together, both in and out of the sandtray.

Releasing the Urge to Fix

It is difficult to witness the suffering of another. It is also difficult to sit with uncertainty about how and when that suffering will diminish. Putting these two challenges together, we might find the origin of our desire for a "quick fix." On top of our own discomfort, there may also be pressure from the one doing the suffering. Caron (Chapter 7) touched on this common dilemma. Jackie and her family desperately wanted things to feel better, as did Caron. But she knew that to really heal, the path would be longer and slower than anyone desired.

In Chapter 2 of this book, I make the distinction between helping and healing. While it may be helpful to offer strategies to relieve current distress, those strategies may not touch the underlying cause of the difficulty. Sometimes pain itself is a necessary teacher. If we reach beyond symptom relief to healing the underlying pain and fear, we are agreeing to go the distance with our clients. We are also agreeing to release any agenda of how long it will take or where the journey will take us.

Embracing

Releasing agendas, strict adherence to protocols, attachment to certainty and predetermined outcomes is synonymous with shifting out of left-hemisphere dominance and embracing the ambiguity and uncertainty of the right hemisphere. The more we experience the power of sandtray for ourselves, the easier it becomes to trust the process and allow sandtray to work its healing magic. Throughout the chapters in this book, we see examples of the power inherent in sandtray therapy. We will revisit some of them here.

Embracing Trust

Releasing agendas for our clients, ourselves, and our work together requires deep trust. Generally, trust increases with experience and feedback that what we are doing is working. Aimee's successful work with Cheryl (Chapter 6) gave her a boost of confidence she appreciated as a new sandtray therapist. Roz (Chapter 8) admits that had Mist come to her earlier in her development as a psychotherapist, she would have been tempted to focus on the presenting problem (hair pulling) and adhere to treatment protocols that target the specific unwanted behavior. Such an approach would have ignored Mist's wholeness and her inner wisdom's capacity to guide her individual healing path. Both Aimee's and Roz's experiences speak to the developmental stages of becoming a therapist and developing trust in the process.

Working in the sandtray can present some additional challenges due to its non-verbal nature. When we are accustomed to connecting through words, it can feel like a leap of faith to embark on a healing journey during which few or no words may be spoken. Fortunately, there is a sure-fire way to develop trust in the power of sandtray therapy: embark on your own personal healing journey with the support of a skilled witness.

To this day, even after witnessing thousands of sandtray sessions, I still find myself wanting to know the details of how the figures in the tray relate to my client's life experiences. Sometimes I arrive at such an understanding, and sometimes I do not. When the latter happens, I take a breath and let go, leaning into my deep trust of sandtray therapy which is grounded in two beliefs: it worked for me; I'm not that special, so it must work for others also. I have experienced deep healing in my personal sandtray process, some of which is described in Chapter 2 of this book. At times, even I didn't have a left-hemisphere understanding of my own work. I only knew something inside me had shifted, and I felt better. If I am able to have such experiences, I can trust the same is true for my clients, regardless of whether or not I have any cognitive understanding of what is happening in the sandtray.

Embracing the Power

Our personal encounter with sandtray therapy is often our first glimpse of the inherent power it offers. The more we journey in the sand, the more we come to understand, respect, and honor that power. Before long, we may feel the urge to adjust our role in the therapeutic encounter, stepping back from any sense of responsibility to direct, and allowing the process to unfold according to the prompting of our client's implicit world. We shift from therapist to witness, from leader to follower, from observer to co-journeyer. We hear the echoes of sandtray's power throughout the stories in this book.

Joanne's work with Aliyah (Chapter 11), an asylum seeker housed in a refugee center, demonstrates the power of sandtray images to transcend protocols, cultural norms, and language barriers. Given that sandtrays were not allowed in the detention center, Joanne had only her collection of figures, and they were ones that were not familiar within Aliyah's culture. In addition, Joanne and Aliyah spoke different languages, necessitating the presence of a translator. Both the sandtray collection and the therapist spoke a different language from Aliyah, and yet she was able to do deep, healing work with unfamiliar toys placed on the floor.

While, as sandtray therapists, we strive to equip our sandtray rooms with the prescribed equipment and a robust "vocabulary" of images, sometimes, environmental constraints make that impossible. The words of my teacher, Gisela De Domenico, come to mind: "Psyche will adjust" (personal communication). Aliyah's pain was great, as was her drive to heal. Within Joanne's warm embrace and surrounded by caring adults, she was able to work within the limitations of the tools available to her and regain a sense of safety and connection.

We see the power of sandtray to bring connection and comfort at times when we need to reach beyond words to convey our most intense experiences in Barbara's chapter on grief (Chapter 9). When words fall short, we can reach for the symbols and images of a sandtray collection to communicate, right hemisphere to right hemisphere, the enormity of what we need to say. Barbara used the sandtray within a process group for children who had experienced the death of a loved one. Instead of talking about the funeral, they were able to select sandtray figures that captured the varied and nuanced experience of their loss and grief. Reflecting on the contributions of other group members, participants felt seen and heard and, perhaps best of all, accompanied in their grief journey by others with a shared experience of loss. Sandtray's invitation to release the left-hemisphere process of finding words, which all too often confines expression, offers a powerful right-hemisphere-based relational experience that can provide comfort in the isolation of profound grief.

Bonnie (Chapter 13) speaks to the powerful influence of the sandtray and collection of images in our counseling rooms, whether or not they are used in what we might consider to be a traditional way. She tells us story after story of the interaction between images on her sandtray shelves and the implicit world of her clients. For Andi, simply approaching the shelves awakened an implicit memory, making it available for healing within the warmth of her relationship with Bonnie. Dierdre needed only the sand. Sylvie chose a single figure, which never made its way into the sand but offered a powerful healing experience.

Arriving

When we arrive to a sandtray session, we bring our whole selves. As we know from the study of neurobiology (Chapter 3), we are constantly sensing one another's autonomic state below the level of conscious awareness. It is neurobiologically impossible to detach ourselves from the encounter, although it is possible to numb the felt sense of the experience by shifting into our left hemisphere or dissociating. While we do our best to be fully present, we also need to hold our efforts with compassion, remembering that our own woundedness may protectively distance us from what is unfolding in the moment. Healing such wounds, which in turn expands our capacity to be present, is the work of a lifetime for a sandtray therapist. When we do arrive in a state of openness, we enter an experience that may touch us in many ways, including physically and emotionally. As we have seen in the stories in this book, such experiences can be gifts, both to our clients and to ourselves.

Arriving Physically

To help us bring our whole selves to the sandtray and the relationship with our clients, we can focus on the physical sensations arising in our bodies. Mirror neurons and resonance circuits, as discussed in Chapter 3 of this book, help us sense one another's bodily states, emotional states, and intentions. Sean (Chapter 6) illustrates the phenomenon of deep interpersonal presence manifesting in physical sensations. During a session with Jackson, Sean noticed the arrival of a pain in his left side and, upon inquiring, discovered Jackson's left leg had been hurt when he was pushed by a bully. Attending to his own body and being curious about an unexpected sensation led Sean to inquire if Jackson was experiencing any pain. Jackson may never have told the story of the bully and his leg injury had Sean not asked. Sometimes the sensations in our bodies reflect our personal reaction to what is happening in session. Aimee (Chapter 6) speaks of the "lightning bolts of anxiety" she experienced while witnessing the purposeful, controlled chaos of Cheryl's dumping. At other times, we may physically sense the back-and-forth within the relationship. MereAnn (Chapter 12) describes the dance of Marti's nervous system with hers as, together, they encountered a difficult truth that had the power to overwhelm either one of them. Connecting through eye gaze and breath, their respective nervous systems were able to find and settle one another. These examples demonstrate the depth and richness that can be mined in a sandtray therapy session when we tune into our own bodies.

Arriving Emotionally

Deep right-hemisphere and body-based presence in a sandtray session asks us to suspend left-hemisphere processes for at least some part of the time. In doing so, we also release the protection from emotional pain that is offered through the relational detachment of the left hemisphere. Roz (Chapter 8) reminds us of this reality as she notes the need to contain her own sadness in response to Mist's grief. Given the intimacy of the therapeutic encounter, it is impossible to expect that our own unhealed implicit pain will not be touched from time to time.

When Asha proclaimed, "My body is against me!" (Chapter 10), the statement reverberated in Elaine with an intensity that caught her attention. Sensing the emotional response stemmed from her own challenges with an aging body, she sought consultation with Jacqueline, and together, they processed her response to Asha's statement in the sandtray. In so doing, Elaine discovered gifts embedded in the experience, including an opportunity to confront the realities of an aging body and the possibility of seeing things a bit differently.

When MereAnn (Chapter 12) recognized that taking Marti on as a client might touch her own grief journey, she sought consultation and support. The work we do as therapists is challenging, and we are not meant to go it alone.

In my work with Monique (Chapter 5), when it became clear that her journey would touch my personal experience of divorce, the mere act of calling my clinical consultant's kind face to mind settled my nervous system. I was comforted with the knowledge that I had a trusted other to help me navigate whatever was to come so I could be my best for Monique.

The Gifts

Reflecting on the experiences of a sandtray therapist, there are many gifts. As we have categorized these experiences into "releasing," "embracing," and "arriving," so too we can view the gifts from this perspective. Releasing brings with it a sense of freedom. As I release the hold of my left hemisphere on needing to control a session or push for a particular outcome, I can settle into true presence and connection. Fed from the experience of the present moment, my left hemisphere may offer ideas or suggestions that are supportive of the healing process. The gift to me as therapist is freedom to respond to the unfolding needs of my client. The gift to my client is being truly seen, held, and honored.

Embracing trust in the power of sandtray often originates from our own experiences of healing through a personal sandtray process, which is a gift in and of itself. Through our work in the sand, we come to know, experientially, the inherent power sandtray offers. To have such a powerful healing tool available to our clients is a gift to everyone involved. The privilege of accompanying another human on their unique journey toward wholeness is a gift beyond measure.

Arriving to a sandtray session with our whole being offers the possibility of deep engagement. Our nervous systems seek connection and ventral presence, which is akin to a relational oasis in the prevailing culture of fast pace and distractions. Such connection is a gift to our clients, who may feel us right there with them as they approach tender territory in their healing work. And, at times, they return the favor by awakening some bit of implicitly held unhealed pain, bringing it into our awareness and inviting us to further our own individual journey toward wholeness.

The themes, reflected in the stories told in this book and summarized in this chapter, are just a small sample among many. Stories of healing are as numerous as the number of people who have trusted sand, water, and symbolic images to invite that which is hidden or elusive into the physical plane and possibly into conscious awareness. The experiences of those who have the privilege to witness such journeys is equally numerous. And the gifts sandtray therapy brings to both client and therapist are impossible to catalog and number, much like the grains of sand in a sandtray!

15 Honoring the Legacy

Keeping Margaret Lowenfeld's Vision Alive in the Future

Theresa Fraser

Dr. Lowenfeld created a model and a method that provided children with a manner in which to communicate feelings and thoughts. She believed that the sand and toys communicated these preverbal thoughts stored in the right brain often even before language was formed.

> Lowenfeld would explain that using the toys in the sand was a form of "picture thinking" and that it was helpful because some ideas and feelings could not easily be expressed in words. She would say, "make whatever comes into your head." (Dr. Margaret Lowenfeld Trust, 2017)

Dr. Gisela De Domenico instructs the builder to "follow their heart" (De Domenico, 2002). When worlds are built, revealed material impacts more than the head and the heart of the builder. The sandtray creates a free and protected space (Kalff, 1991) for the world builder's stories to emerge and be held as sacred by both builder and witness. Dora Kalff states that "it is the therapist's task to give shape to such a space: a free space in which the client feels fully accepted" (Kalff, 1991, para. 11).

Toys are the means of communication, as are the actions, movements, and shared energy. Just as the builder does not need to use spoken language, neither does the witness. Creating connection without spoken language requires attunement, or "feeling felt," that we don't necessarily learn or practice in our counseling education programs. Being cognitively, physically, spiritually, and emotionally present while following the builder's lead requires a therapist to be aware of their head (cortical brain), heart (physiological reactions), and limbic (subcortical) system reactions to co-construct the healing milieu.

Selected toys embody experiences that match the social location of those who use them and the social locations of others. Touching these figures, along with the soft sand, activates thoughts and feelings in a way that talking does not. The figures come to life in the sandtray: Symbols known and sometimes not yet known enter into a dance with one another. The dance is sometimes slow (static worlds), sometimes fast (ever-moving worlds), and

DOI: 10.4324/9781003055808-18

can be so meaningful that tears, anger, joy, fear, or connections become real. With our hands in the sand, we can be anchored in the present while revisiting the past and anticipating the future.

As witness, I have had the privilege of experiencing limbic subcortical countertransference. At those times, I have needed to ground myself and simply notice the implicit memories surfacing while simultaneously holding space for the builder. These personal responses can be taken to the sandtray for my own processing at a later time. This is why each witnessed sandtray is a reciprocal gift between builder and witness. This book has shared story after story of the transformational power of engaging in this sacred, fully instructed process for builders of all ages. It all began with a physician who read a book and adapted what she read into a psychotherapeutic approach that would be used, for the next century and beyond, by therapists and children of all ages the world over. The individuals that were seen in Lowenfeld's Clinic for Nervous and Difficult Children in 1928 were not documented as having eating disorders or gender dysphoria. These were not problems or human conditions that were of concern at the time. However, a child's need to communicate via play was celebrated, and the world technique continues to embrace whatever therapeutic needs arrive.

In our century, Dr. Jessica Stone created the first digital sandtray application utilized by many therapists prior to the world pandemic (known as COVID-19). She and her partner, Chris Ewing, created an app (digital application) where the therapist could bring the power of sandtray into spaces, such as immigration camps or hospitals, where it would otherwise be prohibited. In these settings, the therapist could share a tablet, allowing a builder to access miniatures to create a world with one finger. Throughout the world pandemic, this program became the first sandtray product that supported worlds being shared from the client's physical space to a therapist's office via the Internet while keeping therapist and client safe from sharing a virus. The world technique continues to support healing for persons across the life span, whether used in a face-to-face or virtual space. Thank you, Dr. Lowenfeld.

In our work (and sandtray community), let us honor the legacy of where and how this sacred intervention was birthed. Let us acknowledge that we can't just take a one-day training and use this way of working with clients authentically and ethically. We need to challenge the left-shifted culture that would have us believe true symptom relief can result from brief, solution-focused interventions. We must maintain the distinction between therapies that are helpful and those that actually heal our embodied brains. It is our hope that after reading this book, you will dig deeply into your experience and psyche to reflect on what sandtray means to you. We urge you to marry this reflection with supervision and practice, as well as lots more training, to continue to deepen what you bring to the sandtray experience. Thank you for listening to our stories. We hope someday to hear yours.

References

De Domenico, G. (2002). The sandtray-worldplay method. *Sandtray Network Journal, 6*(1).

Dr. Margaret Lowenfeld Trust. (2017). *The world technique.* https://lowenfeld.org/the-world-technique/

Kalff, D. (1991). Introduction to sandplay therapy. *Journal of Sandplay Therapy, 1*(1).

Index

Note: Page numbers in *italics* indicate a figure on the corresponding page.

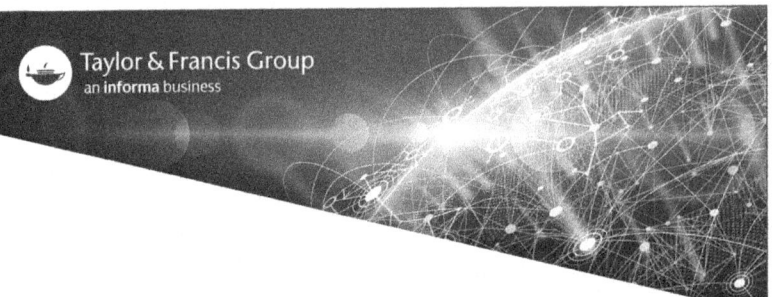
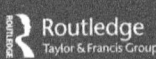
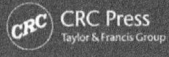

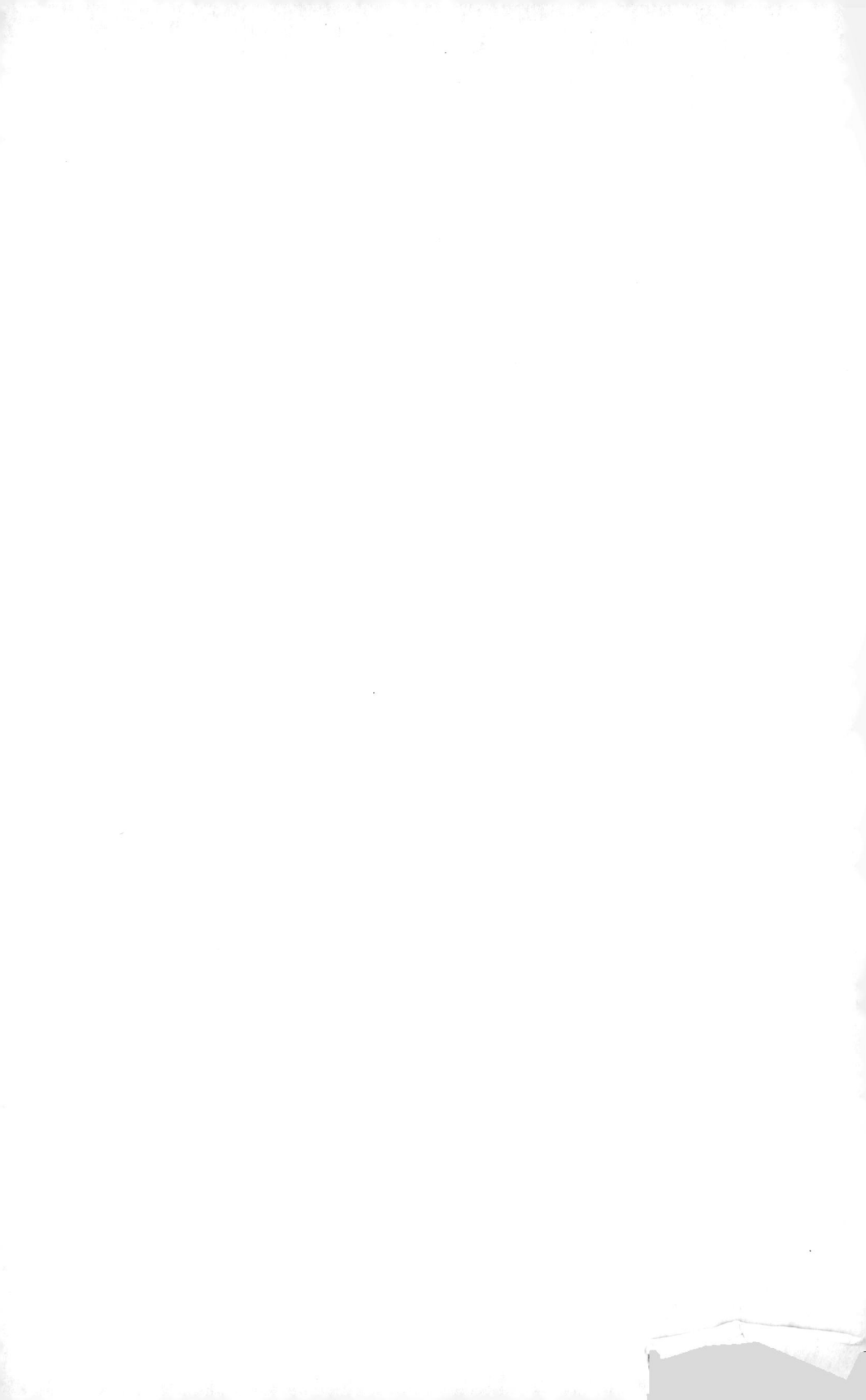